CT and MRI of the Abdomen and Pelvis

A TEACHING FILE

CT and MRI of the Abdomen and Pelvis

A TEACHING FILE

PABLO R. ROS, M.D., FACR

Professor and Associate Chairman
Director, Division of Body Imaging and MRI
Department of Radiology
University of Florida
Gainesville, Florida

SYLVESTER LEE, M.D.

Assistant Professor
Department of Radiology
University of Florida-Jacksonville
Jacksonville, Florida

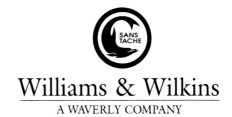

Williams & Wilkins
A WAVERLY COMPANY

BALTIMORE • PHILADELPHIA • LONDON • PARIS • BANGKOK
BUENOS AIRES • HONG KONG • MUNICH • SYDNEY • TOKYO • WROCLAW

Editor: Charles W. Mitchell
Managing Editor: Marjorie Kidd Keating
Marketing Manager: Lorraine A. Smith
Production Coordinator: Raymond E. Reter
Designer: Dan Pfisterer
Illustration Planner: Lorraine Wrzosek
Cover Design: Dan Pfisterer
Typesetter: Peirce Graphic Services, Stuart, Florida
Printer and Binder: R. R. Donnelley & Sons Company, Crawfordsville, Indiana
Digitized Illustrations: Publicity Engravers, Inc., Baltimore, Maryland

Copyright © 1997 Williams & Wilkins

351 West Camden Street
Baltimore, Maryland 21201–2436 USA

Rose Tree Corporate Center
1400 North Providence Road
Building II, Suite 5025
Media, Pennsylvania 19063–2043 USA

Accurate indications, adverse reactions and dosage schedules for drugs are provided in
this book, but it is possible that they may change. The reader is urged to review the
package information data of the manufacturers of the medications mentioned.

Printed in the United States of America

Library of Congress Cataloging-in-Publication Data

Ros, Pablo R.
    CT and MRI of the abdomen and pelvis : a teaching file / Pablo R. Ros, Sylvester
Lee.
        p.   cm.
    Includes bibliographical references and index.
    ISBN 0-683-18218-8
    1. Abdomen—Tomography—Case studies.   2. Abdomen—Magnetic resonance
imaging—Case studies.   3. Pelvis—Tomography—Case studies.   4. Pelvis—
Magnetic resonance imaging—Case studies.   I. Lee, Sylvester.   II. Title.
    [DNLM: 1. Abdomen—pathology—atlases.   2. Digestive System Diseases—
diagnosis—atlases.   3. Pelvis—pathology—atlases.   4. Digestive System—
pathology—atlases.   5. Diagnosis, Differential—atlases.   6. Diagnostic Imaging—
atlases.   WI 17 R788c 1997]
RC944.R674 1997
617.5′507′548—dc21
DNLM/DLC
for Library of Congress   97–1121
                                                                                        CIP

*The publishers have made every effort to trace the copyright holders for borrowed material.
If they have inadvertently overlooked any, they will be pleased to make the necessary
arrangements at the first opportunity.*

To purchase additional copies of this book, call our customer service department at
(800) 638-0672 or fax orders to **(800) 447-8438.** For other book services, including chapter reprints and large quantity sales, ask for the Special Sales department.

Canadian customers should call **(800) 665-1148,** or fax **(800) 665-0103.** For all
other calls originating outside of the United States, please call **(410) 528-4223** or fax
us at **(410) 528-8550.**

Visit *Williams & Wilkins* on the Internet: http://www.wwilkins.com or contact
our customer service department at **custserv@wwilkins.com**. Williams & Wilkins customer service representatives are available from 8:30 am to 6:00 pm, EST, Monday
through Friday, for telephone access.

97 98 99 00 01
2 3 4 5 6 7 8 9 10

To the medical students and residents
who inspired me through the years,
To my friends, parents and colleagues
who were always present with words of encouragement,
To my wife, Donna,
whose love, patience, and understanding made this long journey possible.

SYLVESTER LEE, MD

To all the residents, fellows and medical students I had the privilege to teach, since they
constitute the reason for my academic career and the main source of my professional satisfaction.

PABLO R. ROS, MD, FACR

PUBLISHER'S FOREWORD

Teaching Files are one of the hallmarks of education in Radiology. There has long been a need for a comprehensive series of books, using the Teaching File format, that would provide the kind of personal "consultation with the experts" normally found only in the setting of a teaching hospital. Williams & Wilkins is proud to have created such a series; our goal is to provide the resident and practicing radiologist with a useful resource that answers this need.

Actual cases have been culled from extensive teaching files in major medical centers. The discussions presented mimic those performed on a daily basis between residents and faculty members in all radiology departments.

The format of the books is designed so that each case can be studied as an unknown, if desired. A consistent format is used to present each case. A brief clinical history is given, followed by several images. Then, relevant findings, differential diagnosis, and final diagnosis are given, followed by a discussion of the case. The authors thereby guide the reader through the interpretation of each case.

We hope that this series will become a valuable and trusted teaching tool for radiologists at any stage of training or practice, and that it will also be a benefit to clinicians whose patients undergo these imaging studies.

THE PUBLISHER
WILLIAMS & WILKINS

PREFACE

This book is the fruit of our collaboration that spans at least 6 years, when both of us were in the Department of Radiology at the University of Florida College of Medicine, Gainesville. Although the point-of-view of one of us (Sly) changed from medical student to radiology resident, fellow, and finally attending, we tried to duplicate the experience of reviewing interesting cases presented in the Abdominal Imaging divisional conferences, in "hot seat" sessions for the senior residents, and most importantly, in daily read-out sessions.

Our goal was to select the "best in show" material out of an archive of over 5,000 teaching file cases and put it in book format. The Abdominal Imaging teaching file at the University of Florida College of Medicine contains primarily cases that have been performed at Shands Hospital at the University of Florida and also cases originating from the Armed Forces Institute of Pathology, Washington, D.C. It also includes cases collected in visiting professorships in the United States and Canada, as well as other countries in Europe, Central and South America, and Asia, cases that have been presented in film-reading panels in national and international meetings, and cases that have been brought by visitors to the department. All cases entered into the teaching file have to be proven by either surgery, biopsy, laboratory data, or clinical and/or radiologic follow-up. Cases with an obvious pathognomonic imaging diagnosis (e.g., pneumoperitoneum) are also included. From this pool, we selected the best ones and divided them into chapters according to the traditional abdominal sections: liver and biliary tree, pancreas, spleen, gastrointestinal tract, kidney, retroperitoneum and adrenal, mesentery and omentum, and pelvis. We also added a chapter called "Unknowns and Aunt Minnies," which contains a potpourri of cases with a short differential diagnosis.

The format for each case is the same. A brief clinical history is followed by two to four images, which by definition are either computed tomography, magnetic resonance imaging scans, or a combination of both. Then, pertinent findings, differential diagnosis, final diagnosis, and a brief discussion follow.

This format is designed so that cases can be taken as unknowns. A simple piece of paper will cover the entire information given on each case. If the reader wants to know the findings or the differential diagnosis before knowing the final diagnosis, this can be easily accomplished by removing the paper.

To make this book reflect real life, we took actual cases from an extensive teaching file and recreated the discussions performed on a daily basis in hundreds of departments of radiology between residents and faculty members. We duplicated our discussions at the viewbox, emphasizing a practical approach. The cases in each chapter are not presented with traditional divisions (congenital, inflammatory, neoplastic, vascular, etc), but are all mixed up, again mimicking real life. The end result, we hope, is that radiologists at any stage in their training or careers will benefit from reading this book.

We had fun selecting the cases, going over differential diagnosis lists, and trying to summarize a pertinent discussion for each case. We hope the reader will also enjoy going over them and learning more about diseases of the abdomen and pelvis using computed tomography and magnetic resonance imaging as diagnostic tools.

PABLO R. ROS, MD, FACR
SYLVESTER LEE, MD

ACKNOWLEDGMENTS

This book would not have been possible if it were not for the efforts of two outstanding radiology departments: University of Florida at Gainesville and Jacksonville. Talented technologists obtained these images through the years, especially Tony Litwiller and Mary Ellen Bentham. Kai Woods worked tirelessly at preparing this manuscript. Dr. Baird and Dr. Luis Ros contributed outstanding cases to this book. In addition, the staff at Williams & Wilkins, particularly Charles Mitchell and Margie Keating, offered their endless support for this project.

We would like to acknowledge all of the members of the Division of Body Imaging and Magnetic Resonance Imaging at the University of Florida, including Pat Abbitt, Sharon Burton, Juri V. Kaude, Gladys Torres, and Patricia Mergo. All of them have directly or indirectly participated in this book by either contributing cases for our teaching file or by presenting the differential diagnoses when these cases were initially read. Special thanks go to Frederick Vines and Edward V. Staab, Professor and Chairman. Their encouragement helped to initiate and complete this project.

We would like to thank all the residents and medical students we have known through the years. Their curiosity and thirst for knowledge has continually challenged us to learn and teach what we have learned to others. Hopefully, this book can start to repay them for the lifetime of inspiration they have given us.

SYLVESTER LEE, MD
PABLO R. ROS, MD, FACR

I would like to personally thank my many mentors at the University of Florida: Walt Drane, Jim Grantham, and all the members of the Division of Body Imaging and Magnetic Resonance Imaging. In their own ways, each taught me about radiology and life. In particular, two individuals have been my greatest inspiration as a radiologist: Patricia Abbitt and my coauthor Pablo Ros. Their undying love for teaching and learning has touched the lives of countless people who have had the good fortune to work with them.

I must recognize two people who spawned the idea for this textbook: Karl Weingarten and Margaret Weeks. Karl first came up with the notion of a teaching file textbook after seeing a stack of cases in Pat Abbitt's office. Mags encouraged me to do a textbook on the abdomen and pelvis over a cold beer in Chapel Hill, North Carolina. The greatest ideas often come when you least expect them.

Finally, I thank my close friends and family—Cathy Johnson, Dave Bulley, Joe and Nicole Kim, Ron Fisher, Mark Renfro, Andy Pedersen, Kelley and Fred Trent, and my wife, Donna. Over the past 6 years, they provided me with love, friendship, and support, which allowed me to accomplish this task. Most importantly, they taught me something that can never be taught in any textbook—the importance of friendship, family, living life to the fullest, and just plain, having fun. From the immortal words of Jimmy Buffett, "If we couldn't laugh, we would all go insane."

SYLVESTER LEE, MD

CONTENTS

chapter 1

LIVER AND BILIARY
SYSTEM

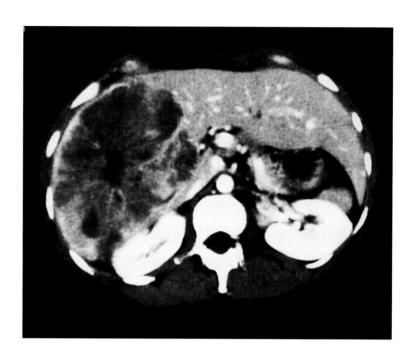

CASE 1

Clinical History: 49-year-old woman with right upper quadrant pain.

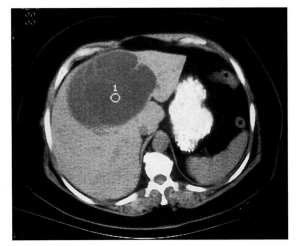
Figure 1.1 A

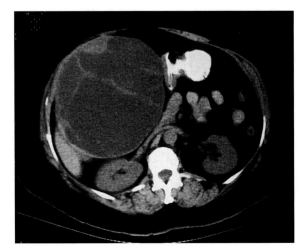
Figure 1.1 B

Findings: CECT demonstrates a large septated cystic lesion involving the left lobe of the liver.

Differential Diagnosis: Echinococcal cyst, hepatic abscess, necrotic neoplasm.

Diagnosis: Biliary cystadenoma.

Discussion: Biliary cystadenoma is a slow-growing cystic neoplasm occurring predominantly in women. It can be complicated by hemorrhage, infection, rupture, and malignant transformation into cystadenocarcinomas. Typically biliary cystadenoma is almost entirely cystic with very little solid component present. These septated cystic neoplasms may be indistinguishable from echinococcal cysts. Appropriate history is often necessary to distinguish the two entities. Calcifications can occur in the wall of the biliary cystadenoma. The presence of thick calcifications and a large solid component should raise the possibility of a cystic hepatic neoplasm (cystadenocarcinoma). Both hepatic abscesses and necrotic metastases have a different CT appearance than a typical biliary cystadenoma with a thick irregular enhancing wall rather than thin well-defined septated cysts.

CASE 2

Clinical History: 59-year-old man with history of bacterial endocarditis.

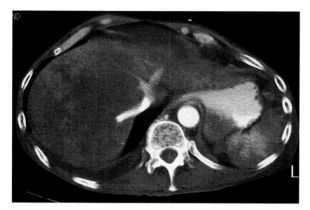

Figure 1.2 A

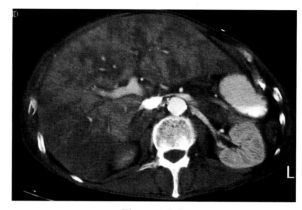

Figure 1.2 B

Findings: CECT demonstrates diffuse areas of low attenuation within the liver and multiple wedge-shaped defects in the spleen.

Differential Diagnosis: Diffuse metastatic disease, intrahepatic cholangiocarcinoma.

Diagnosis: Hepatic and splenic infarction.

Discussion: Hepatic infarction is thought to be a rare process secondary to the dual blood supply to the liver from the portal vein and hepatic artery. Although this is true, infarctions are seen when either a portal branch or hepatic arterial branch is occluded. The areas of infarction are usually hypodense and do not demonstrate enhancement with contrast. They appear either well circumscribed and wedge shaped or ill defined and diffuse as is seen in this example. Causes of hepatic infarction include emboli (usually from the heart), occlusion of the hepatic artery or portal vein from a mass, thrombosis of the hepatic artery, atherosclerosis, and vasculitides.

The key to the diagnosis in this example is the history of endocarditis and the multiple wedge-shaped infarcts of the spleen. This suggests the diagnosis of hepatic and splenic infarcts from emboli originating from the heart. Intrahepatic cholangiocarcinoma can also have this appearance but enhancement on CECT is typically present.

CASE 3

Clinical History: 60-year-old female with history of cirrhosis.

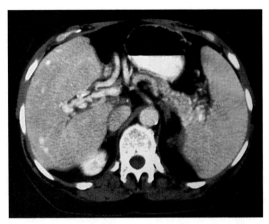

Figure 1.3 A

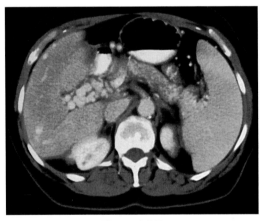

Figure 1.3 B

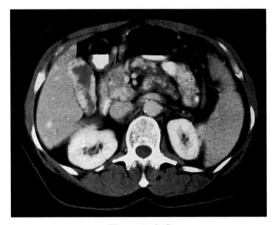

Figure 1.3 C

Findings: CECT demonstrates multiple serpiginous collateral vessels in the expected location of the portal vein. There is splenomegaly and enhancement of serpiginous vessels in the gallbladder wall.

Differential Diagnosis: None.

Diagnosis: Cavernous transformation of the portal vein with pericholecystic collateral vessels.

Discussion: Portal vein thrombosis can be secondary to multiple causes including malignancies (HCC, cholangiocarcinoma, pancreatic neoplasms), trauma, hematologic disorders, and phlebitis from sepsis. In up to 50% of the cases, the etiology is unknown. Portal vein thrombosis can either be intrahepatic or extrahepatic with cirrhosis being the most common cause for intrahepatic thrombosis. Cavernous transformation of the portal vein is the formation of multiple periportal collaterals in the expected location of the portal vein. This can often alter the enhancement pattern of the liver because of compensatory arterial blood flow to the liver. The collateral vessels are thought to represent the recanalized periportal venous plexus rather than true recanalization of the thrombosed portal vein. These collateral vessels can often extend to the wall of the gallbladder as well as in the porta hepatis as in this example.

CASE 4

Clinical History: 64-year-old man with a history of alcoholism, weight loss, and abnormal liver function tests.

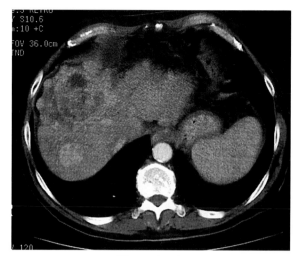

Figure 1.4 A

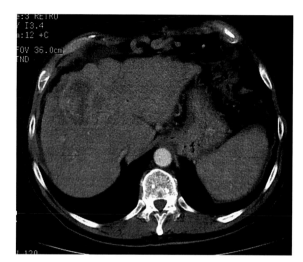

Figure 1.4 B

Findings: CECT shows a 6-cm heterogeneous enhancing lesion in the right lobe of the liver close to the diaphragm. Multiple small enhancing nodules surround the lesion causing nodularity of the liver surface. There is also enlargement of the left and caudate lobes and a recanalized paraumbilical vein is present.

Differential Diagnosis: Multifocal hepatocellular carcinoma, metastases.

Diagnosis: Hepatocellular carcinoma with regenerating and adenomatous hyperplastic nodules (dysplastic nodules).*

Discussion: Hepatocellular carcinoma is thought to arise from at least two different pathways. The first is in patients without any underlying liver disease. In one series, 40% of non-Asian patients with HCC did not have any underlying liver disease. The second is in patients who have a background of regenerating nodules and chronic liver disease. It is thought that the regenerating nodule is the first lesion in a spectrum of lesions leading to hepatocellular carcinoma. The multi-step progression ranges from small regenerating nodules, large regenerating nodules, adenomatous hyperplasia, atypical adenomatous hyperplasia with early HCC to early advanced HCC and finally advanced HCC. This case demonstrates a hepatocellular carcinoma amidst multiple regenerating nodules and adenomatous hyperplastic nodules. With time, these lesions will progress to a hepatocellular carcinoma. Multiple hypervascular metastasis could be a possible diagnosis but they do not usually enhance as homogeneously as is seen here. In a setting of cirrhosis and portal hypertension, hepatocellular carcinoma is the most likely diagnosis.

---

*New term for regenerating and adenomatous hyperplastic nodule.

CASE 5

Clinical History: 60-year-old woman with history of hepatitis and cirrhosis.

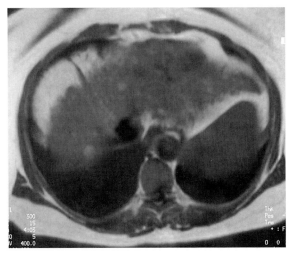

Figure 1.5 A

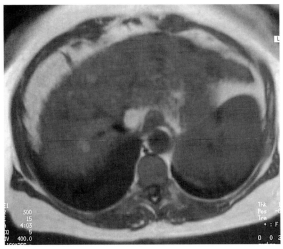

Figure 1.5 B

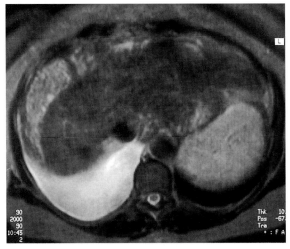

Figure 1.5 C

Findings: (A, B) T1-weighted image of the liver demonstrates multiple small round nodules of increased signal intensity; (C) the T2-weighted images demonstrate these same lesions to be of decreased signal intensity.

Differential Diagnosis: Focal fat, hemorrhage, or hemorrhagic metastases.

Diagnosis: Adenomatous hyperplastic nodule versus regenerating nodules (dysplastic nodule).

Discussion: Few lesions will appear bright on T1-weighted images such as fat, blood, and melanin. Therefore, any lesion that contains any of these components can appear bright on a T1-weighted image. HCC, hepatocellular adenoma, and metastatic liposarcoma can potentially contain fat pathologically. These lesions, however, are usually bright on T2-weighted images. Blood products in hematomas or hemorrhagic metastases can have a variety of MR signal characteristics based on the stage of evolution of the blood. Regenerating nodules and adenomatous hyperplastic nodules are of low signal intensity on T2-weighted imaging and of slight increased signal intensity on T1-weighted images. This is the opposite of the typical signal characteristics of a hepatocellular carcinoma. Many people believe that the signal characteristics of regenerating nodules and adenomatous hyperplastic nodules are due to the presence of hemosiderin within the lesion.

CASE 6

Clinical History: 48-year-old woman with symptoms of flushing and diarrhea.

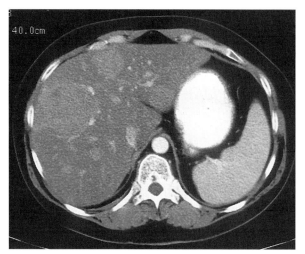

Figure 1.6 A

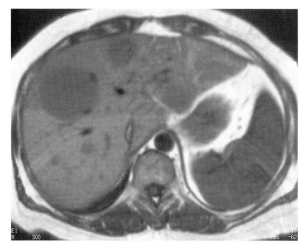

Figure 1.6 B

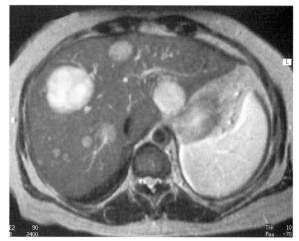

Figure 1.6 C

Findings: (A) CECT demonstrates three large round areas of increased attenuation in the liver measuring 5 cm, 3 cm, and 2 cm. The liver appears diffusely fatty in density; (B) T1WI demonstrates these lesions to be hypointense; (C) T2WI demonstrates these lesions to be hyperintense.

Differential Diagnosis: Focal areas of fatty sparing, multifocal hepatocellular carcinoma.

Diagnosis: Multiple metastases from carcinoid tumor.

Discussion: These metastases on CECT have a unique appearance. Because there is a background of fatty liver, the metastases appear to be of slightly higher attenuation than the surrounding liver. This could have been confused for areas of focal sparing of fat except for the mass effect demonstrated by the lesions. There are no vessels coursing through the lesions, and the vessels are actually displaced by the lesion. Because carcinoid metastases are hypervascular, the lesions enhanced fairly homogeneously simulating normal hepatic parenchyma. The MRI demonstrates these lesions to be hypointense on the T1WI and hyperintense on the T2WI. This is typically seen in many neoplasms, ruling out normal liver with focal sparing in a diffusely fatty liver.

CASE 7

Clinical History: Abnormal liver function tests and abdominal pain.

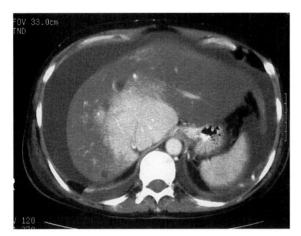

Figure 1.7 A

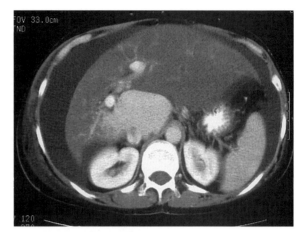

Figure 1.7 B

Findings: CECT reveals hypertrophy of the caudate lobe, which has normal contrast enhancement and diffuse low attenuation in the remainder of the liver. No hepatic veins or intrahepatic IVC is seen. Ascites and bilateral effusions are present.

Differential Diagnosis: None.

Diagnosis: Budd-Chiari syndrome.

Discussion: Budd-Chiari syndrome results from the occlusion of the hepatic veins, the inferior vena cava, or both. Various conditions have been associated with the obstruction of hepatic venous drainage including idiopathic, hypercoagulable states from pregnancy, oral contraceptives, polycythemia vera, trauma, tumors involving or obstructing the IVC or hepatic veins, and webs in the IVC. This leads to stasis and increased postsinusoidal pressure in the liver, which decreases portal blood flow. The caudate lobe has a separate venous drainage directly into the IVC and therefore is not affected by this process. The caudate actually enlarges secondary to the shunted portal blood flow. This case demonstrates the typical findings of chronic Budd-Chiari syndrome with lack of enhancement of most of the liver with sparing and hypertrophy of the caudate lobe. There is also lack of visualization of the hepatic veins. The poorly enhanced portions of the liver are due to decreased portal flow, venous congestion, and rarely infarcts. Delayed imaging can often show washout from the normally enhanced caudate lobe and slow filling in of the remainder of the liver.

CASE 8

Clinical History: 57-year-old woman with history of alcohol abuse.

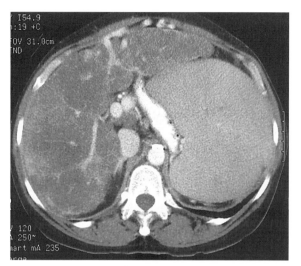

Figure 1.8 A

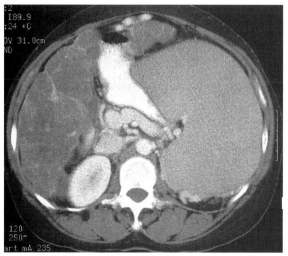

Figure 1.8 B

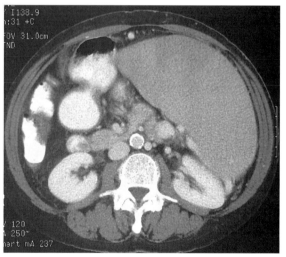

Figure 1.8 C

Findings: CECT demonstrates the liver to be of diffuse low attenuation and patchy areas of higher attenuation. There is also massive splenomegaly and collateral vessels on the anterior surface of the liver.

Differential Diagnosis: Diffuse metastatic disease, intrahepatic cholangiocarcinoma.

Diagnosis: Cirrhosis with fatty liver and recanalized paraumbilical vein.

Discussion: Cirrhosis can produce many findings by CT. These include an enlarged caudate lobe, nodular contour, fatty liver, portal hypertension (with ascites, collaterals and splenomegaly), increased density of the mesenteric fat, and regenerating nodules. Fatty liver is a common early finding of cirrhosis and often precedes other CT findings. As atrophy and fibrosis occur in conjunction with the formation of regenerating nodules, the contour of the liver becomes nodular. In this example, there is diffuse low density to the liver, which could be confused for a diffuse neoplastic process or even intrahepatic cholangiocarcinoma. The key to the differentiation is the lack of mass effect by these low areas of attenuation. The vessels are seen to have a normal course through the liver without displacement. Other findings of cirrhosis are present including a recanalized paraumbilical vein and massive splenomegaly both the result of the portal hypertension.

CASE 9

Clinical History: 70-year-old man with history of meningioma resection in the distant past.

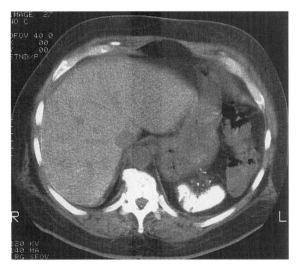

Figure 1.9 A

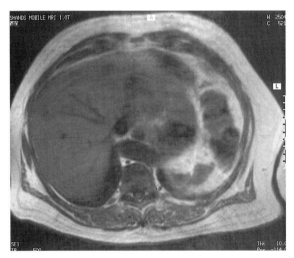

Figure 1.9 B

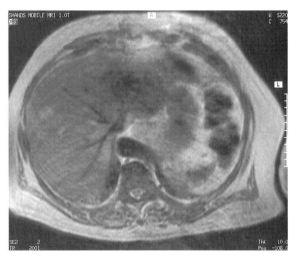

Figure 1.9 C

Findings: (A) NECT demonstrates the liver to be of high attenuation and the spleen is small and very dense; (B) T1-weighted image demonstrates a small hypointense lesion in the anterior segment of the right lobe of the liver; (C) this is hyperintense on the postgadolinium image.

Differential Diagnosis: Intrahepatic cholangiocarcinoma, hepatocellular carcinoma.

Diagnosis: Angiosarcoma in a patient s/p Thorotrast administration.

Discussion: Thorotrast was a radiographic contrast agent developed in the late 1920s and used until the late 1950s primarily in cerebral angiography. Thorotrast is picked up by the reticuloendothelial system of the liver, spleen, lymph nodes and bone marrow. It was later discovered that Thorotrast decayed by means of alpha, beta and gamma emission. The mean dose to the liver was approximately 700 rads in a 30 year period. Thorotrast trapped in the RES of the liver and spleen caused them to be of high attenuation on a NECT. The spleen will be small due to the fibrosis induced by the Thorotrast and markedly dense in appearance. The radiation from the Thorotrast results in the formation of several solid organ neoplasms. These include, in the liver, angiosarcoma, cholangiocarcinoma, and hepatocellular carcinoma. The appearance of angiosarcoma on MRI is that of a nonspecific nodule. It is hypointense on the T1 image and hyperintense on the postgadolinium image. The key to the diagnosis is the finding of prior Thorotrast administration.

CASE 10

Clinical History: 36-year-old woman with history of oral contraceptive use presents with abdominal pain and hypotension.

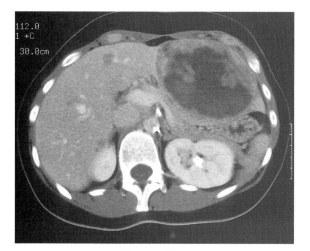

Figure 1.10 A

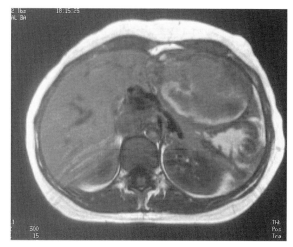

Figure 1.10 B

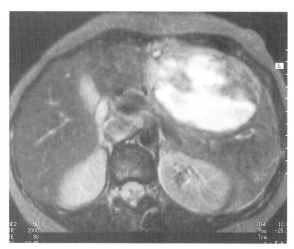

Figure 1.10 C

Findings: (A) CECT demonstrates a 9-cm lesion with an enhancing rim in the left lobe of the liver. A second lesion is in the medial segment. (B) T1-weighted image demonstrates a large isointense lesion with a hyperintense rim seen posteriorly. (C) T2-weighted image demonstrates this lesion to be moderately hyperintense with markedly hyperintense areas posteriorly. There is a second lesion in the caudate lobe.

Differential Diagnosis: Metastases, multiple hepatocellular carcinomas, abscesses.

Diagnosis: Multiple hepatocellular adenomas with areas of hemorrhage.

Discussion: Large hepatocellular adenomas will often rupture and can lead to massive and often fatal hemoperitoneum. Because of this possible grave complication, these lesions are often surgically removed prophylactically. In this example, the rim of increased signal intensity on the T1-weighted image represent hemorrhage from a prior bleed. This area is even more apparent on the T2-weighted image. The large size of the lesion, presence of hemorrhage, age of the patient, and history of oral contraceptive use makes hepatocellular adenoma the best diagnosis. Multiple hepatocellular adenomas are rare and would raise the possibility of abscesses and metastases in this case. Multiple hepatocellular adenomas are associated with glycogen storage diseases.

CASE 11

Clinical History: 35-year-old woman who is taking oral contraceptives.

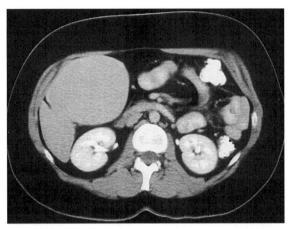
Figure 1.11 A

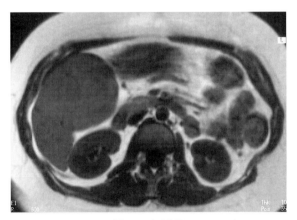
Figure 1.11 B

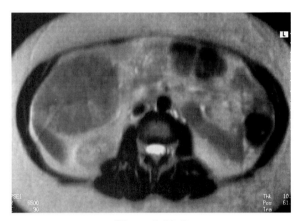
Figure 1.11 C

Findings: (A) CECT demonstrates an isodense lesion in the right lobe of the liver; (B) T1WI demonstrates the mass to be isointense; (C) this lesion is of increased signal intensity on the T2WI. No necrosis or hemorrhage is seen.

Differential Diagnosis: Focal nodular hyperplasia, hepatocellular carcinoma.

Diagnosis: Hepatocellular adenoma.

Discussion: Hepatocellular adenomas are benign neoplasm of the liver, composed of sheets of hepatocytes without veins or ducts. Oral contraceptive use is thought to lead to the development of adenomas as well as increase the risk for hemorrhage by the tumor. Although seen predominantly in females of childbearing age, males on anabolic steroids also have an increased risk. Glycogen storage disease is associated with multiple hepatocellular adenomas. Large adenomas are usually hypointense or isointense on T1WI and slightly to moderately hyperintense on the T2WI. This case is unusual in that large adenomas usually demonstrate areas of hemorrhage and necrosis, which this lesion does not. Areas of fat can also be found in adenomas. By MR characteristics, this lesion could be an FNH although no central scar is seen. A hepatocellular carcinoma would be less likely because no cirrhosis or peritumoral halo is seen. The age and sex of the patient with the history of oral contraceptive use makes hepatocellular adenoma the best choice. Further workup could be done with nuclear medicine studies.

CASE 12

Clinical History: 29-year-old man with history of leukemia presents with fevers.

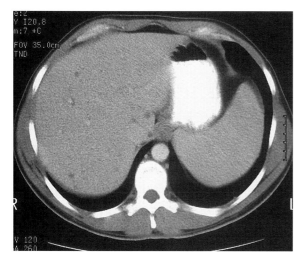

Figure 1.12 A

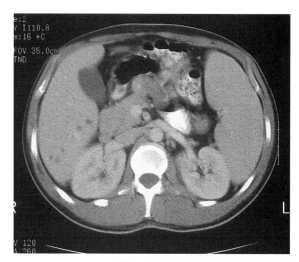

Figure 1.12 B

Findings: Multiple low attenuation lesions seen throughout the liver. Splenomegaly is also present.

Differential Diagnosis: Metastatic disease, infections (fungal), septic emboli, von Meyenburg complex.

Diagnosis: Hepatic candidiasis.

Discussion: Candidiasis is the most common fungal infection encountered in immunocompromised hosts and with the increase of AIDS, it is becoming even more prevalent. In autopsy series, hepatic candidiasis is found in approximately 50% of patients with acute leukemia and lymphoma. The diagnosis is often difficult clinically secondary to the nonspecific signs and symptoms of fever, abdominal pain, and hepatomegaly. The CT appearance of hepatic candidiasis varies depending on the phase of the infection. During the acute phase, there are multiple, small low attenuation lesions throughout the liver and spleen. After treatment with antifungal therapy, there can be calcifications within the lesions as well as areas of high attenuation on the nonenhanced images due to the fibrosis. Other fungal infections such as aspergillus, cryptococcus, and *Pneumocystis carinii* can mimic the healing phase of hepatic candidiasis with multiple hepatic and visceral calcifications. This case demonstrates the acute phase of hepatic candidiasis with multiple low attenuation lesions within the liver and splenomegaly secondary to leukemia.

Clinical History: 65-year-old man with weight loss.

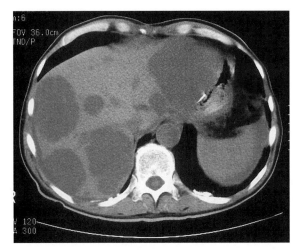

Figure 1.13 A

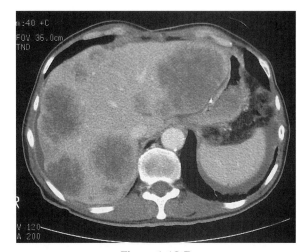

Figure 1.13 B

Findings: (A) NECT demonstrates multiple large, round, hypodense lesions within the liver. There is a small amount of perihepatic ascites; (B) CECT demonstrates enhancement throughout the lesions although they remain hypodense relative to liver.

Differential Diagnosis: Multifocal hepatocellular carcinoma, lymphoma.

Diagnosis: Multiple liver metastases from gastric adenocarcinoma.

Discussion: Assessing the liver for metastatic disease is crucial for the staging and prognosis of the patient. Approximately 24–36% of patients who die of a malignancy will demonstrate liver metastasis at autopsy. Neoplasms arising from the gastrointestinal tract, in particular, have a propensity to metastasize to the liver secondary to the drainage through the portal vein. Approximately 45% of patients with gastric carcinoma have metastasis to the liver at the time of diagnosis. The appearance of multiple, large, round, hypodense lesions in the liver is most commonly due to metastatic disease. Abscesses would be unlikely in this case because they would not demonstrate central enhancement as is seen in these lesions. Multifocal hepatocellular carcinoma is a possibility but the size, number, and lack of cirrhosis would make this diagnosis less likely. A search for a primary lesion in the gastrointestinal tract would be necessary in the workup of this patient.

CASE 14

Clinical History: 45-year-old woman with abdominal pain and elevated liver function tests.

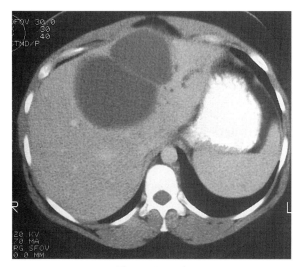

Figure 1.14 A

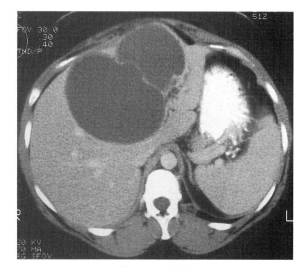

Figure 1.14 B

Findings: CECT demonstrates a large septated cystic mass arising from the left lobe of the liver. Note mild intrahepatic biliary dilatation.

Differential Diagnosis: Echinococcal cyst, abscess, necrotic metastasis, or primary neoplasm.

Diagnosis: Biliary cystadenoma.

Discussion: Biliary cystadenoma is a rare benign tumor of the liver with malignant potential, which is thought to arise from hamartomatous bile ducts. They are more commonly seen in females. They are usually intrahepatic but can be extra-hepatic presenting commonly with jaundice. Biliary cystadenomas resemble mucinous cystic neoplasms of the pancreas. They are typically cystic in appearance and can have multiple septations. There is often a thin rim of calcification within the wall of the lesion as well as a solid component. The thicker the calcification and larger the solid component, the more likely it is a malignant cystadenocarcinoma. This lesion has the typical findings of a biliary cystadenoma with a thin wall and septations. Necrotic metastases and abscesses tend to have a thicker enhancing wall than in this case. Echinococcal cyst would be a good second choice if there was a history of travel to an endemic area with exposure to sheep and dogs.

CASE 15

Clinical History: 14-month-old boy presents with increasing abdominal girth.

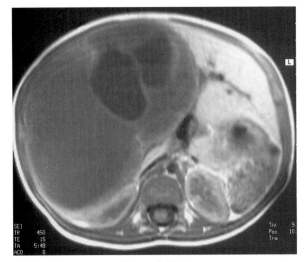

Figure 1.15 A

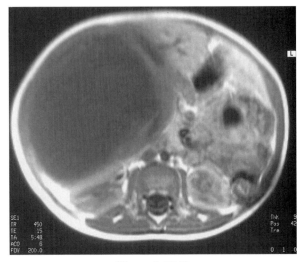

Figure 1.15 B

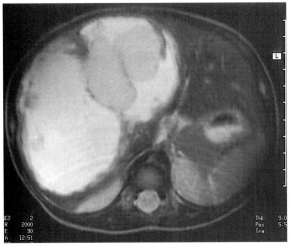

Figure 1.15 C

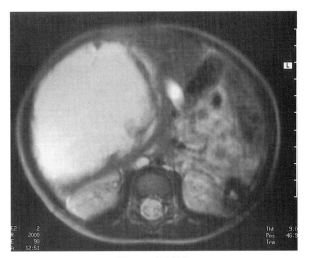

Figure 1.15 D

Findings: (A, B) T1-weighted images demonstrates a low signal intensity lesion replacing the right lobe of the liver. Note the normal gallbladder and an adjacent cystic structure of similar intensity; (C, D) T2 image demonstrates these same lesions to be hyperintense following the signal characteristics of simple fluid.

Differential Diagnosis: Undifferentiated embryonal sarcoma, infantile hemangioendothelioma, hepatoblastoma, metastases.

Diagnosis: Mesenchymal hamartoma.

Discussion: Mesenchymal hamartomas is a cystic mass of the liver thought to be developmental in origin. It usually grows slowly to a very large size before discovery. Rapid growth can occur as fluid accumulates in the hamartoma's lobules. The MR signal characteristics of mesenchymal hamartoma reflect its cystic nature. The signal follows that of fluid with varied appearance of the cysts in a given patient, indicating the variable accumulation of proteinaceous material in the cysts. In this age group, the other hepatic masses would include an infantile hemangioendothelioma, hepatoblastoma, metastases (most commonly from neuroblastoma), and mesenchymal hamartoma. Mesenchymal hamartoma is typically a cystic mass, whereas the other lesions tend to be solid except for occasional areas of necrosis. Undifferentiated embryonal sarcoma is commonly cystic from necrosis due to its rapid growth and aggressive nature. UESs, however, usually occur in late childhood. A large cystic lesion in an infant is most likely to be a mesenchymal hamartoma.

CASE 16

Clinical History: 59-year-old female with a history of alcohol abuse.

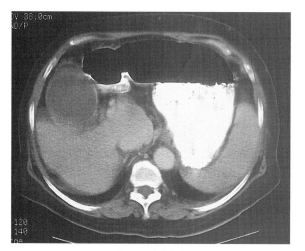

Figure 1.16 A

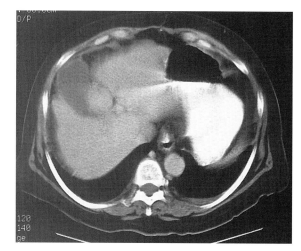

Figure 1.16 B

Findings: CECT demonstrates a small liver with an enlarged caudate lobe. Note the dilated gallbladder.

Differential Diagnosis: None.

Diagnosis: Cirrhosis.

Discussion: Cirrhosis is a chronic disease of the liver that can be caused by a variety of etiologies—with alcohol being the most common in the United States. Other etiologies include hepatitis, inheritable diseases such as Wilson's disease, tyrosinemia, glycogen-storage disease, primary biliary cirrhosis, and chronic right-sided heart failure. There are many CT findings in cirrhosis. This case demonstrates an enlarged caudate lobe with atrophy of the rest of the liver. There are several theories for this finding. One suggests that the fibrosis and regeneration of the liver impairs the normal venous drainage leading to atrophy. The caudate lobe, which has a separate drainage into the IVC, is less affected by this process. Blood is, therefore, preferentially shunted to the caudate lobe causing it to hypertrophy while the rest of the liver atrophies. Budd-Chiari syndrome can also cause caudate lobe hypertrophy by the same mechanism but no other findings of Budd-Chiari are seen in this patient.

CASE 17

Clinical History: 43-year-old woman with abdominal discomfort.

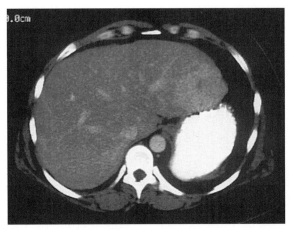

Figure 1.17 A

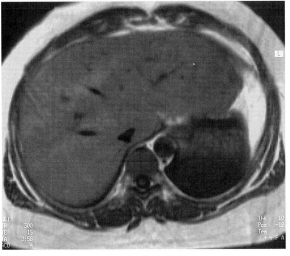

Figure 1.17 B

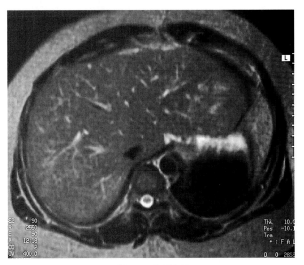

Figure 1.17 C

Findings: (A) CECT shows a 5-cm slightly hyperdense lesion in the left lobe of the liver. Note the low-density central scar; (B, C) T1-weighted image demonstrates a slightly hypointense lesion that is slightly hyperintense on the T2-weighted image. There is increased signal seen in the central scar on the T2 image.

Differential Diagnosis: Metastasis, hepatocellular adenoma, hepatocellular carcinoma.

Diagnosis: Focal nodular hyperplasia.

Discussion: Focal nodular hyperplasia tends to be isointense on most MR sequences making it difficult to detect. Because the lesion in this case is slightly hypointense on the T1 images and slightly hyperintense on the T2 images, its appearance is nonspecific. The presence of the central scar, however, makes the diagnosis of focal nodular hyperplasia most likely. The central scar can often aid in the diagnosis because it will be hypointense on the T1-weighted images and hyperintense on the T2-weighted images relative to the liver. This is in distinction to the central scar seen in fibrolamellar hepatocellular carcinoma, which tend to be hypointense on both the T1- and T2-weighted sequences. The increased signal of the central scar in the FNH may be related to the slow flowing blood and bile within the vascular channels and bile ducts found within the septa of the collagenous scar. In fibrolamellar HCC, however, the central scar is poorly vascularized and its MR characteristics are more typical for that of collagen. These MRI findings of FNH and fibrolamellar HCC can overlap making the diagnosis difficult. The central scar, lack of cirrhosis, and age of the patient makes focal nodular hyperplasia the best diagnosis.

CASE 18

Clinical History: 4-month-old boy with elevated alpha fetoprotein and irritability.

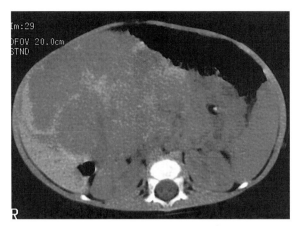

Figure 1.18 A

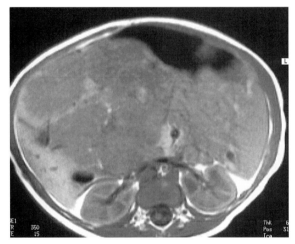

Figure 1.18 B

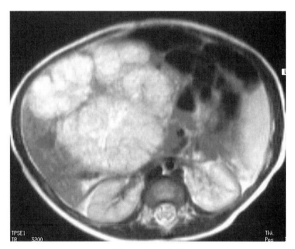

Figure 1.18 C

Findings: (A) NECT demonstrates a 10-cm lesion in the liver with septations; (B) T1-weighted image demonstrates a hypointense mass with linear areas of increased signal intensity; (C) T2-weighted image demonstrates this lesion to be hyperintense. The linear areas noted on T1 are hypointense on the T2 image. Round areas of hemorrhage are present.

Differential Diagnosis: Infantile hemangioendothelioma, metastatic neuroblastoma, mesenchymal hamartoma, hepatocellular carcinoma.

Diagnosis: Hepatoblastoma.

Discussion: The findings of hepatoblastoma on MRI are similar to those seen in a hepatocellular carcinoma. Both neoplasms will frequently produce an elevated level of alpha fetoprotein. Hepatoblastoma, however, usually occurs in patients younger than 5 years of age whereas HCC in those older than 5 years of age. Like HCC, hepatoblastomas will be hypointense on T1-weighted images and hyperintense on the T2-weighted images. The linear areas seen in this example represent fibrous septa found in mixed hepatoblastomas. Although hemorrhage and necrosis is rare in small hepatoblastomas, they can occasionally occur in very large lesions such as in this case. However, cystic transformation of a hepatoblastoma almost never occurs. These areas of hemorrhage and necrosis are not nearly as large as those typically seen in undifferentiated embryonal sarcoma and mesenchymal hamartoma. Both infantile hemangioendothelioma and metastatic neuroblastoma can have similar MR appearance to hepatoblastoma but will rarely produce an elevated alpha fetoprotein. Metastatic neuroblastomas, like most metastases, tend to be multiple.

CASE 19

Clinical History: A young child with fevers and swollen axillary lymph nodes.

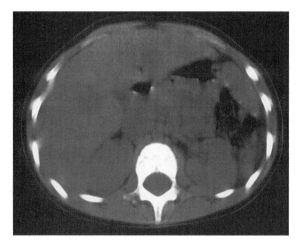

Figure 1.19 A

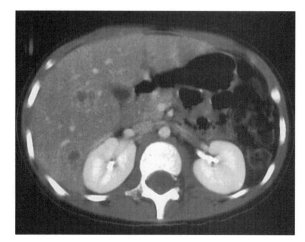

Figure 1.19 B

Findings: (A) NECT demonstrates multiple moderately sized hypodense lesions throughout the liver. (B) On the CECT, these same lesions appear smaller with marked peripheral enhancement.

Differential Diagnosis: Granulomatous disease (sarcoid, tuberculosis), fungal infection, pyogenic abscesses, hypervascular metastasis.

Diagnosis: Cat scratch disease of the liver.

Discussion: The etiology of cat-scratch disease is unknown but is thought to be secondary to a gram-negative bacteria. It usually occurs in children or adolescents who present with fever and unilateral, asymmetric lymphadenitis. Approximately 90% of the patients report scratches or close contact to cats. Diagnosis can be made with a skin test and is often a diagnosis of exclusion based on history and lymph node biopsy. This case demonstrates the classic findings of cat scratch disease in the liver consisting of multiple hypodense lesions ranging in size from 3 mm to 2 cm in size. On the enhanced images, the lesions appear smaller due to contrast enhancement and can even become isodense to normal liver. Subtle peripheral enhancement helps to delineate these lesions. The true prevalence of this disease in the liver and spleen is difficult to know but is thought to be very rare. The disease is usually self-limited and normally resolves in 4–8 weeks. Aspiration of a peripheral suppurative lymph node can be performed to relieve pain if necessary and to aid in the diagnosis.

CASE 20

Clinical History: 19-year-old woman status post right-chest tube placement.

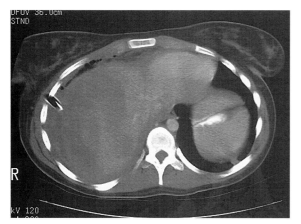

Figure 1.20 A

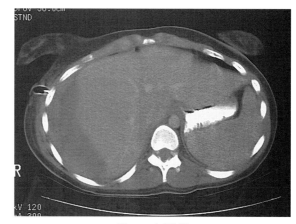

Figure 1.20 B

Findings: CECT demonstrates a large subcapsular fluid collection with areas of high attenuation within it. Note the chest tube coursing through the fluid collection. A small amount of free air is seen in the fluid collection along the anterior surface of the liver

Differential Diagnosis: None.

Diagnosis: Large subcapsular hematoma secondary to chest tube placement.

Discussion: Hepatic trauma can result in perihepatic, intrahepatic, or subcapsular fluid collections. Hematomas tend to be hypodense relative to liver parenchyma but can have areas of higher attenuation representing clotted blood. As the hematoma matures, it will become lower in attenuation in the range of uncomplicated fluid. Unclotted blood is often difficult to distinguish from ascitic fluid because its higher attenuation can be very subtle. Subcapsular hematomas tend to indent the liver parenchyma and deform the liver contour as is seen in this case. This differentiates it from perihepatic fluid collections that will flow into the dependent portions of the abdomen and pelvis such as the paracolic gutters and pelvis. Subcapsular hematomas can be due to trauma, iatrogenic causes, and intrahepatic neoplasms, such as a hepatocellular adenoma, which can rupture causing hemorrhage. If a history of trauma or prior procedure is not found, then a search for a hepatic neoplasm is necessary.

Clinical History: 32-year-old man with the presumptive diagnosis of biliary stricture and cholangitis. The patient has undergone an ERCP.

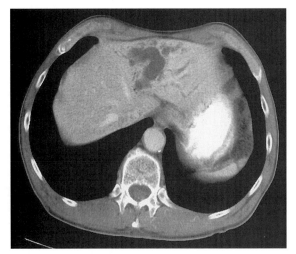

Figure 1.21 A

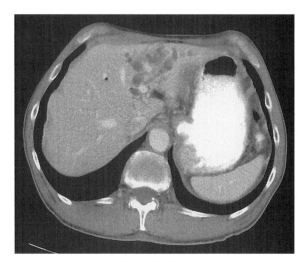

Figure 1.21 B

Findings: CECT demonstrates focal saccular dilatation of the biliary tree in the left lobe of the liver. Note pneumobilia s/p ERCP.

Differential Diagnosis: Biliary stricture, recurrent pyogenic cholangitis, cholangiocarcinoma.

Diagnosis: Focal Caroli disease.

Discussion: Focal Caroli disease is often difficult to diagnose. This patient had several admissions for cholangitis and as a result of these infections was thought to have a biliary stricture causing biliary dilatation. ERCP was performed and demonstrated no strictures or dilated extrahepatic biliary tree excluding the diagnosis of biliary strictures and recurrent pyogenic cholangitis. The diagnosis of Caroli disease was confirmed after resection of the affected segment. Besides recurrent infections and sepsis, other complications of Caroli disease include biliary strictures and stasis, which further worsens the primary disease. Cholangiocarcinomas can complicate Caroli disease, foreshortening its course. Because of the association with congenital fibrosis, portal hypertension is often found in these patients, which can lead to GI hemorrhage.

CASE 22

Clinical History: 73-year-old male with blood per rectum.

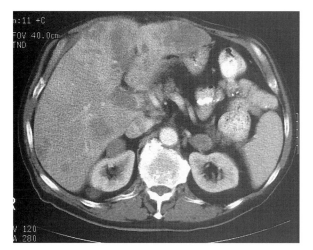

Figure 1.22 A

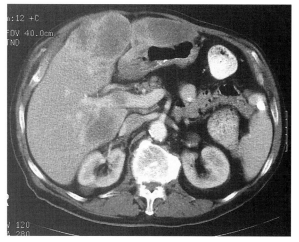

Figure 1.22 B

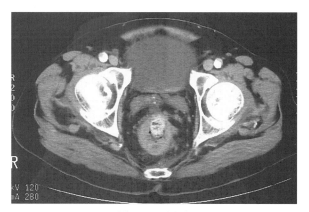

Figure 1.22 C

Findings: CECT demonstrates multiple large low attenuation lesions in both lobes of the liver with the largest being in the left lobe. There is also a soft tissue mass seen within the portal vein. Bilateral adrenal masses are also present. Image of the pelvis demonstrates thickening of the rectal wall.

Differential Diagnosis: Multifocal hepatocellular carcinoma, multiple abscesses.

Diagnosis: Metastatic rectal carcinoma to the liver with a bland thrombus in the portal vein.

Discussion: Portal vein thrombosis can be idiopathic or secondary to multiple etiologies such as tumor invasion, intraabdominal infection with phlebitis, or hypercoaguable states. Portal vein thrombosis secondary to tumor invasion usually enlarges the portal vein and flow can often be demonstrated within the thrombus by ultrasound, enhancement on CECT, or angiography. Tumor invasion of the portal vein can be seen frequently in hepatocellular carcinoma, and rarely in pancreatic carcinoma, and gastric carcinoma. Metastasis will rarely invade the portal vein. This case demonstrates multiple metastases from a rectal carcinoma and a thrombus within the portal vein. Colorectal metastases, as stated previously, rarely invade the portal vein. The thrombus does not appear to be enlarging the portal vein and there is no streaky enhancement as is typically seen in a tumor thrombus. The thrombus in this example is a bland thrombus from either partial obstruction of the portal vein or from the hypercoaguable state caused by the tumor.

Clinical History: 25-year-old woman with history of polycythemia vera.

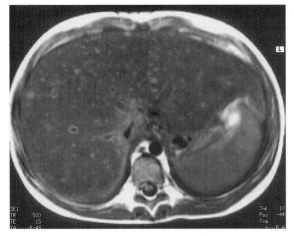

Figure 1.23 A

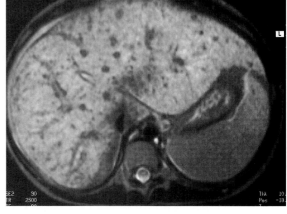

Figure 1.23 B

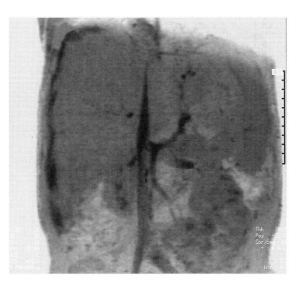

Figure 1.23 C

Findings: (A) T1-weighted MRI demonstrates multiple punctate areas of increased signal intensity without demonstrable hepatic veins; (B) T2-weighted MRI at the same level demonstrates multiple punctate areas of low signal intensity corresponding to those seen on the T1 weighted image. Again no hepatic veins are seen; (C) MR angio demonstrates the IVC to be patent but attenuated without visualization of the hepatic veins.

Differential Diagnosis: None.

Diagnosis: Budd-Chiari syndrome.

Discussion: MR is very useful to detect Budd-Chiari syndrome. The typical findings on CT of an enlarged caudate, ascites, and hepatomegaly are readily seen on MR. MR also adds the ability to image in multiple planes as well as MRA to evaluate the hepatic veins and IVC. Intrahepatic and extrahepatic collateral circulation are easily seen on MR. Patent collaterals, as are most vessels, are seen as structures with flow voids on standard spin echo techniques that have high signal intensity on gradient echo imaging. In this example, there was no evidence of flow in the hepatic veins. The multiple punctate areas seen throughout the liver correspond to intrahepatic collaterals, which have formed due to the hepatic venous outflow obstruction. These findings are typical of Budd-Chiari syndrome.

CASE 24

Clinical History: 52-year-old woman with cirrhosis.

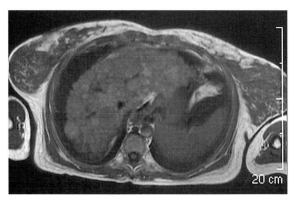

Figure 1.24 A

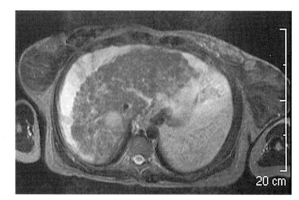

Figure 1.24 B

Findings: (A) T1-weighted image demonstrates a small shrunken, nodular liver with multiple nodules of slightly increased signal intensity. There is a single hypointense lesion in the right lobe; (B) T2-weighted image demonstrates the nodules to be of low signal intensity, and the previously noted hypointense lesion is now hyperintense.

Differential Diagnosis: Metastases.

Diagnosis: HCC and regenerating nodules in a cirrhotic liver (dysplastic nodule).

Discussion: This case demonstrates the spectrum of focal lesions that can occur in a cirrhotic liver. In a cirrhotic liver, there will be regenerating nodules that can progress to adenomatous hyperplastic nodules and finally become hepatocellular carcinoma. This progression is continuous and is thought to eventually occur in every regenerating nodule. Therefore, resection of an HCC is not curative because other regenerating nodules will eventually lead to other hepatocellular carcinomas. Definitive treatment for cirrhotic livers is transplantation. The signal characteristics of a regenerating nodule and adenomatous hyperplastic nodule are essentially the same. They will both be iso- to hyperintense on the T1-weighted images and iso- to hypointense on the T2-weighted images. A hepatocellular carcinoma, on the other hand, will act like most malignancies and be hypointense on T1 and hyperintense on T2-weighted images. This distinguishes HCC from regenerating nodules and adenomatous hyperplastic nodules.

CASE 25

Clinical History: 44-year-old woman with diabetes.

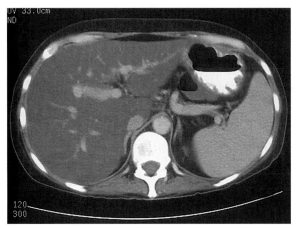

Figure 1.25 A

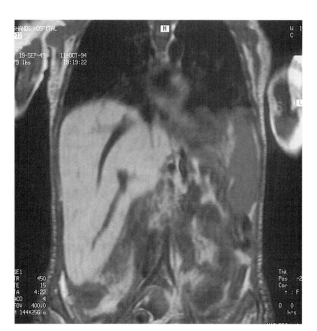

Figure 1.25 B

Findings: (A) CECT demonstrated diffuse low attenuation of the liver without displacement of the hepatic vessels; (B) Coronal T1WI demonstrates the liver to be diffusely hyperintense relative to the spleen.

Differential Diagnosis: None.

Diagnosis: Diffuse fatty liver.

Discussion: There is a multitude of disorders that can lead to fatty liver. The most common cause in the United States is alcoholic liver disease. Other causes include diabetes, parenteral nutrition, steroids, obesity, and chemotherapeutic drugs. Fatty liver can produce hepatomegaly and rarely causes significant elevation of liver function tests. The diagnosis is usually made incidentally.

The diagnosis of fatty liver is easily made on CT scans. The spleen is normally 8–10 HU lower in attenuation than the liver on a NECT. A reversal of this relationship leads to the diagnosis of fatty liver. Because of the variability in enhancement of the liver and spleen, mild fatty change may be difficult to detect on a CECT. On CECT, a difference of 25 HU suggests fatty liver. No mass effect is caused by the fatty liver so the vessels are normal in appearance. MRI demonstrates the liver to be of similar signal intensity to the surrounding fat. A fat suppression image could also be performed to confirm the diagnosis.

CASE 26

Clinical History: 50-year-old man with malaise and fatigue.

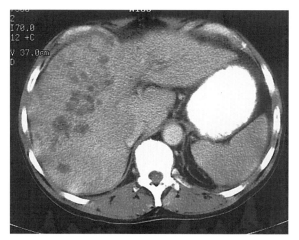

Figure 1.26 A

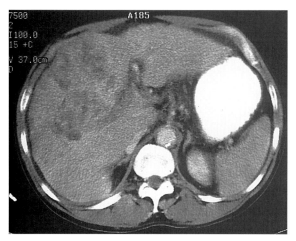

Figure 1.26 B

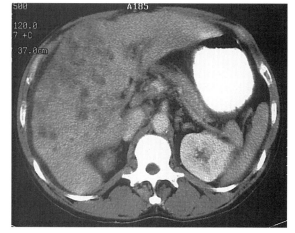

Figure 1.26 C

Findings: CECT demonstrates multiple small hypodense foci that are seen diffusely in the right lobe of the liver. The portal vein is thrombosed. Changes of cirrhosis are present with enlargement of the caudate lobe and the left lobe of the liver.

Differential Diagnosis: Metastasis, intrahepatic cholangiocarcinoma.

Diagnosis: Hepatocellular carcinoma.

Discussion: Hepatocellular carcinoma can present in three different ways on imaging studies: 1) a single solitary lesion (expansile HCC), which is often very large; 2) multifocal HCC, which is comprised of multiple separate nodules; 3) cirrhotomimetic or diffuse HCC, which is composed of multiple tiny indistinct nodules. This case is an example of the cirrhotomimetic or diffuse form of hepatocellular carcinoma. This diagnosis is suggested by the underlying cirrhosis and the portal vein invasion, which is seen in approximately 70% of cases of HCC. The streaks of contrast in the region of the portal vein most likely represents enhancement of the periportal venous plexus. Cholangiocarcinoma usually does not cause portal vein thrombosis but instead will surround and encase vessels. Metastases will rarely cause a tumor thrombus occurring in less than 20% of cases.

CASE 27

Clinical History: 65-year-old woman with left lower quadrant pain.

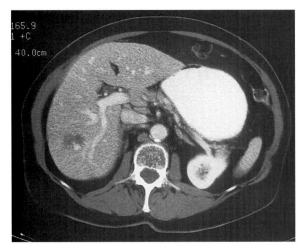

Figure 1.27 A

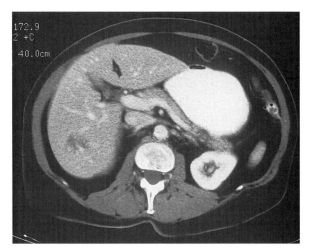

Figure 1.27 B

Findings: CECT demonstrates a low attenuation lesion in the right lobe of the liver, which demonstrates puddling of contrast in the periphery of the lesion.

Differential Diagnosis: Metastasis.

Diagnosis: Hemangioma.

Discussion: Hemangiomas are the most common liver tumors. They are more commonly seen in women than men (5:1). They are typically asymptomatic and found incidentally except when hemorrhage is present. They are often subcapsular in location but can also be pedunculated.

Dynamic contrast administration demonstrates dense thick peripheral enhancement of the lesion with sequential filling in of the lesion over time. This can take minutes to hours to occur. Eventually the contrast will wash out of the liver but at a much faster rate than the hemangioma, which will be hyperdense relative to the liver. Puddling of contrast in the periphery of the lesion is also characteristic for a hemangioma and is only seen in a minority of metastases. This is demonstrated well in this example. Without a history of a primary malignancy, a solitary metastasis is unlikely in this case, making a hemangioma the best diagnosis.

CASE 28

Clinical History: 57-year-old man with diverticulitis involving the sigmoid colon.

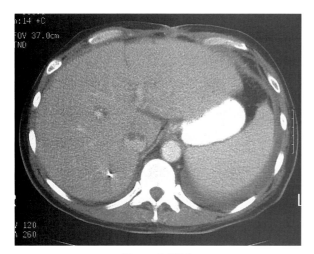

Figure 1.28 A

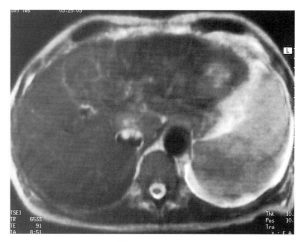

Figure 1.28 B

Findings: CECT demonstrates a low attenuation thrombus within the anterior portion of the inferior vena cava. T2-weighted MRI reveals the same lesion in the inferior vena cava as well as a hyperintense lesion just anterior to the inferior vena cava and a second lesion in the left lobe of the liver.

Differential Diagnosis: Metastasis.

Diagnosis: Multiple pyogenic liver abscesses with secondary inferior vena cava thrombus.

Discussion: Most hepatic abscesses in the United States are pyogenic in origin but with the increase in immunocompromised patients from chemotherapy, organ transplants, and AIDS, fungal abscesses are also increasing. In one series, approximately 60% of the abscesses were hypointense on the T1-weighted images and 72% were hyperintense on the T2-weighted images; 35% of the abscesses demonstrated increased signal intensity on the T2 images around the lesion, which is thought to represent perilesional edema. This case was unusual in that the lesions were not very apparent on the CECT images except for the involvement of the inferior vena cava. MRI, however, easily demonstrated the lesions and the effect on the inferior vena cava. The increased signal on the T2 image, the multifocality of the lesions, and history of diverticulitis makes abscesses most likely. Metastases could also have this appearance and an obstructing colon cancer causing the diverticulitis must be excluded. Diagnosing these lesions is crucial because antibiotic therapy is often not sufficient for treatment and aspiration and drainage is necessary for total resolution. In this case, multiple aspirations and drainages were performed using ultrasound guidance.

CASE 29

Clinical History: 35-year-old woman with pure red cell aplasia requiring multiple transfusions.

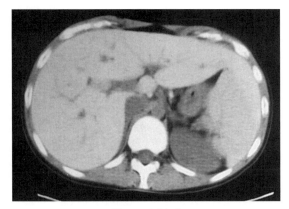

Figure 1.29 A

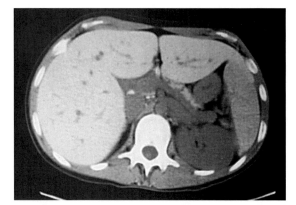

Figure 1.29 B

Findings: NECT demonstrates increased attenuation to the liver and spleen.

Differential Diagnosis: Glycogen storage disease, drugs (chemotherapy, gold, amiodarone) Thorotrast, Wilson's disease.

Diagnosis: Secondary hemochromatosis.

Discussion: Secondary hemochromatosis, which is related to multiple transfusions predominantly affects the reticuloendothelial system. This leads to the deposition of iron in the liver and spleen causing them to be dense on NECT. The normal density of the liver is 30–60 HU, reaching 75–130 HU with hemochromatosis. Other causes of increased liver density include glycogen storage disease, drugs, and occasionally Wilson's disease. These, however, usually do not affect the spleen as is seen in this case. Thorotrast, however, does affect the spleen. Thorotrast was a contrast agent introduced in 1928 but its use was discontinued in the mid 1950s when it was found to lead to the development of angiosarcomas and other visceral neoplasms. It would be unlikely that a patient of this age would have been exposed to this agent.

CASE 30

Clinical History: 34-year-old woman with hepatomegaly and abdominal pain.

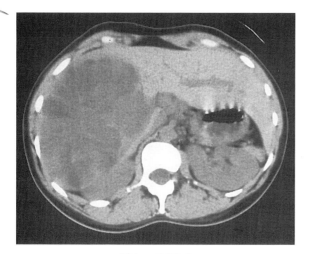

Figure 1.30 A

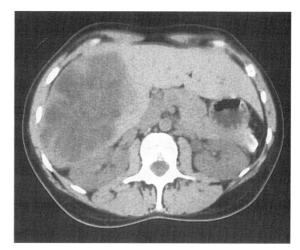

Figure 1.30 B

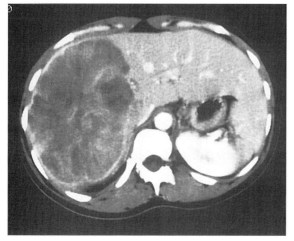

Figure 1.30 C

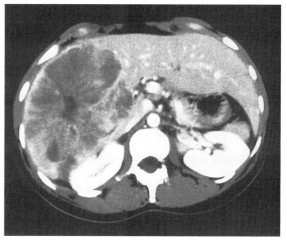

Figure 1.30 D

Findings: (A, B) NECT demonstrates a 10-cm low attenuation mass in the right lobe of the liver; (C, D) CECT reveals this lesion to have heterogeneous enhancement with a central area without enhancement.

Differential Diagnosis: Hepatic adenoma, focal nodular hyperplasia.

Diagnosis: Fibrolamellar hepatocellular carcinoma.

Discussion: Fibrolamellar hepatocellular carcinoma differs from a typical HCC in that there is no underlying liver disease (cirrhosis), the alpha fetoprotein level is usually normal, and the age of onset is typically under 40 years of age. The prognosis for fibrolamellar HCC is better than typical HCC.

CT findings include an enhancing mass with a non-enhancing fibrous central scar, well seen in this example. The lesion is typically solitary and can have calcifications within the lesion. Both hepatic adenoma and focal nodular hyperplasia could have a similar appearance by CT. Hepatic adenoma does not usually have a scar and a history of oral contraceptive use is usually present. Fibrolamellar HCC will often have gallium uptake, which can aid in the diagnostic workup.

Clinical History: 49-year-old woman with right upper quadrant pain and a palpable mass.

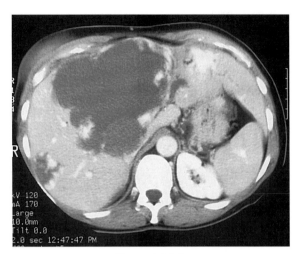

Figure 1.31 A

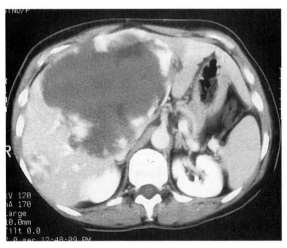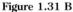

Figure 1.31 B

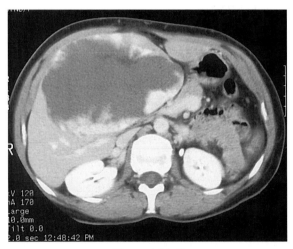

Figure 1.31 C

Findings: CECT demonstrates a 12-cm mass replacing the entire left lobe of the liver. There is peripheral globular enhancement with a low attenuation center. A second smaller lesion is seen in the right lobe.

Differential Diagnosis: Hypervascular metastasis.

Diagnosis: Giant hemangioma of the liver.

Discussion: Hemangiomas are the most common liver tumors. They are usually found incidentally unless they become symptomatic from hemorrhage or large size. They tend to be small and are multiple in about 10% of cases. Punctate and coarse calcifications can occur especially in giant hemangiomas. CT findings include intense globular peripheral enhancement of the lesion with centripetal filling in of the lesion over time. There can be areas of necrosis and cyst formation within the lesion, especially with giant hemangiomas. This case is typical of giant hemangiomas. There is intense puddling of contrast in the periphery of the lesion after bolus injection of contrast. This enhancement is much more intense than in hypervascular neoplasms or abscesses. In addition, the enhancement pattern of hypervascular neoplasms and abscesses tend to be ringlike rather than globular. The lack of history for fever or elevated white blood cell count makes abscess unlikely. No evidence of cirrhosis to suggest HCC and the enhancement pattern is atypical for metastases.

CASE 32

Clinical History: 15-year-old girl with right upper quadrant pain and elevated liver enzymes.

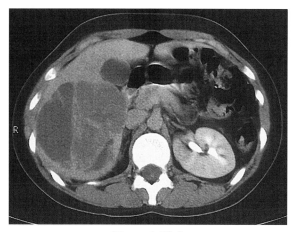

Figure 1.32 A

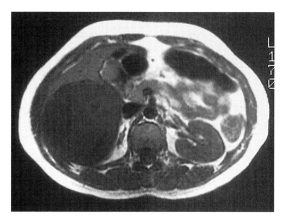

Figure 1.32 B

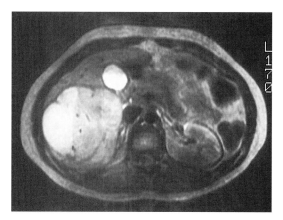

Figure 1.32 C

Findings: (A) CECT demonstrates a complex cystic lesion in the right lobe of the liver; (B) T1-weighted image demonstrates the lesion to be hypointense. Note the subtle area of lower signal intensity seen on the right side of the lesion; (C) This same lesion is hyperintense on the T2-weighted image. Note the higher area of signal intensity on the right side of the lesion representing necrosis.

Differential Diagnosis: Mesenchymal hamartoma, hepatocellular carcinoma, hepatic adenoma, necrotic metastases.

Diagnosis: Undifferentiated embryonal sarcoma.

Discussion: Undifferentiated embryonal sarcoma (UES) is an uncommon malignant neoplasm of mesenchymal origin composed of spindle-shaped sarcomatous cells. About 90% of these lesions occur before the age of 15, with most occurring in older children (6–12 years). Even with surgery, chemotherapy, and radiotherapy, the prognosis is poor with life expectancy of less than 12 months. UES is typically a large mass with areas of hemorrhage and necrosis. The lesion will, therefore, appear as a combination of large cystic and solid areas. The only good differential diagnosis for this appearance in the pediatric patient is the benign mesenchymal hamartoma. Other possibilities such as a HCC and HCA are much less likely in the pediatric patient. UESs are typically hypointense on T1 and hyperintense on T2 images with the areas of necrosis having the signal characteristics of water. The solid component of UES enhances after gadolinium administration.

CASE 33

Clinical History: 69-year-old man with weight loss and history of hemochromatosis.

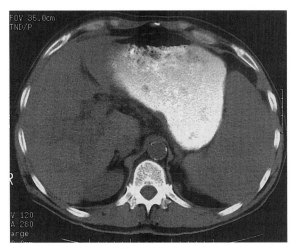

Figure 1.33 A

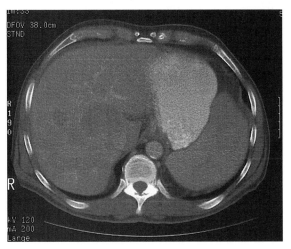

Figure 1.33 B

Figure 1.33 C

Findings: (A) NECT demonstrates subtle diffuse increased attenuation of the liver with an enlarged right portal vein; (B) CECT demonstrates two low-density lesions within the liver; (C) CECT also shows right portal vein thrombosis.

Differential Diagnosis: Metastases.

Diagnosis: Hemochromatosis with hepatocellular carcinoma and portal vein invasion.

Discussion: The subtle increase in attenuation of the liver is secondary to iron deposition within the liver parenchyma in this patient with a known history of hemochromatosis. Patient's with hemochromatosis have an increased incidence of hepatocellular carcinoma, which has a propensity to invade the portal vein as in this case. Metastases are less likely to occur in patients with cirrhosis due to the altered blood flow to the liver. They are also less likely to cause portal vein invasion as is seen in this example. The invasion of the portal vein, the multifocal nature, and history of hemochromatosis make hepatocellular carcinoma the most likely diagnosis in this patient.

CASE 34

Clinical History: 30-year-old man with nausea, vomiting, and abdominal pain.

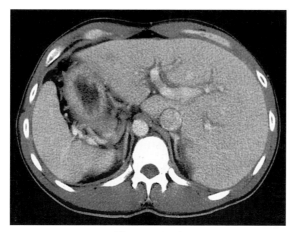

Figure 1.34 A

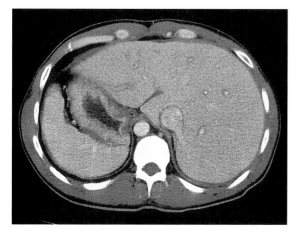

Figure 1.34 B

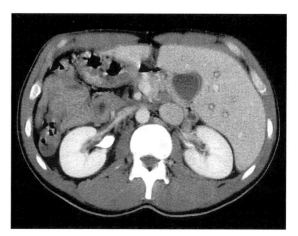

Figure 1.34 C

Findings: CECT demonstrates periportal lucency, mild hepatomegaly, and thickened gallbladder wall.

Differential Diagnosis: AIDS, trauma, congestive heart failure, liver transplant rejection.

Diagnosis: Viral hepatitis.

Discussion: Hepatitis can be viral, bacterial, or fungal in origin. In most cases, hepatitis refers to viral hepatitis, which accounts for the majority of the fulminant hepatic failures from hepatitis. It can be acute or chronic in nature. If the inflammatory changes last for more than 6 months, the patient is thought to have chronic hepatitis. The findings on CT are nonspecific. These include hepatomegaly, which can lead to abdominal pain, portal lymphadenopathy, and gallbladder wall thickening. Periportal edema can be seen as lucency surrounding the portal branches. Other causes for periportal edema include AIDS, trauma, CHF, and liver transplant rejection. In this patient, there was no history of trauma or a liver transplant and the patient had no symptoms of CHF. AIDS is a possibility especially in a younger patient, but the other abdominal findings for AIDS such as lymphadenopathy, AIDS nephritis, and AIDS cholangitis were not present in this case.

CASE 35

Clinical History: 44-year-old man with right upper quadrant pain. Patient has a history of foreign travel.

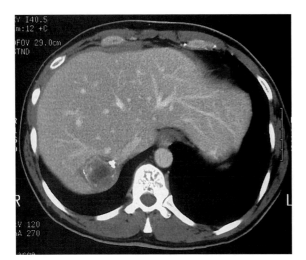

Figure 1.35 A

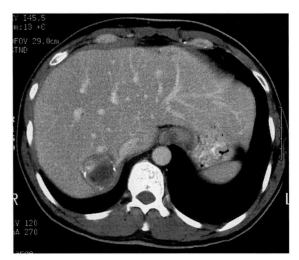

Figure 1.35 B

Findings: 3-cm low-density lesion in the right lobe of the liver with peripheral enhancement and calcifications.

Differential Diagnosis: Old hematoma, pyogenic abscess, calcified necrotic metastasis (sarcomas, mucinous neoplasms), biliary cystadenoma/carcinoma.

Diagnosis: Echinococcal cyst of the liver.

Discussion: Hydatid disease is endemic to many parts of the world where sheep are raised such as Australia, Africa, South America, and in the Middle East. The United States is also seeing an increase in the number of cases most likely due to the influx of immigrants and travelers from these endemic countries. Patients usually present with symptoms that mimic choledocholithiasis such as recurrent jaundice, colicky right upper quadrant pain, and fevers. This case demonstrates many of the classic findings found in echinococcal disease of the liver. The lesion is usually round or oval with a low-density center. As in this case, peripheral calcifications can occur in approximately 10–20% of the time; 75% of the lesions occur in the right lobe of the liver and can demonstrate peripheral enhancement. Enhancement is thought to be secondary to compression of the surrounding liver parenchyma and the adjacent inflammatory response. In one series, the detection rate with computed tomography was as high as 98%.

CASE 36

Clinical History: 64-year-old woman with weight loss.

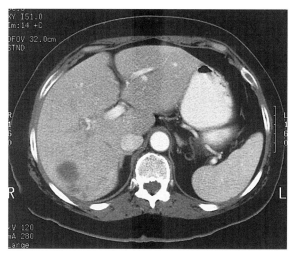

Figure 1.36 A

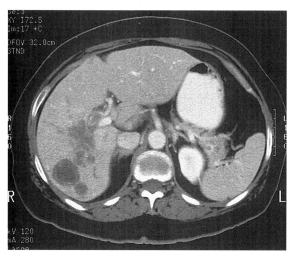

Figure 1.36 B

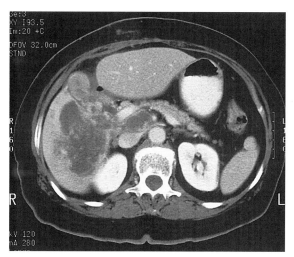

Figure 1.36 C

Findings: Large ill-defined low-density lesion in the right lobe of the liver with smaller satellite lesions adjacent to it. Necrotic periportal adenopathy is also present. Note the mildly dilated intrahepatic ducts and the encasement of the portal vein without invasion.

Differential Diagnosis: Hepatocellular carcinoma, metastasis.

Diagnosis: Intrahepatic cholangiocarcinoma (I-CAC).

Discussion: Intrahepatic cholangiocarcinoma originates in the small intrahepatic bile ducts and is the second most common primary malignant hepatic tumor after hepatocellular carcinoma. Only 10% of all cholangiocarcinomas are intrahepatic. There is an increased incidence of I-CAC seen in patients with chronic biliary obstruction and infection, such as in patients with Caroli's disease, sclerosing cholangitis, inflammatory bowel disease, and clonorchis infection. Although it is often impossible to differentiate I-CAC from metastases and hepatocellular carcinoma, certain findings can be helpful. Intrahepatic cholangiocarcinoma commonly causes biliary dilatation because it arises and spreads via the biliary system. It will also encase the portal vein rather than invade it as seen in this example. HCC, on the other hand, frequently invades the portal vein and underlying cirrhosis is usually present. It is also uncommon to have biliary dilatation secondary to metastases making them less likely in this case. Clinically, alpha fetoprotein levels may be helpful because they tend to be normal in patients with intrahepatic cholangiocarcinoma and metastases and will be elevated in HCC.

CASE 37

Clinical History: 14-year-old girl who underwent liver biopsy.

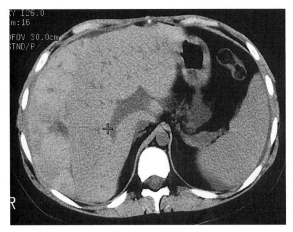

Figure 1.37 A

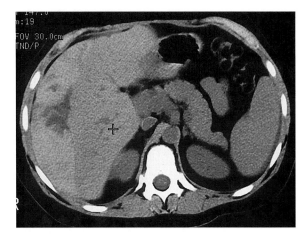

Figure 1.37 B

Findings: NECT demonstrates a large subcapsular high attenuation fluid collection around the liver. Note the areas of low attenuation within the fluid.

Differential Diagnosis: None.

Diagnosis: Large subcapsular hematoma.

Discussion: Blood in an acute stage will be hyperdense on a NECT. The hemorrhage in this example is actually of higher attenuation than the liver and almost mimics liver parenchyma in appearance. This represents clotted blood and will eventually become lower in attenuation as the clot matures. In the very acute stage of a hemorrhage on a CECT, contrast can sometimes be seen flowing into a fluid collection indicating active bleeding. This fluid causes mass effect on the liver because it is subcapsular rather than extracapsular. This can sometimes be beneficial to the patient because it may tamponade the bleeding, obviating surgical intervention.

CASE 38

Clinical History: 76-year-old male with elevated liver function.

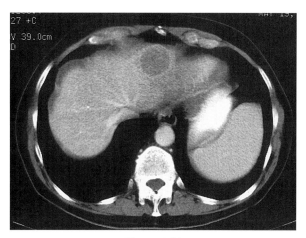

Figure 1.38

Findings: A 3.5-cm well-circumscribed low attenuation lesion is seen in the left lobe of the liver with an enhancing rim on a CECT.

Differential Diagnosis: Metastasis, hepatocellular adenoma.

Diagnosis: Hepatocellular carcinoma, encapsulated.

Discussion: Hepatocellular carcinoma has a variable incidence based on geographic location. In low-incident areas such as the United States, this lesion is seen most commonly in the elderly population with cirrhosis related to alcohol consumption. The onset is usually slow and insidious with symptoms of abdominal pain and occasionally fever and malaise. In high-incident areas, such as the Far East and sub-Sahara Africa, hepatocellular carcinoma is seen in middle-aged patients and tends to have a more rapid onset with abdominal pain, fever, and weight loss. The etiology in the high-incident areas is thought to be secondary to hepatitis B. This case demonstrates the encapsulated form of hepatocellular carcinoma. These lesions tend to have a better prognosis because of the greater ease in resection than the nonencapsulated form. The fibrous capsule tends to be hyperdense on the contrast-enhanced images as in this example. The enhancing center of the lesion makes the diagnosis of an abscess unlikely. A metastasis, however, is a possibility although they are more commonly multiple. The patient's age and gender would be unlikely for an hepatic adenoma, and the enhancement pattern would be atypical for a hemangioma.

CASE 39

Clinical History: 46-year-old man with right upper quadrant pain.

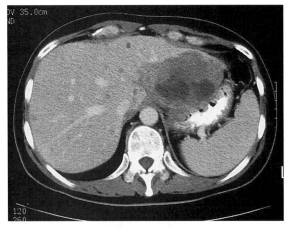

Figure 1.39 A

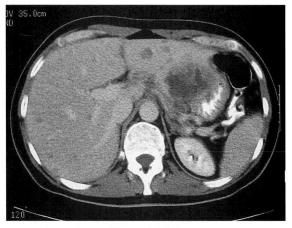

Figure 1.39 B

Findings: CECT demonstrates a large low attenuation mass in the left lobe of the liver with central necrosis. Multiple small satellite nodules of low attenuation are also seen.

Differential Diagnosis: Metastases, hepatocellular carcinoma, multiple abscesses.

Diagnosis: Primary lymphoma of the liver.

Discussion: Lymphoma of the liver can be either primary or secondary. Secondary involvement with lymphoma is fairly common being seen in 50–60% of patients with Hodgkin's and non-Hodgkin's disease at autopsy, although is detected in only 15–25% of the cases by imaging. Secondary lymphoma of the liver is especially common in patients with AIDS. Primary lymphoma is rare and is usually of the large cell type. It presents most often as a large multilobulated mass often with areas of necrosis and hemorrhage. There is usually minimal enhancement with intravenous contrast.

This case demonstrates not only a large mass of lymphoma, but also multiple small nodules scattered throughout the liver. This pattern is nonspecific and could be secondary to metastases, abscesses, and multifocal primary neoplasms (HCC, I-CAC and angiosarcoma). A search for a source in the GI tract would be warranted in the workup of this patient. Multiple hepatocellular carcinomas would be less likely because no evidence of cirrhosis is seen.

CASE 40

Clinical History: 42-year-old man with right upper quadrant pain and fever. No history of foreign travel.

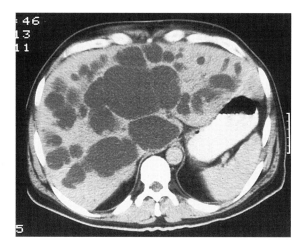

Figure 1.40 A

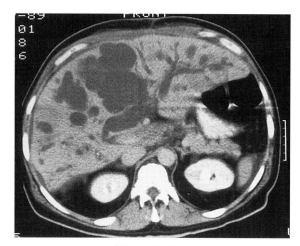

Figure 1.40 B

Findings: CECT demonstrates multiple cystic lesions within the liver, which appear to communicate with the biliary tree.

Differential Diagnosis: Polycystic liver disease, multiple hepatic abscesses, recurrent pyogenic cholangitis.

Diagnosis: Caroli disease (diffuse form).

Discussion: Caroli disease is defined as congenital nonobstructive cystic dilatation of the intrahepatic biliary tree. It can be diffuse, as is seen in this example or localized. It is believed that Caroli disease is part of the spectrum of fibrocystic diseases that range from congenital hepatic fibrosis to choledochal cyst. Caroli disease can be associated with medullary sponge kidney and autosomal recessive polycystic kidney disease or present as an isolated phenomenon and not associated with other entities. The key to the diagnosis of Caroli disease is recognizing that the saccular dilatations are in communication with the biliary tree. The saccular dilatations in Caroli disease tend to radiate toward the porta hepatis following the path of the portal vein branches. This is in contradistinction to polycystic liver disease and abscesses, which are randomly dispersed in the liver. The saccular dilatations in Caroli disease tend to be irregularly shaped, a feature that also helps to distinguish it from polycystic liver disease and abscesses. These tend to be spherical and vary in size. Recurrent pyogenic cholangitis usually does not produce saccular dilatation as in this case and involvement is frequently extrahepatic.

CASE 41

Clinical History: 30-year-old man with acute onset of abdominal pain, nausea, and vomiting.

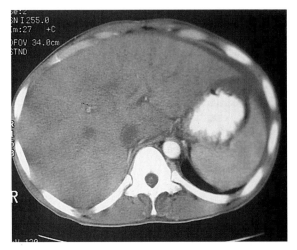

Figure 1.41 A

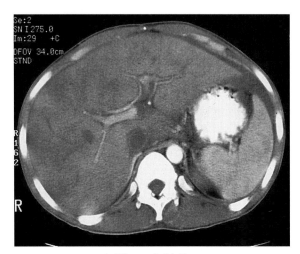

Figure 1.41 B

Findings: CECT demonstrates hepatomegaly without contrast seen in the hepatic veins or IVC. Note the ascites around the left lobe of the liver and poor enhancement of the spleen.

Differential Diagnosis: None.

Diagnosis: Budd-Chiari syndrome.

Discussion: Budd-Chiari syndrome is defined as partial or complete obstruction of the hepatic veins or IVC. Obstruction to hepatic venous flow can occur at different anatomic levels accounting for the various presentations and manifestations of Budd-Chiari syndrome. The reduced hepatic venous flow causes ascites, hepatomegaly, collateral vessel formation, and splenomegaly. This case demonstrates many of the classic findings of Budd-Chiari syndrome. There is no contrast enhancement in the hepatic veins or IVC, which is diagnostic of Budd-Chiari syndrome. Because of the impaired venous outflow, there is often hepatomegaly as well as portal hypertension, which leads to the formation of ascites and collateral vessels. The portal hypertension also causes poor enhancement of the spleen as seen in this example leading to splenic infarcts. Thrombolysis and anticoagulant therapy has limited success in Budd-Chiari syndrome with portosystemic shunting or liver transplant as therapeutic alternatives.

CASE 42

Clinical History: 27-year-old woman with weight loss.

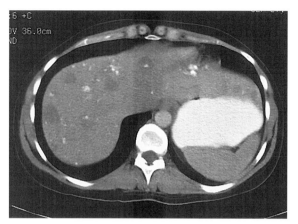

Figure 1.42 A

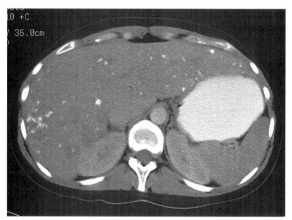

Figure 1.42 B

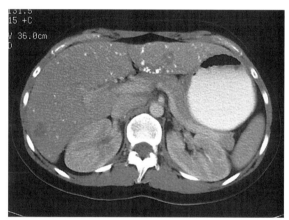

Figure 1.42 C

Findings: CECT shows multiple small nodular calcifications and multiple small low attenuation lesions seen diffusely throughout the liver.

Differential Diagnosis: Untreated calcified metastasis, treated hepatic candidiasis, granulomatous disease, Caroli's disease, oriental cholangiohepatitis, *pneumocystis carinii* (PCP).

Diagnosis: Calcified metastases of small cell carcinoma of the lung after chemotherapy.

Discussion: Some liver metastases are calcified. This includes mucinous carcinoma of the GI tract, osteosarcoma, leiomyosarcoma, papillary serous ovarian cystadenocarcinoma, medullary carcinoma of the thyroid, and breast carcinoma. Treated metastasis from any primary, granulomatous disease and PCP can also calcify. This case is extremely unusual in that the patient was young to have developed small cell carcinoma of the lung. Calcified metastases from medullary carcinoma of the thyroid, osteosarcoma, and treated lymphoma would have been other good considerations for the diagnosis. Granulomatous disease would have not accounted for the low attenuation lesions in the liver and there were no dilated ducts to consider Caroli's disease or oriental cholangiohepatitis.

CASE 43

Clinical History: 45-year-old woman with weight loss.

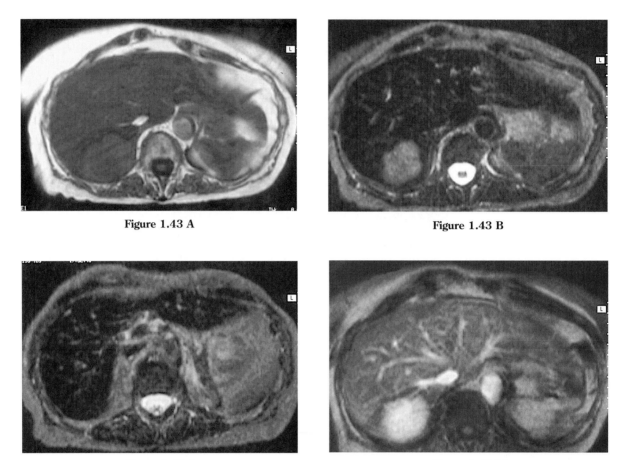

Figure 1.43 A

Figure 1.43 B

Figure 1.43 C

Figure 1.43 D

Findings: (A) T1-weighted image demonstrates a slightly hyperintense 4-cm lesion in the right lobe of the liver; (B, C) T2-weighted images demonstrate diffuse hypointensity to the liver and pancreas relative to muscle. The lesion is hyperintense on the T2 image; (D) Post gadolinium image demonstrates enhancement of this lesion.

Differential Diagnosis: Metastasis, hepatic adenoma.

Diagnosis: Primary hemochromatosis with a hepatocellular carcinoma.

Discussion: Hemochromatosis can be divided into primary idiopathic hemochromatosis versus iron overload states from multiple blood transfusions. Parenchymal deposition seen in primary hemochromatosis causes decreased T2 signal in both the liver and pancreas as is seen in this case. This decreased signal can be measured against the signal seen in adjacent skeletal muscles. On the other hand, transfusional hemochromatosis, which involves the reticuloendothelial system causes decreased T2 signal within the liver and spleen with sparing of the pancreas. This case also demonstrates a hyperintense lesion within the liver, which by itself is nonspecific. Approximately 20% of patients with hemochromatosis develop hepatocellular carcinoma. Taking into account the finding of primary hemochromatosis, hepatocellular carcinoma is the most likely diagnosis for this focal lesion. A single metastasis would be uncommon and without a fever or elevated white blood cell count, an abscess would be unlikely. A hemangioma is unlikely due to the uniform enhancement pattern seen on the post gadolinium image.

CASE 44

Clinical History: 64-year-old woman with 2-month history of weight loss and abdominal pain. The patient is known to have gallstones.

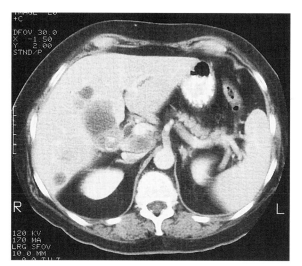

Figure 1.44 A

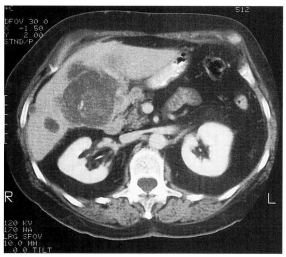

Figure 1.44 B

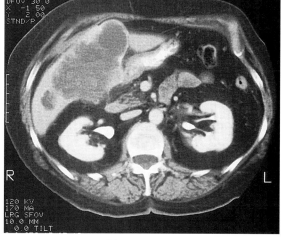

Figure 1.44 C

Findings: CECT demonstrates multiple low attenuation lesions within the liver as well as portal adenopathy. There is a large low attenuation lesion involving the posterior portion of the gallbladder with extension into the liver. Note the small satellite lesion.

Differential Diagnosis: Metastases, multiple abscesses, hepatocellular carcinoma.

Diagnosis: Gallbladder adenocarcinoma with liver metastases.

Discussion: Gallbladder cancer is an uncommon malignancy. Histologically, gallbladder cancer is usually an adenocarcinoma although other cell types such as squamous cell carcinoma, anaplastic carcinoma, and sarcomas have been reported. Gallstones are present in more than 70% of the cases of gallbladder cancer with a slight female predominance. Gallbladder adenocarcinoma can present as a focal or diffuse thickening of the gallbladder wall, a polypoid lesion, or a mass replacing the gallbladder. Metastases are present at the time of diagnosis in approximately 75% of cases. This case demonstrates many findings of gallbladder carcinoma. There is typically an ill-defined low attenuation mass involving the galbladder wall and invading the liver parenchyma. Multiple liver metastases are often present and account for the poor prognosis. These findings along with the history of gallstones makes gallbladder carcinoma the best diagnosis.

CASE 45

Clinical History: 31-year-old woman with weight loss.*

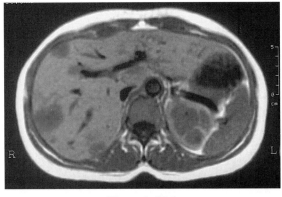

Figure 1.45 A

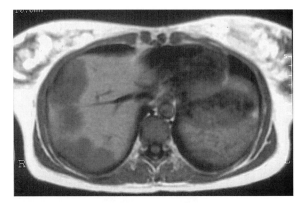

Figure 1.45 B

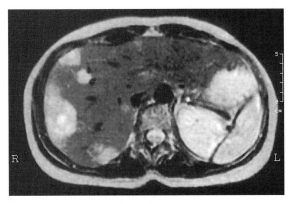

Figure 1.45 C

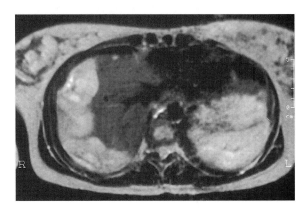

Figure 1.45 D

Findings: (A, B) T1-weighted images demonstrate multiple large peripheral hypointense masses in the right lobe of the liver; (C, D) T2-weighted images show these same areas to be of high signal intensity.

Differential Diagnosis: Metastases.

Diagnosis: Hepatic epithelioid hemangioendothelioma (EHE)-diffuse form.

Discussion: Epithelioid hemangioendothelioma is a slow-growing vascular malignancy that can arise in other parts of the body including the lung. The prognosis varies from 2 to 20 years. They have a slight female predominance and present in the fourth through sixth decades. There are two forms of EHE: nodular and diffuse. The two forms can coexist because the nodules can enlarge and coalesce simulating the diffuse form. The nodular form is hard to distinguish from multiple metastases and can be both central and peripheral in location. The diffuse form, as in this case, is typically peripheral in location and will not usually deform the liver contour. The peripheral location is thought to be due to the spread of the neoplasm through the portal and hepatic veins. The liver will classically appear to have a rind of tumor along its periphery and hypertrophy of the uninvolved segments due to shunted blood.

*Case courtesy of Luis Ros, MD, Zargoza, Spain.

Clinical History: 54-year-old man status post subtotal gastrectomy presenting with fever and elevated white cell count.

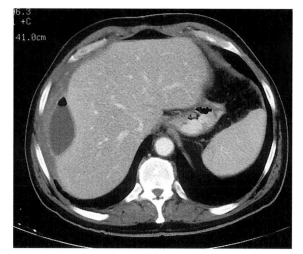

Figure 1.46 A

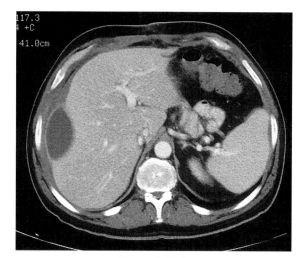

Figure 1.46 B

Findings: CECT demonstrates a low attenuation elliptical subcapsular fluid collection that contains air. Higher attenuation fluid surrounds the liver as well.

Differential Diagnosis: Hematoma, infected necrotic neoplasm, post-op fluid and air.

Diagnosis: Subcapsular abscess.

Discussion: There is a limited differential diagnosis for a fluid collection that contains air. The air could be due to a gas-forming organism in an abscess or an infected necrotic neoplasm. The infecting organism can reach the fluid collection by way of direct spread or hematogenously. The air can also come from an outside source such as fistulization from a loop of bowel or introduced by a prior procedure (i.e., biopsy, surgery, drain placement). This patient has a history of a prior surgery with a postoperative abscess. The higher attenuation fluid around the liver represented postoperative blood. Diagnosis was made by aspiration of the fluid percutaneously.

CASE 47

Clinical History: 59-year-old woman with idiopathic cardiomyopathy and congestive heart failure.

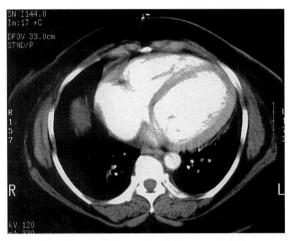

Figure 1.47 A

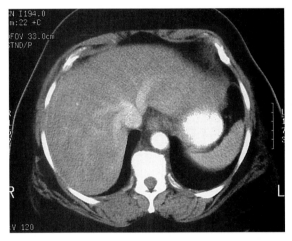

Figure 1.47 B

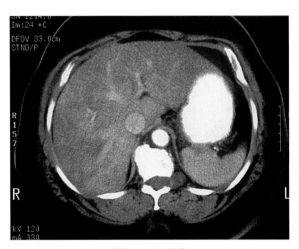

Figure 1.47 C

Findings: CECT demonstrates heterogeneous enhancement of the liver with areas of low and high attenuation. Note the dilated IVC and hepatic veins as well as cardiomegaly.

Differential Diagnosis: Fatty liver, diffusely infiltrating neoplasm.

Diagnosis: Hepatic congestion from right-sided heart failure.

Discussion: Patients who have right-sided cardiac dysfunction from a myocardial infarction or cardiomyopathy will develop right-sided congestive failure. As blood begins to pool in the IVC and hepatic veins from vascular stasis, these vessels will begin to dilate. This will in turn cause heterogeneous enhancement of the liver because of the inability of the blood and contrast from the portal vein and hepatic artery to pass through the liver and back to the heart. Grossly, hepatic congestion secondary to cardiac failure has a characteristic mottled appearance referred to as a "nutmeg liver" since it resembles the appearance of a sectioned nutmeg. This case demonstrates the typical findings in hepatic congestion. There is dilatation of both the IVC and hepatic veins and heterogeneous enhancement of the liver. A diffusely infiltrating neoplasm such as HCC would be unlikely because there is no mass effect. A heterogeneous fatty liver is a possibility because there is no displacement of the vessels found in this entity. The history of a cardiomyopathy as well as the dilated IVC and hepatic veins makes hepatic congestion the best diagnosis.

CASE 48

Clinical History: 43-year-old Asian woman presenting with jaundice and fever.

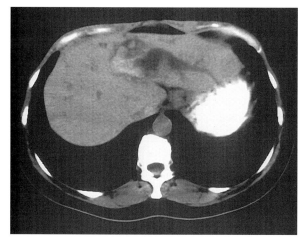

Figure 1.48 A

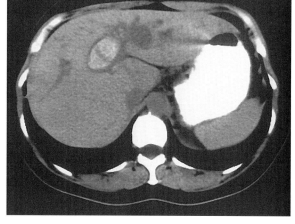

Figure 1.48 B

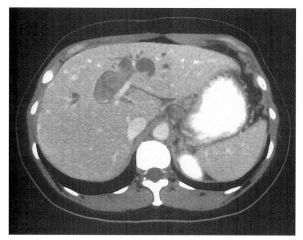

Figure 1.48 C

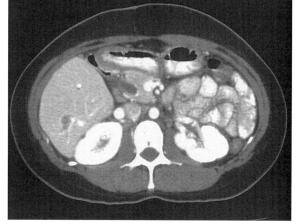

Figure 1.48 D

Findings: (A, B) NECT demonstrates intrahepatic biliary dilatation with a calcified foci within the dilated duct; (C, D) CECT again demonstrates the dilated ducts and the calcified foci. Note the dilated common bile duct.

Differential Diagnosis: Caroli disease.

Diagnosis: Oriental cholangiohepatitis (recurrent pyogenic cholangitis).

Discussion: Recurrent pyogenic cholangitis is a disease that is endemic to the Far East and is thought to be secondary to infestation by *Clonorchis sinensis*. The parasite is thought to either cause direct damage to the biliary ducts or act as a focus for the formation of stones. This results in biliary dilatation and cholangitis. The patients present with intermittent bouts of jaundice, fever, and right upper quadrant pain. Radiologically, recurrent pyogenic cholangitis presents with intrahepatic and often extrahepatic biliary dilatation. The intrahepatic dilatation is often found centrally, and multiple areas of strictures are seen on cholangiograms. Stone formation and sludge is commonly seen in these patients. This case demonstrates intrahepatic and extrahepatic biliary dilatation, stone formation, and a clinical history that helps to make the diagnosis almost certain. Caroli disease with abscess formation is another diagnostic possibility but the extrahepatic biliary dilatation is uncommon in Caroli disease.

Clinical History: 78-year-old man without history of cirrhosis.

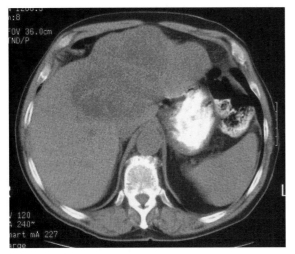

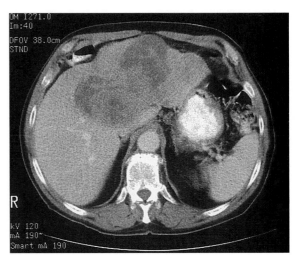

Figure 1.49 A   **Figure 1.49 B**

Findings: (A) NECT demonstrates a large mass that involves almost the entire left lobe of the liver. The lesion also extends outside the expected contour of the liver; (B) CECT demonstrates heterogeneous enhancement in the mass. The portal vein is displaced posteriorly.

Differential Diagnosis: Metastasis, cholangiocarcinoma.

Diagnosis: Hepatocellular carcinoma.

Discussion: There are many different etiologies for hepatocellular carcinoma, which can be divided into three main categories: chronic hepatitis B, cirrhosis, and carcinogens. Cirrhosis in the United States is most commonly due to alcoholism and hepatocellular carcinomas occur in approximately 3% of these patients. Other causes of cirrhosis that can lead to hepatocellular carcinoma include hemochromatosis and less commonly inborn errors of metabolism such Wilson's disease, glycogen storage disease, and alpha-1-antitrypsin deficiency. Carcinogens found to be associated with hepatocellular carcinoma include aflatoxins produced by the fungus *Aspergillus fumigatus,* siderosis from high dietary iron, and Thorotrast. This case is unusual in that there is no radiographic or laboratory evidence for cirrhosis in this patient. Although uncommon, hepatocellular carcinoma can occur without evidence for cirrhosis. The heterogeneous appearance of the lesion and the bulging of the tumor from the surface of the liver is suggestive of a hepatic malignancy. Cholangiocarcinoma would be less likely because they do not normally bulge from the surface of the liver but actually cause contraction secondary to desmoplastic reaction. Metastases would be a good choice for this case although they tend to be multiple instead of solitary.

CASE 50

Clinical History: 56-year-old woman with abdominal pain and weight loss.

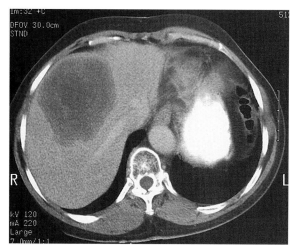

Figure 1.50 A

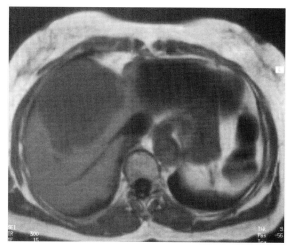

Figure 1.50 B

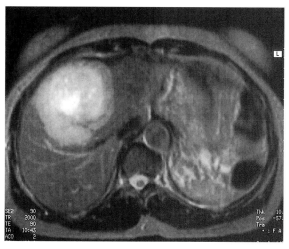

Figure 1.50 C

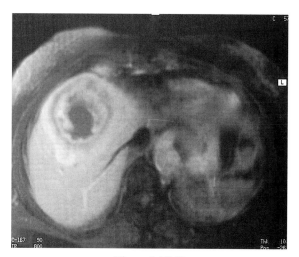

Figure 1.50 D

Findings: (A) CECT demonstrates a 9-cm enhancing lesion in the liver; (B) T1WI demonstrates this lesion to be hypointense producing displacement of the middle hepatic vein; (C) On the T2WI, there is an area of increased signal intensity in the center of the lesion representing necrosis. There is a halo of increased signal intensity surrounding this central region; (D) Fat saturation T1WI post gadolinium demonstrates peripheral enhancement.

Differential Diagnosis: Hepatic adenoma, abscess, hepatocellular carcinoma.

Diagnosis: Metastases from a sarcoma.

Discussion: MR imaging can be helpful in characterizing liver lesions. In one series, 98% of colorectal metastases were hyperintense on the T2WI. Histologically, these were found to represent areas of necrosis and desmoplasia. Initially, it was thought that the peripheral rim of increased T2 signal around the lesion represented edema in the surrounding parenchyma. In one series, the entire lesion seen on the T2WI, including the "halo" of increased peripheral signal, represented tumor. This case demonstrates a large necrotic metastasis from a sarcoma with a halo of increased signal intensity on the T2WI. Any necrotic lesion could have a similar appearance such as a hepatocellular carcinoma or hepatic adenoma. There is, however, no evidence for cirrhosis to suggest an HCC nor is this a good age group for a hepatic adenoma. An abscess would be a good consideration in this case.

CASE 51

Clinical History: 54-year-old man with endstage cirrhosis.

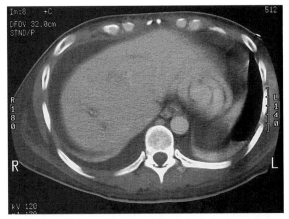

Figure 1.51 A

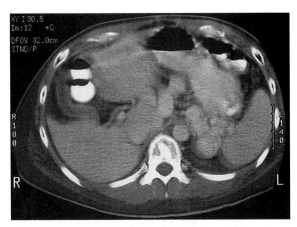

Figure 1.51 B

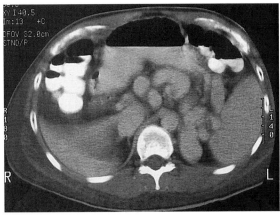

Figure 1.51 C

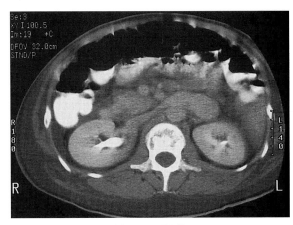

Figure 1.51 D

Findings: CECT demonstrates a cirrhotic liver with extensive collateral vessels. Collateral vessels are seen near the gastric fundus and leading from the splenic hilum to the left kidney. Also note the ascites and bilateral effusions.

Differential Diagnosis: Collateral vessels mimic opacified bowel.

Diagnosis: Cirrhosis and portal hypertension leading to massive collateral vessel formation including gastric varices and a splenorenal shunt.

Discussion: There are multiple causes for portal hypertension, the most common being cirrhosis. These causes can be divided into three categories: intrahepatic, extrahepatic presinusoidal, and extrahepatic postsinusoidal. Intrahepatic causes are more common and include cirrhosis, schistosomiasis, hepatitis, and neoplasms. Extrahepatic presinusoidal causes include portal vein thrombosis and extrahepatic postsinusoidal causes include pericarditis and CHF. Portal hypertension leads to the formation of portosystemic shunts to bypass the liver as is seen in this case. There is enlargement of the coronary vein and short gastric veins as the blood gets directed from the portal vein through these vessels into the azygous vein and finally the SVC. This case demonstrates how large these collaterals can become and how these can impress on the fundus of the stomach and simulate a mass on UGI series. A large splenorenal shunt is also present which could be confused with normal opacified bowel if the entire scan is not viewed carefully.

CASE 52

Clinical History: 17-year-old man with history of multiple UGI bleeds and autosomal recessive polycystic kidney disease (ARPCKD).

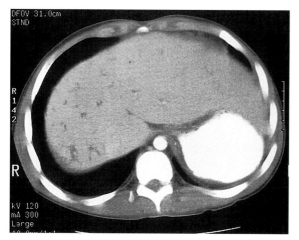

Figure 1.52 A

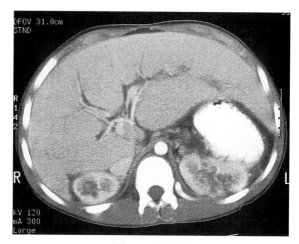

Figure 1.52 B

Findings: CECT demonstrates an enlarged liver with multiple linear areas of low attenuation. The intrahepatic vessels are attenuated and there is periportal lucency. The kidneys demonstrate findings of ARPCKD (see ARPCKD).

Differential Diagnosis: Hepatitis, cirrhosis, hepatic schistosomiasis.

Diagnosis: Congenital hepatic fibrosis with ARPCKD.

Discussion: The variable presentations of ARPCKD have a component of congenital hepatic fibrosis. In patients who have the mild renal form of ARPCKD, congenital hepatic fibrosis predominates. These patients will present with liver failure and symptoms of portal hypertension such as UGI bleedings from esophageal varices. Congenital hepatic fibrosis can also be an isolated phenomenon or be associated with other entities such as Caroli disease and medullary sponge kidney. Some of the common CT findings of congenital hepatic fibrosis are present in this example. There is commonly hepatomegaly with areas of fibrosis that appear as linear low attenuation areas on CT. In this example, these low attenuation areas are seen in the dome of the liver. Periportal fibrosis is present as periportal lucency. Periportal lucency can also be due to edema as in hepatitis or CHF. The fibrotic liver causes the vessels to be markedly attenuated leading to portal hypertension.

CASE 53

Clinical History: 60-year-old man with nonspecific abdominal pain.

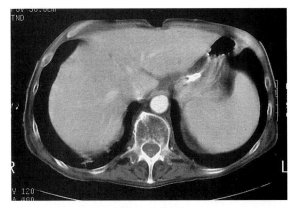

Figure 1.53 A

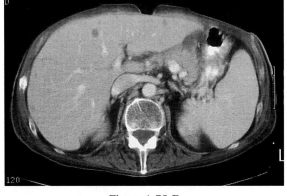

Figure 1.53 B

Findings: Multiple small, nonenhancing low-density lesions throughout the liver.

Differential Diagnosis: Metastasis, lymphoma/leukemia, infection(fungal), multiple cysts.

Diagnosis: Bile duct hamartoma (von Meyenburg complex).

Discussion: Bile duct hamartomas (von Meyenburg complexes) are dilated clusters of biliary ducts that are lined by a single layer of cuboidal epithelium within a fibrous stroma. These clusters are filled with proteinaceous material and biliary fluid. They can be single or multiple in its presentation. They are part of the spectrum of fibropolycystic hepatorenal diseases and are therefore associated with polycystic liver disease, polycystic kidney disease, congenital hepatic fibrosis, and Caroli disease. As is seen in this case, the lesions are usually small (<5 mm) and have low attenuation. Some lesions up to 2 cm in size can occasionally be seen. Typically, they are adjacent to the portal area or subcapsular in location. Because they can be multiple, they can be confused with metastatic disease or disseminated infections often requiring biopsy to confirm the diagnosis.

CASE 54

Clinical History: 64-year-old man with weight loss and bright red blood per rectum.

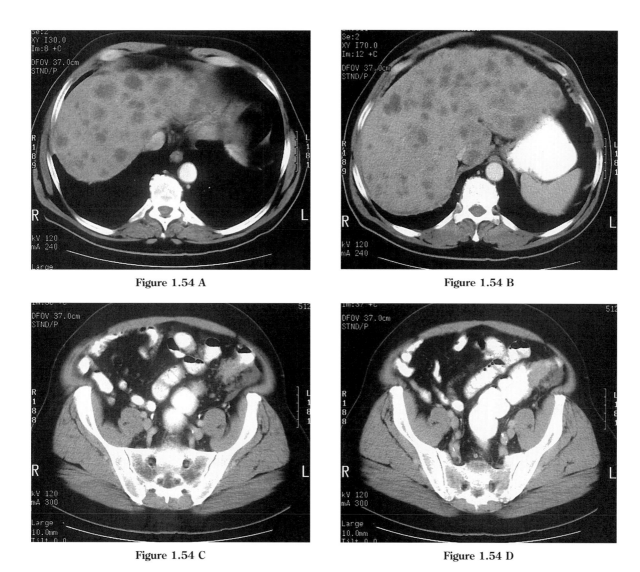

Figure 1.54 A

Figure 1.54 B

Figure 1.54 C

Figure 1.54 D

Findings: CECT demonstrates multiple low attenuation lesions involving all segments of the liver. The lesions range in size from <1 cm to almost 2 cm. CECT of the pelvis reveals a soft tissue mass in the sigmoid colon.

Differential Diagnosis: Multiple abscesses (pyogenic, Candida), lymphoma.

Diagnosis: Liver metastases from adenocarcinoma of the colon.

Discussion: Metastatic disease to the liver involves both the right and left lobes of the liver in 77% of the cases. If only one lobe is involved with metastatic disease, it is more commonly the right lobe. Hepatic metastases from colorectal cancer are present in 24% of patients at the time of diagnosis but in 71% of patients at time of autopsy. The spread pattern of colon cancer is via the portal vein. It is, therefore, very uncommon to see colon metastases to lung or other extra-abdominal sites without liver involvement. The differential diagnosis for multiple focal hepatic lesions would have to include multiple abscesses such as Candidiasis, especially if the patient was immunocompromised. The finding of a sigmoid lesion makes the diagnosis of metastatic colon cancer almost certain. Although unlikely, the sigmoid lesion could represent diverticulitis and the liver lesions could represent abscesses. A barium enema or colonoscopy would be necessary to confirm the diagnosis of colon cancer.

CASE 55

Clinical History: 2½-year-old girl with abdominal distension and CHF. Patient had normal alpha fetoprotein levels.

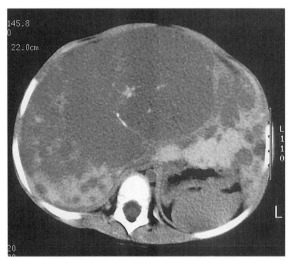

Figure 1.55 A

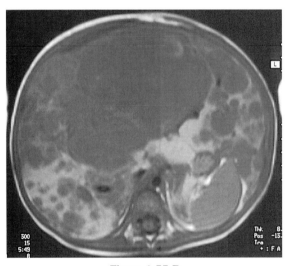

Figure 1.55 B

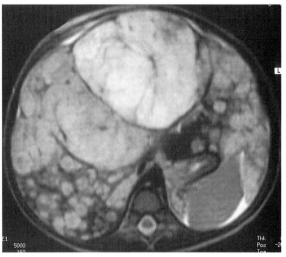

Figure 1.55 C

Findings: (A) NECT demonstrates a massive hypodense lesion in the left lobe with multiple smaller lesions. Fine linear calcifications are present. (B) T1-weighted image demonstrates the lesions to be hypointense. Note the area of necrosis in the left lobe. (C) On T2-weighted image, this lesion is markedly hyperintense.

Differential Diagnosis: Hepatoblastoma, metastases, mesenchymal hamartoma.

Diagnosis: Infantile hemangioendothelioma (IHE).

Discussion: Infantile hemangioendotheliomas are vascular tumors derived from endothelial cells. They are considered benign but can occasionally show aggressive features and distant metastasis. The majority present in children younger than 6 months of age and spontaneously regress after 18 months. Some have been reported to persist into adulthood. The lesions can range in size from a few millimeters up to 10–15 cm in size and are usually multiple. Calcifications, when they occur, tend to be fine and granular rather than coarse as is seen in this case. Infantile hemangioendotheliomas tend to be intensely bright on T2 images like hemangiomas. They can also be inhomogeneous on both T1 and T2-weighted images due to the areas of hemorrhage, necrosis, and scarring. A large area of necrosis is seen in this case. This differentiates IHE from hepatoblastomas, which rarely have large areas of necrosis. Mesenchymal hamartomas are typically not multiple and rarely have a large solid component. The large area of necrosis, the multiple lesions and history of CHF makes infantile hemangioendothelioma the best diagnosis.

CASE 56

Clinical History: 59-year-old man with weight loss.

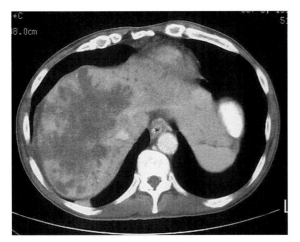

Figure 1.56 A

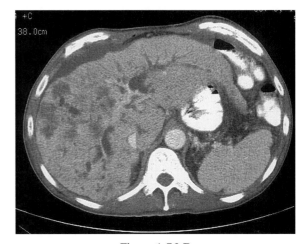

Figure 1.56 B

Findings: Large infiltrating low attenuation mass in the right lobe of the liver. Note the associated dilated biliary ducts.

Differential Diagnosis: Metastasis, hepatocellular carcinoma.

Diagnosis: Intrahepatic cholangiocarcinoma, massive.

Discussion: There are two forms of intrahepatic cholangiocarcinoma: massive and diffuse. Massive cholangiocarcinoma presents as a round well-defined mass with peripheral enhancement. Occasionally, it can appear as an ill-defined mass. The enhancement of the lesion may be equal to or greater than the normal liver. I-CAC can produce mucin and calcifications. The diffuse or sclerotic cholangiocarcinoma usually does not have a demonstrable mass but will present with thickened bile duct walls on CT scans. This can lead to intrahepatic biliary dilatation. This case demonstrates intrahepatic biliary dilatation associated with an ill-defined mass. This is typically seen in massive I-CAC. No evidence for cirrhosis is seen to suggest a hepatocellular carcinoma. It is also unlikely for HCC or metastases to cause intrahepatic biliary dilatation to such a degree. Metastasis also more commonly present as multiple well-defined low-density lesions rather than an infiltrating mass.

CASE 57

Clinical History: 61-year-old man with fevers and right upper quadrant pain.

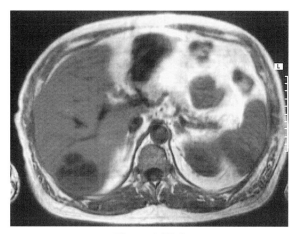

Figure 1.57 A

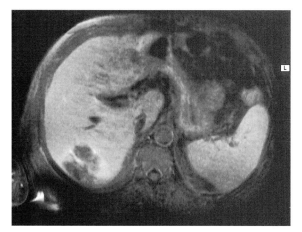

Figure 1.57 B

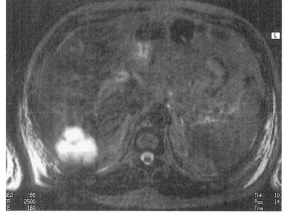

Figure 1.57 C

Findings: (A) T1WI demonstrates a 4-cm hypointense lesion in the right lobe of the liver. (B) Post gadolinium T1WI demonstrates peripheral rim enhancement as well as enhancement of the septations in the lesion; (C) T2WI reveals the lesion to be hyperintense.

Differential Diagnosis: Pyogenic or fungal abscess, necrotic metastasis, hepatocellular carcinoma.

Diagnosis: Amebic abscess.

Discussion: Amebic abscesses are caused by the parasite *Entamoeba histolytica*. Amebiasis is more commonly seen in the GI tract (amebic colitis) rather than the liver. Spread to the liver occurs through the portal system and therefore involves the right lobe greater than the left secondary to preferential blood flow to the right lobe. The liver is the most common extraintestinal organ involved by amebiasis followed by lung and brain. Amebic abscesses tend to occur in the dome of the liver and can be complicated by intraperitoneal rupture with subsequent peritonitis. Conservative treatment with metronidazole and chloroquine is effective in most cases with percutaneous drainage reserved for larger abscesses and for those adjacent to the heart. The finding on MRI of a rim-enhancing lesion is nonspecific and can be seen with any type of abscess or necrotic tumor. Enhancing septations, however, are less commonly seen with necrotic tumors and suggest an abscess. The lack of evidence for cirrhosis would make hepatocellular carcinoma less likely. An abscess of a different etiology or cystic metastases cannot be excluded in this case.

CASE 58

Clinical History: 22-year-old man with multiple subcutaneous soft tissue nodules.

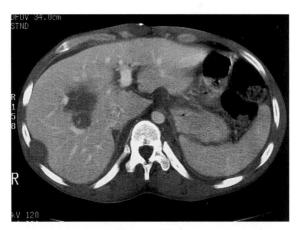

Figure 1.58 A

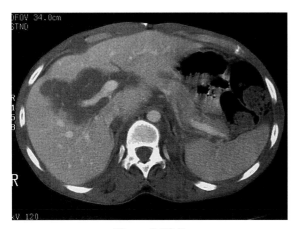

Figure 1.58 B

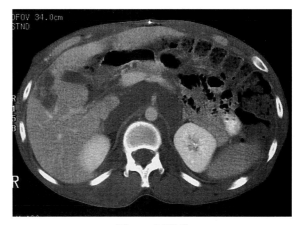

Figure 1.58 C

Findings: CECT demonstrates a low attenuation soft tissue mass surrounding the portal vein and involving the retroperitoneum, and chest wall.

Differential Diagnosis: Lymphoma, metastases.

Diagnosis: Plexiform neurofibromatosis involving the liver.

Discussion: Von Recklinghausen disease or neurofibromatosis type 1 is the most common form of neurofibromatosis. It is often referred to as peripheral neurofibromatosis because many of the most striking findings include lesions outside the intracranial central nervous system. These include cafe-au-lait spots, neurofibromas, and skeletal anomalies. The neurofibromas are typically round or spherical. Plexiform neurofibromas, on the other hand, are tortuous masses of enlarged peripheral nerves. The autonomic innervation of the biliary system arises from the celiac plexus and travels with the biliary tract. Therefore, hepatic neurofibromas will often be located along the path of the portal vein. Neurofibromas and plexiform neurofibromas are usually low in attenuation and tend to surround adjacent vessels and organs without significant obstruction or invasion. In this case, the portal vein is completely encased by the mass and yet there is no obstruction of the vessel or signs of portal hypertension. This mass is not causing biliary dilatation either. The key to the diagnosis is the involvement of the neurofibroma of the retroperitoneum and a rib causing rib notching. The typical location of these masses in the periportal region, retroperitoneum, and inferior surface of the rib without obstruction of the portal vein and biliary system makes neurofibromatosis the most likely diagnosis.

CASE 59

Clinical History: 45-year-old asymptomatic woman.

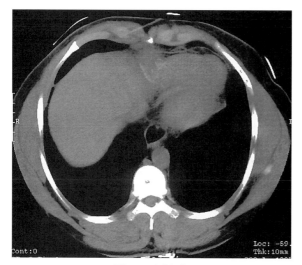

Figure 1.59 A

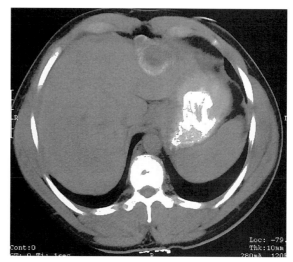

Figure 1.59 B

Findings: NECT demonstrates a 4-cm lesion in the lateral segment of the left lobe of the liver with a calcified rim.

Differential Diagnosis: Echinococcal cyst, old hematoma, old abscess, calcified metastasis.

Diagnosis: Calcified pericardial cyst.

Discussion: Pericardial cysts are found commonly in asymptomatic males. They are usually on the right side near the cardiophrenic angle and less commonly in the mediastinum. They tend to be round or ovoid in shape. This lesion appears to be intrahepatic in location but on careful examination the origin of this lesion is seen to be the right pericardium. This pericardial cyst is actually indenting on the surface of the liver simulating a hepatic lesion. Like cysts in the liver, pericardial cysts can calcify especially after hemorrhage.

CASE 60

Clinical History: 81-year-old man with fevers and elevated white blood cell count.

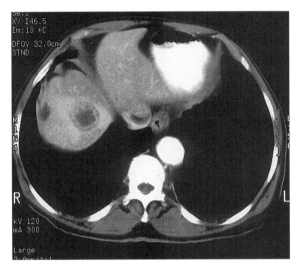

Figure 1.60 A

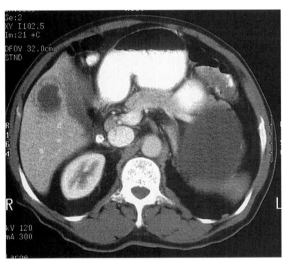

Figure 1.60 B

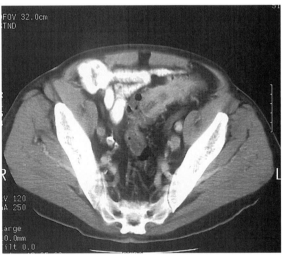

Figure 1.60 C

Findings: There are several irregular low attenuation lesions within the liver surrounded by a concentric hyperdense rim then by a hypodense ring on a dynamic CECT. The surrounding parenchyma also demonstrates increased attenuation. Image of the pelvis demonstrates diverticulitis.

Differential Diagnosis: Hypervascular metastasis, hepatic adenomas, hepatocellular carcinomas.

Diagnosis: Pyogenic abscesses of the liver.

Discussion: Pyogenic abscesses are most commonly due to gram-negative bacilli with *E. coli* most commonly cultured in adults. Approximately 50% of pyogenic abscesses are due to anaerobic or a mixture of aerobic and anaerobic organisms. The infection can reach the liver by several routes: 1) via the portal vein (appendicitis, diverticulitis, or infected colon cancer); 2) via the biliary system (cholangitis); 3) via direct extension (peptic ulcer disease or pyelonephritis); 4) via the hepatic artery (endocarditis, or arterial catheters); and 5) trauma. Typically, the abscesses are low in attenuation and multiple although they may be single. This lesion is highly suggestive of a pyogenic abscess because of its "double target sign" appearance on the dynamic CT. This consists of a hypodense center surrounded by a hyperdense rim followed by a hypodense ring. In one series this was seen in 30% of the patients. In addition, the surrounding liver parenchyma demonstrates increased attenuation from the arterioportal shunting often seen in pyogenic abscesses. The age and sex of the patient would make an hepatic adenoma unlikely and with the lack of findings to suggest cirrhosis, a hepatocellular carcinoma would also be unusual.

CASE 61

Clinical History: 1-year-old boy presents with a palpable abdominal mass.

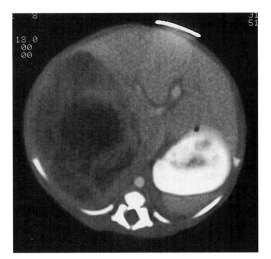

Figure 1.61 A

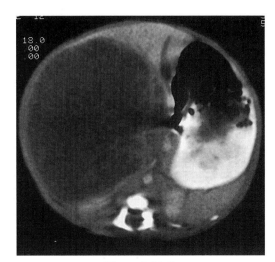

Figure 1.61 B

Findings: CECT demonstrates a large 9-cm low attenuation, predominantly cystic mass in the right lobe of the liver. There is displacement of the portal vein.

Differential Diagnosis: Undifferentiated embryonal sarcoma, infantile hemangioendothelioma, hepatoblastoma, metastases.

Diagnosis: Mesenchymal hamartoma.

Discussion: Mesenchymal hamartomas is a benign cystic lesion of the liver that is thought to arise from the mesenchymal tissue surrounding the portal tracts. The patients typically are between 1–2 years of age but some cases have been reported in older patients up to their teen years.

　　The lesions are typically large and composed of multiple cysts. There is a variable amount of solid component but the cystic component usually predominates. Occasionally, the cysts are small and the lesion can appear solid. Both infantile hemangioendotheliomas and hepatoblastomas rarely have a large cystic component and the age of the patient makes undifferentiated embryonal sarcoma unlikely. Metastases from neuroblastoma tend to be multiple and solid rather than cystic.

CASE 62

Clinical History: 65-year-old man with abnormal liver function tests.

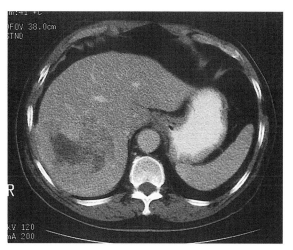

Figure 1.62 A

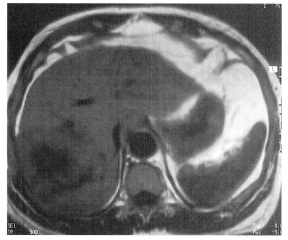

Figure 1.62 B

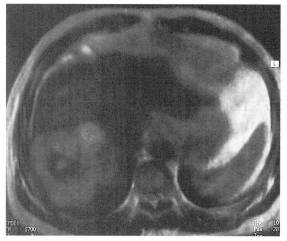

Figure 1.62 C

Findings: (A) CECT demonstrates an enhancing lesion in the right lobe of the liver. (B) T1WI demonstrates a hypointense lesion. This lesion hyperintense on the T2WI (C).

Differential Diagnosis: Abscess, hypervascular metastasis.

Diagnosis: Hepatocellular carcinoma.

Discussion: MR imaging characteristics for hepatocellular carcinoma vary depending on the amount of fibrosis, fat, necrosis, and hemorrhage present within the lesion. Hepatocellular carcinoma is most commonly hypointense on the T1WI but can be isointense or hyperintense as well. This is due in part to the amount of fat present in the tumor, which will have increased signal on the T1WI. Hepatocellular carcinoma is predominantly hyperintense on the T2WI and demonstrates enhancement with gadolinium administration.

CASE 63

Clinical History: 33-year-old man from Tunisia admitted for right upper quadrant pain and fevers.

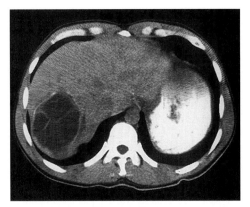

Figure 1.63 A

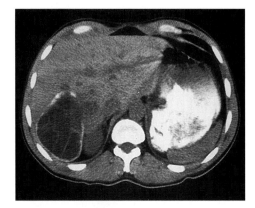

Figure 1.63 B

Findings: NECT demonstrates a cystic well-defined lesion in the right lobe of the liver with multiple septations. Calcifications are noted in the wall of this lesion.

Differential Diagnosis: Old hematoma, pyogenic abscess, necrotic metastasis, biliary cystadenoma.

Diagnosis: Echinococcal cyst.

Discussion: Echinococcus granulosus is the most common of the various forms of echinococcus infections. Human disease follows the ingestion of the ova by humans in regions where people herd sheep and have close contact with dogs. Hepatic echinococcosis can have complications such as intracystic infection, rupture of the cyst, bile duct communication, and right pleural effusion. Because these lesions can be large, they can compress adjacent vascular structures and cause portal hypertension or IVC occlusion. This case is typical of an echinococcal cyst with wall calcifications and septations. The presence of other lesions may make us consider the diagnosis of metastases, but in this case the mass is solitary. Biliary cystadenoma and hematoma would not account for the patient's fever and pain unless the lesion was superinfected. Pyogenic abscesses tend to have thicker walls and higher density fluid within the lesion. The appearance and history of being from an endemic area makes echinococcal cyst the most likely diagnosis.

CASE 64

Clinical History: 62-year-old female with history of well-controlled seizures.

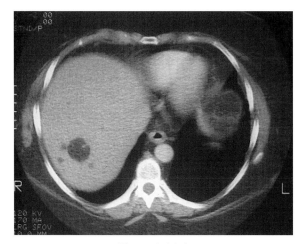

Figure 1.64 A

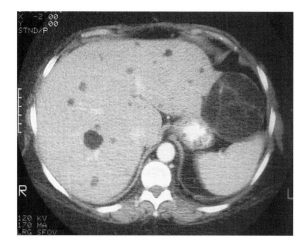

Figure 1.64 B

Findings: CECT demonstrates multiple low attenuation lesions that are of fat density in the liver. There is a large 7-cm fatty lesion with septations seen extending off the left lobe of the liver.

Differential Diagnosis: Lipomas, myelolipomas, metastatic liposarcoma, focal fatty change.

Diagnosis: Multiple hepatic angiomyolipomas in a patient with tuberous sclerosis.

Discussion: Lipomatous tumors of the liver include simple lipomas that are purely fat and lesions which contain fat and soft tissues such as adenolipomas, angiomyolipomas, and angiolipomas. Angiomyolipomas of the liver are often associated with renal angiomyolipomas and tuberous sclerosis. They can be solitary or multiple. Lipomas of the liver are of fat density measuring about −30 HU. They do not typically demonstrate contrast enhancement. In this case the septations seen in the left lobe lesion have contrast enhancement ruling out a simple lipoma. Other lesions in the liver that contain fat include liposarcoma metastases, hepatocellular carcinoma, and hepatic adenoma. Metastases from malignant teratomas will frequently contain fat but almost always contain calcium as well. The history of seizures with fatty lesions in the liver is diagnostic of multiple angiomyolipomas associated with tuberous sclerosis.

CASE 65

Clinical History: 5-month-old boy with elevated alpha fetoprotein levels.

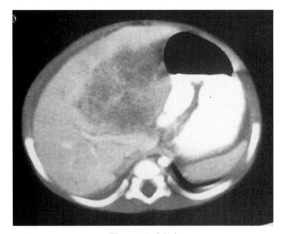

Figure 1.65 A

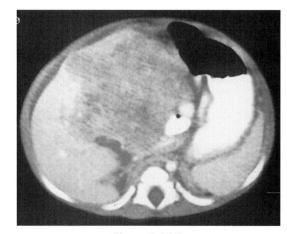

Figure 1.65 B

Findings: CECT demonstrates a large 6-cm solid mass involving most of the left lobe of the liver. The lesion has areas of enhancement centrally.

Differential Diagnosis: Infantile hemangioendothelioma, metastatic neuroblastoma, mesenchymal hamartoma.

Diagnosis: Hepatoblastoma.

Discussion: Hepatoblastoma is the third most common abdominal malignancy in children following Wilm's tumor and neuroblastoma. They are typically found in children less than 3 years of age with the peak age being less than 18 months. Histologically, hepatoblastomas may be composed of epithelial cells or be of mixed cellularity (epithelial and mesenchymal components). Mixed hepatoblastomas frequently have coarse calcifications due to osseous or cartilaginous mesenchymal elements. In a child of 4 months of age, the main differential diagnosis for a hepatic lesion is either a hepatoblastoma, infantile hemangioendothelioma, or metastatic neuroblastoma. An elevated AFP almost ensures the diagnosis of hepatoblastoma. Hepatocellular carcinomas may occur in children but they tend to be older than 5 years of age. On CT, hepatoblastomas are usually low in attenuation in both CECT and NECT. Although the lesion does enhance slightly on CECT, it still enhances less than the adjacent normal liver. As stated previously coarse calcifications occur and the lesion is predominantly solid. This differentiates it from a mesenchymal hamartoma, which has large cystic areas within the lesion.

CASE 66

Clinical History: 54-year-old female with progressive jaundice and weight loss.

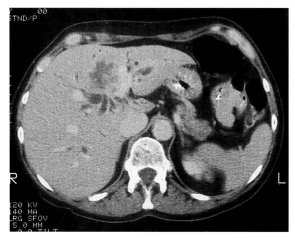

Figure 1.66 A

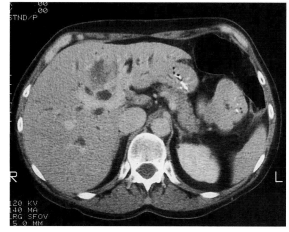

Figure 1.66 B

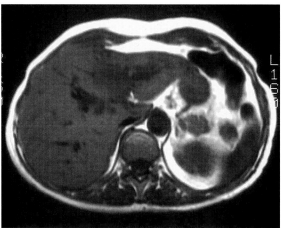

Figure 1.66 C

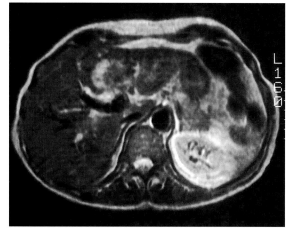

Figure 1.66 D

Findings: (A, B) CECT demonstrates left and right intrahepatic biliary dilatation. There is an enhancing mass in the medial segment of the left lobe of the liver near the confluence of the hepatic ducts. (C) T1WI demonstrates a mass corresponding to the CT of decreased signal intensity. (D) This is of increased signal intensity on the T2WI.

Differential Diagnosis: Hepatocellular carcinoma, metastasis.

Diagnosis: Cholangiocarcinoma (Klatskin tumor).

Discussion: Cholangiocarcinoma (CAC) is a malignant neoplasm of the bile ducts, which has an increased incidence in patients with sclerosing cholangitis, inflammatory bowel disease, and gallstones. CACs occur most commonly in the larger extrahepatic ducts with more than 90% occurring at the confluence of the ducts or more distally. Although extrahepatic cholangiocarcinomas often present early with jaundice secondary to biliary obstruction, the prognosis is still very poor. A Klatskin tumor is a cholangiocarcinoma at the bifurcation of the left and right hepatic ducts. This will cause biliary dilatation in both lobes of the liver. Because the bile ducts are small, a tumor mass is often not seen by imaging when the patients present with jaundice. This case demonstrates not only the biliary dilatation, but also the tumor mass invading into the liver. When a tumor mass is seen, it typically enhances on CT and demonstrates increased signal on T2-weighted images as in this example. Neither HCC nor metastases frequently cause biliary dilatation, making them less likely in this case.

CASE 67

Clinical History: 65-year-old female with history of melanoma resection.

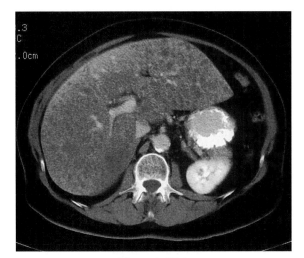

Figure 1.67 A

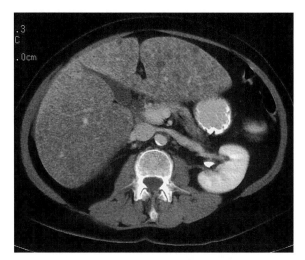

Figure 1.67 B

Findings: CECT demonstrates diffuse involvement of the liver by multiple less than 1-cm low attenuation lesions.

Differential Diagnosis: Disseminated infection (Candidiasis), fatty infiltration.

Diagnosis: Diffuse melanoma metastases.

Discussion: Many factors have also been implicated in the spread of metastases. In the liver, the structure of the endothelial lining plays a role in making the liver susceptible to metastatic disease. The endothelial cells of the sinusoids have small perforations that measure 0.1 μm in diameter. No basal lamina is present at the sites of these perforations. Therefore, the normal barriers to metastatic disease are not present in the liver, allowing metastases to enter from the sinusoids into the extracellular matrix of the space of Disse. This case is difficult because the lesions are so numerous and diffuse they are difficult to appreciate. Fatty infiltration is usually more geographic in appearance and not punctate as in this case. Disseminated fungal infection is a good possibility especially if the patient is immunocompromised.

CASE 68

Clinical History: 55-year-old man with fever and right upper quadrant pain.

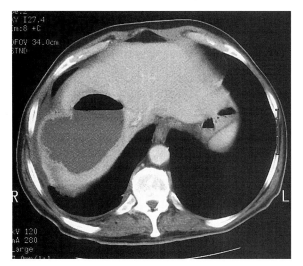

Figure 1.68 A

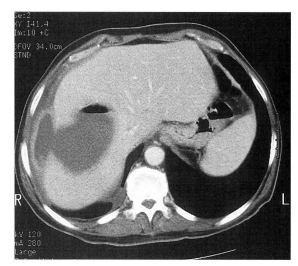

Figure 1.68 B

Findings: 8-cm low density lesion is seen in the right lobe of the liver with an air-fluid level within it. The lesion appears to extend outside the liver capsule. A small amount of fluid is also seen around the liver.

Differential Diagnosis: Instrumentation, trauma.

Diagnosis: Pyogenic abscess.

Discussion: Pyogenic abscesses tend to be multiple in 50–60% of the cases with a predilection for the right lobe of the liver. This is thought to be secondary to the preferential flow of blood from the superior mesenteric vein into the portal vein and into the right lobe. The presence of gas within this lesion is suggestive of either communication with a hollow viscus, prior trauma or instrumentation, or a gas-forming organism. This lesion is within the liver and does not appear to communicate with bowel nor is there air within any portion of the biliary tree to account for the air-fluid level. Without a history of trauma or previous manipulation, the diagnosis of a pyogenic abscess is almost certain. The rim enhancement seen around the fluid collection extending outside the liver contour is also suggestive of an infectious etiology which has broken through the liver capsule. Although less likely, a solitary, infected, necrotic metastasis, or primary liver tumor could also have this appearance.

CASE 69

Clinical History: 28-year-old man with recurrent fever and right upper pain.*

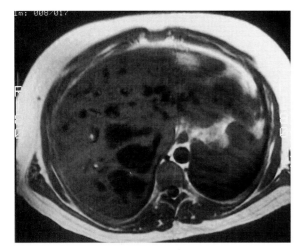

Figure 1.69 A

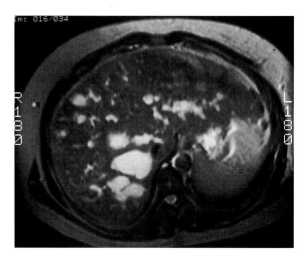

Figure 1.69 B

Findings: (A) T1-weighted image demonstrates round irregular areas of low-signal intensity predominantly in the right lobe of the liver; (B) These same areas are of high signal intensity on the T2-weighted image.

Differential Diagnosis: Polycystic liver disease, multiple abscesses, recurrent pyogenic cholangitis.

Diagnosis: Caroli disease (segmental form).

Discussion: Caroli disease can be either localized or diffuse in its presentation. When localized, it tends to involve the left lobe more often than the right. Bile inspissation in Caroli disease results in cholelithiasis and biliary stasis, which can lead to ascending cholangitis and cholecystitis. Recurrent episodes of cholangitis are common and can lead to stenosis of the ducts requiring percutaneous drainage and antibiotics. Surgical resection of the involved segment can be of benefit and is often curative. As one would expect, the MR findings of Caroli disease parallels that of CT. There are multiple cystic spaces that are irregularly shaped and communicate with the biliary tree. They radiate toward the porta hepatis and follow the portal branches. This case is unusual since the right side is preferentially involved rather than the left. Multiple abscesses from recurrent pyogenic cholangitis could easily have a similar appearance and would be difficult to distinguish.

*Case courtesy of Dr. Steven Harms, Little Rock, Arkansas.

CASE 70

Clinical History: 68-year-old female with history of colon cancer resection without evidence of liver metastasis at the time of surgery.

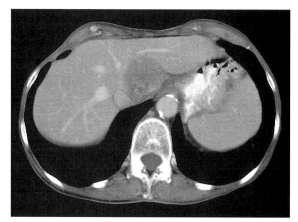

Figure 1.70 A

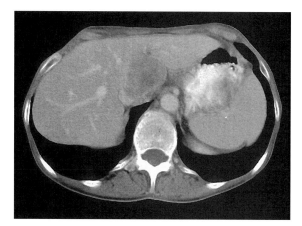

Figure 1.70 B

Findings: CECT demonstrates a solitary 4-cm hypodense lesion in the liver with mass effect on the IVC.

Differential Diagnosis: Hepatocellular carcinoma, abscess.

Diagnosis: Solitary metastasis from colon cancer.

Discussion: Metastatic disease is almost always multiple with solitary metastasis occurring in only 2% of cases. Often, however, small metastasis can be missed due to poor technique or their small size. Most hepatic metastasis are hypovascular and therefore will be hypodense on CECT. This is especially true for colorectal adenocarcinoma metastases. Scanning for these metastases is best performed during the portal phase of contrast injection. Our typical protocol is that of 150 ml of 60% contrast medium injected at 2 cc/sec with the initiation of scanning at 70 seconds after injection. Detection of metastases is excellent with dynamic scanning except for subcentimeter lesions where the sensitivity decreases. This case is unusual in that the initial presurgical CT did not demonstrate any metastasis but the follow-up CT post surgery demonstrated a single large metastatic lesion. Because of a negative prior CT, metastasis and abscess are the most likely diagnoses ruling out primary benign and malignant tumors. The enhancement in the central portion of the lesion makes an abscess unlikely.

Clinical History: 45-year-old woman with abdominal discomfort.

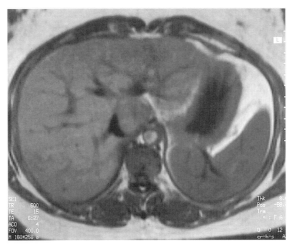

Figure 1.71 A

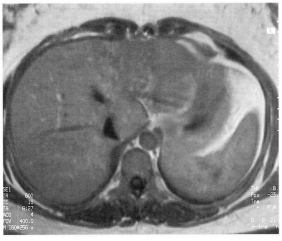

Figure 1.71 B

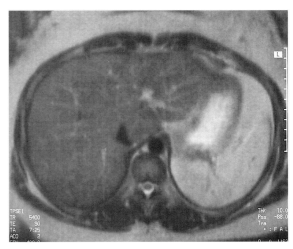

Figure 1.71 C

Findings: (A) 3-cm mass in the caudate lobe, which is isointense to liver on the T1-weighted image with a central low intensity spiculated area; (B) This central area enhances on the post gadolinium images; (C) This lesion is isointense on T2 sequences with a hyperintense scar. There is mass effect on the IVC.

Differential Diagnosis: Normal liver.

Diagnosis: Focal nodular hyperplasia.

Discussion: FNH is a benign tumor-like condition in the liver, which is composed of abnormally arranged nodules of normal liver separated by fibrous septa. Bile ductules are often present within the fibrous septa or between the hepatocytes. These lesions are unencapsulated and lack the presence of central veins and portal triads. Because of the nature of the FNH, 1/3 of these lesions tend to be isointense and similar in appearance to the normal liver parenchyma on T1- and T2-weighted images often making it difficult to detect. Approximately ⅔ of FNH are either slightly bright on the T2 images or slightly dark on the T1 images or both. As can be seen in this example, this lesion could easily be confused for normal liver parenchyma. A clue to its presence is the mass effect seen on the inferior vena cava and the surrounding vasculature. In addition, the central scar enhances on the post gadolinium image and is bright on the T2 image which is seen in focal nodular hyperplasia. Because this lesion demonstrates mass effect and is isointense to liver with an enhancing scar, focal nodular hyperplasia would be the most likely diagnosis.

SUGGESTED READINGS

Hepatic Neoplasms

Baker ME, Pelly R. Hepatic metastases: basic principles and implications for radiologists. Radiology 1995;197:329–337.

Bankoff MS, Tuckman GA, Scarborough D. CT appearance of liver mestastases from medullary carcinoma of the thyroid. J Comput Assist Tomogr 1987;11:1102–1103.

Berman MM, Libbey NP, Foster JH. Hepatocellular carcinoma. Cancer 1980; 46:1448–1455.

Boechat MI, Kangarloo H, Ortega J, et al. Primary liver tumors in children: comparison of CT and MR imaging. Radiology 1988;169:727–732.

Dachman AH, Lichtenstein JE, Friedman AC, et al. Infantile hemangioendothelioma of the liver: a radiologic-pathologic-clinical correlation. AJR 1983;140:1091–1096.

Ebara M, Masao O, Yoshirou W. Diagnosis of small hepatocellular carcinoma: correlation of MR imaging and tumor histologic studies. Radiology 1986;159:371–377.

Eisenberg D, Lawrence H, Albert CY. CT and sonography of multiple bile-duct hamartomas simulating malignant liver disease (case report). AJR 1986;147:279–280.

Fechner RE, Roehm JOF. Angiographic and pathologic correlations of heptic focal nodular hyperplasia. Am J Surg Pathol 1977;1:217–224.

Freeny PC, Baron RL, Teefey SA. Hepatocellular carcinoma: reduced frequency of typical findings with dynamic contrast-enhanced CT in a non-asian population. Radiology 1992;182:143–148.

Freeny PC, Marks MM. Patterns of contrast enhancement of benign and malignant hepatic neoplasms during bolus dynamic and delayed CT. Radiology 1986;160:613–618.

Friedman AC, Dachman AH. Radiology of the liver, biliary tract and pancreas. St. Louis: Mosby, 1994.

Furui S, Yuji I, Yamauchi T. Hepatic epithelioid hemangioendothelioma: report of five cases. Radiology 1989;171:63–68.

Ishak KG, Rabin L. Benign tumors of the liver. Med Clin North Am 1975;59:995–1013.

Itai Y, Nisikawa J, Tasaka A. Computed tomography in the evaluation of hepatocellular carcinoma. Radiology 1979;131:165–170.

Itai Y, Shin O, Kuni O, et al. Regenerating nodules of liver cirrhosis: MR imaging. Radiology 1987;165:419–423.

Kassianides C, Kew MC. The clinical manifestations and natural history of hepatocellular carcinoma. Gastro Clin North Am 1987;16:553–562.

Korobkin M, Kirks D, Sullivan D, et al. Computed tomography of primary liver tumors in children. Radiology 1981;13:431–435.

Matsui O, Masumi K, Tomiaki K. Benign and malignant nodules in cirrhotic livers: distinction based on blood supply. Radiology 1991;178:493–497.

Mattison G, Glazer G, Quint L, et al. MR imaging of hepatic focal nodular hyperplasia: characterization and distinction from pirmary malignant hepatic tumors. AJR 1987;148:711–715.

Mergo PJ, Ros P. Diagnostic imaging of diffuse liver disease. BUMC Proc 1996;9:9–13.

Murakami T, Chikazumi K, Taro M, et al. Regenerating nodules in hepatic cirrhosis: MR findings with pathologic correlation. AJR 1990;155:1227–1231.

Outwater E, Tomaszewski J, Daly J, et al. Hepatic colorectal metastases: correlation of MR imaging and pathologic appearance. Radiology 1991;180:327–332.

Quinn SF, Benjamin GG. Hepatic cavernous hemangiomas: simple diagnostic sign with dynamic bolus CT. Radiology 1992;182:545–548.

Radin DR, Craig JR, Colletti PM, et al. Hepatic epithelioid hemangioendothelioma. Radiology 1988;169:145–148.

Ros PR, Zachary DG, Ishak KG, et al. Mesenchymal hamartoma of the liver: radiologic-pathologic correlation. Radiology 1986;158:619–624.

Rustgi VK. Epidemiology of hepatocellular carcinoma. Gastro Clin North Am 1987;16:545–551.

Sanders LM, Botet JF, Straus DJ, et al. CT of primary lymphoma of the liver. AJR 1989;152:973–976.

Schiebler ML, Kressel HY, Saul SH, et al. MR imaging of focal nodular hyperlasia of the liver. J Comput Assist Tomogr 1987;11:651–654.

Seltzer SE, Holman BL. Imaging hepatic metastases from colorectal carcinoma: identification of candidates for partial hepatectomy. AJR 1989;152:917–923.

Stanley P, Hall TR, Wolley MM, et al. Mesenchymal hamartomas of the liver in childhood: sonographic and CT findings. AJR 1986;147:1035–1039.

Stocker JT, Ishak KG. Undifferentiated (embryonal) sarcoma of the liver. Cancer 1978;42:336–348.

Takayasu K, Hiroyoshi F, Wakao Y, et al. CT diagnosis of early hepatocellular carcinoma: sensitivity, findings, and CT-pathologic correlation. AJR 1995;164:885–890.

Takayyasu K, Yukio M, Hiroyoshi F, et al. Early hepatocellular carcinoma: appearance at CT during arterial portography and CT arteriography with pathologic correlation. Radiology 1995;194:101–105.

Winter T, Kenichi T, Yukio M, et al. Early advanced hepatocellular carcinoma: evaluation of CT and MR appearance with pathologic correlation. Radiology 1994;192:379–387.

Wong LK, Link DP, Frey CF, et al. Fibrolamellar hepatocarcinoma: radiology, management, and pathology. AJR 1982;139:172–175.

Wu T, Boitnott J. Dysplastic nodules: a new term for premalignant hepatic nodular lesions. Radiology 1996;201:21–22.

Yoshikawa J, Matsui O, Takashima T, et al. Fatty metamorphosis in hepatocellular carcinoma: radiologic features in 10 cases. AJR 1988;15:717–720.

Biliary Disease

Chan F, Man S, Leong LL, et al. Evaluation of recurrent pyogenic cholangitis with CT: analysis of 50 patients. Radiology 1989;170: 165–169.

Ishak KG, Willis GW, Cummins SD, et al. Biliary cystadenoma and cystadenocarcinoma. Cancer 1977;38:322–338.

Gore RM, Levin MS, Laufer I. Textbook of gastrointestinal radiology. Philadelphia, WB Saunders, 1994.

Korobkin M, Stephens DH, Lee JKT, et al. Biliary cystadenoma and cystadenocarcinoma: CT and sonographic findings. AJR 1989;153: 507–511.

Yeh H. Ultrasonography and computed tomography of carcinoma of the gallbladder. Radiology 1979;133:167–173.

Weiner SN, Koenigsberg M, Morehouse H, et al. Sonography and computed tomography in the diagnosis of carcinoma of the gallbladder. AJR 1984;142:735–739.

Miscellaneous

Adler D, Glazer G, Silver T. Computed tomography of liver infarction. AJR 1984;142:315–318.

Kaiser J, Mall J, Salmen B, et al. Diagnosis of caroli disease by computed tomography: report of two cases. Radiology 1979;132:661–664.

Koslin DB, Stanley, RJ, Shin MS, et al. Hepatic perivascular lymphedema: CT appearance. AJR 1988;150:111–113.

Mathieu D, Vasile N, Menu Y, et al. Budd-Chiari syndrome: dynamic CT. Radiology 1987;165:409–413.

Neiderau C, Fischer R, Sonnenberg A, et al. Survival and causes of death in cirrhotic and in noncirrhotic patients with primary hemochromatosis. N Engl J Med 1985;313:1256–1262.

Siegelman E, Mitchell D, Rubin R, et al. Parenchymal versus reticuloendothelial iron overload in the liver: distinction with MR imaging. Radiology 1991;179:361–366.

Stark D, Hahn P, Trey C, et al. MRI of the Budd-Chiari syndrome. AJR 1986;146:1141–1148.

Vogelzang R, Anschuetz S, Gore R. Budd-Chiari syndrome: CT observations. Radiology 1987;163:329–333.

Infection

Acunas B, Izzet R, Levent C, et al. Purely cystic hydatid disease of the liver: treatment with percutaneous aspiration and injection of hypertonic saline. Radiology 1992;182:541–543.

Beggs I. The radiology of hydatid disease. AJR 1985;145:639–648.

Choliz J, Olaverri FJ, Casas T, et al. Computed tomography in hepatic echinococcosis. AJR 1982;139:699–702.

Elizondo G, Weissleder R, Stark D, et al. Amebic liver abscess: diagnosis and treatment evaluation with MR imaging. Radiology 1987;165:795–800.

Francis I, Glazer G, Amendola A, et al. Hepatic abscesses in the immunocompromised patient: role of CT indesection, diagnosis, management, and follow-up. Gastrointest Radiol 1986;11:257–262.

Mathieu D, Vasile N, Pierre-Louis F, et al. Dynamic CT features of hepatic abscesses. Radiology 1985;154:749–752.

Mendez R, Schiebler M, Outwater E, et al. Hepatic abscesses: MR imaging findings. Radiology 1994;190:431–436.

Ralls P, Barnes P, Johnson M, et al. Medical treatment of hepatic amebic abscess: rare need for percutaneous drainage. Radiology 1987;165:805–807.

Ralls P, Henley D, Colletti P, et al. Amebic liver abscess: MR imaging. Radiology 1987;165:801–804.

Rappaport D, Cumming W, Ros P. Disseminated hepatic and splenic lesions in cat-scratch disease: imaging features. AJR 1991;156: 1227–1228.

Shirkhoda A. CT findings in hepatosplenic and renal candidiasis. J Comput Assist Tomogr 1987;11:795–798.

chapter 2

PANCREAS

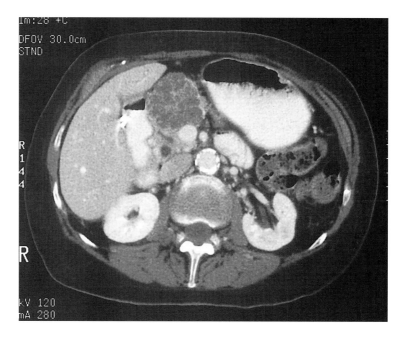

CASE 1

Clinical History: 15-year-old girl with abdominal pain.

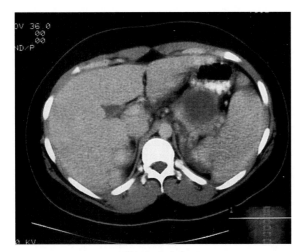

Figure 2.1 A

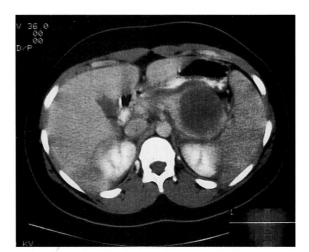

Figure 2.1 B

Findings: CECT demonstrates a 6-cm mass in the tail of the pancreas with central necrosis.

Differential Diagnosis: Pseudocyst, abscess, metastasis.

Diagnosis: Solid and papillary neoplasm.

Discussion: Solid and papillary neoplasm is an uncommon tumor of the pancreas found most commonly in young females. The lesion is typically large and well demarcated because it is encapsulated. A thick rind of tissue is usually present with areas of necrosis centrally. Small nodules of soft tissue can often be seen protruding into the center of the lesion. Solid and papillary neoplasm is mildly hypervascular, and the thick wall demonstrates mild contrast enhancement. The differential diagnosis for a large cystic mass in a young female is pancreatitis, abscess, and a necrotic metastasis. The patient is too young for a nonfunctioning islet cell tumor or mucinous cystic neoplasm. Treatment for this lesion is surgery, which is commonly curative.

CASE 2

Clinical History: 51-year-old man with weight loss and hemoptysis.

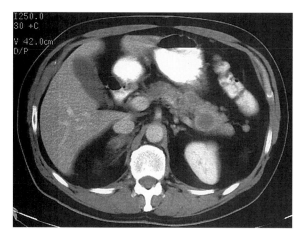

Figure 2.2 A

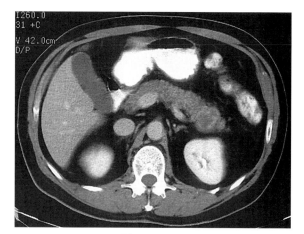

Figure 2.2 B

Findings: CECT demonstrates two low attenuation lesions in the tail of the pancreas with rim enhancement.

Differential Diagnosis: Islet cell tumor, lymphoma.

Diagnosis: Metastatic lung carcinoma.

Discussion: Metastasis to the pancreas is rare but does occur in tumors that spread hematogenously such as lung, breast, and melanoma. Metastasis can also occur to the peripancreatic nodes from any source which can subsequently invade the pancreas. This is often difficult to distinguish from a primary pancreatic neoplasm. The finding of multiple pancreatic lesions is a limited differential. Besides metastases, primary islet cell tumors of the pancreas can also be multiple. Gastrinomas can be multiple in up to 50% of cases especially if associated with MEN I. Lymphoma of the pancreas can present as multiple solid masses or can diffusely involve the pancreas and simulate pancreatitis. The key to the diagnosis is that pancreatic metastases usually occur in advanced stages of the disease, in which a primary malignancy is already known.

CASE 3

Clinical History: 70-year-old man presents with weight loss.

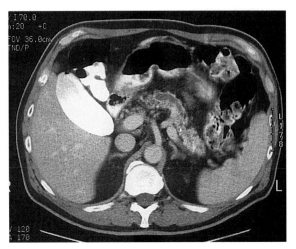

Figure 2.3 A

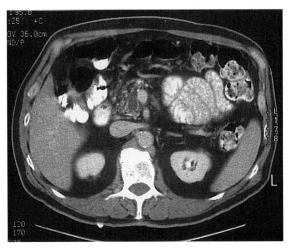

Figure 2.3 B

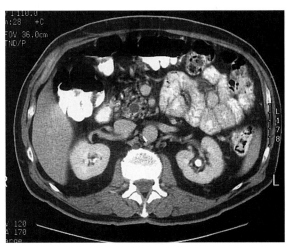

Figure 2.3 C

Findings: CECT demonstrates a dilated pancreatic duct extending to the uncinate process of the pancreas. No mass is identified. No history of pancreatitis or significant alcohol intake.

Differential Diagnosis: Chronic pancreatitis, ampullary carcinoma.

Diagnosis: Ductectatic mucinous cystadenocarcinoma.

Discussion: Ductectatic mucinous cystadenocarcinoma is characterized by grapelike cystic dilatation of a side branch of the pancreatic duct almost always affecting the uncinate process. This lesion is mucin secreting and can involve the entire pancreatic duct. An identifiable mass is rarely seen by CT. Often the only finding is dilatation of the pancreatic duct and small cysts that communicate with the main duct. Without a history of alcohol ingestion and recurrent pancreatitis, chronic pancreatitis would be unlikely. Other findings of chronic pancreatitis such as calcifications are also absent. An ampullary carcinoma can cause dilatation of the pancreatic duct but it is usually associated with dilatation of the common bile duct.

CASE 4

Clinical History: 60-year-old man with vague abdominal pain and arthritis.

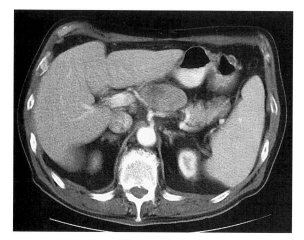

Figure 2.4 A

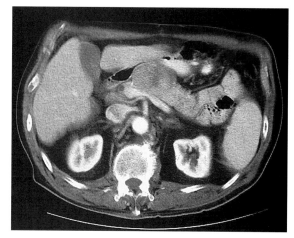

Figure 2.4 B

Findings: CECT demonstrates a 5-cm mass in the body of the pancreas with a small area of low attenuation in the center.

Differential Diagnosis: Pancreatic adenocarcinoma, islet cell tumor, metastasis.

Diagnosis: Acinar cell carcinoma.

Discussion: Acinar cell carcinoma is a rare malignant neoplasm with poor prognosis due to the frequent liver metastases at the time of diagnosis. They are seen in elderly patients with a mean age of 65 years old. Systemic lipase secretion by acinar cell neoplasms leads to distant fat necrosis in the skin, bone, and joints. This results in an erythematous rash, lytic bone lesions, and polyarthralgias in these patients. By CT, acinar cell carcinomas tend to be larger than the typical adenocarcinoma measuring up to 15 cm and are usually well circumscribed with little desmoplastic reaction. Because of their larger size, acinar cell neoplasms can have central necrosis as is seen in this case. A nonfunctioning islet cell tumor would be a good differential diagnosis for this case because those lesions tend to be larger as well.

CASE 5

Clinical History: 43-year-old woman with left upper quadrant discomfort.

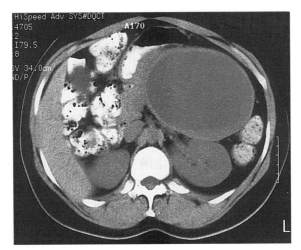

Figure 2.5 A

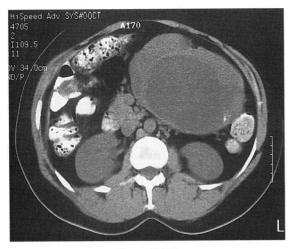

Figure 2.5 B

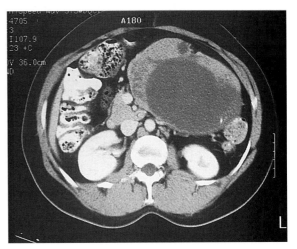

Figure 2.5 C

Findings: (A, B) NECT demonstrates a large 10-cm cystic mass arising from the body and tail of the pancreas. (C) CECT demonstrates an enhancing soft tissue rind that surrounds the central cystic component.

Differential Diagnosis: Mucinous cystic neoplasm, pseudocyst, nonfunctioning islet cell tumor.

Diagnosis: Solid and papillary epithelial neoplasm of the pancreas.

Discussion: Solid and papillary epithelial neoplasm of the pancreas is a rare low-grade malignancy seen most commonly in young women. The mean age of presentation is in the 20s ranging between the 2nd and 6th decades of life. Surgical resection is often curable. The lesions typically present as a large thick-walled cystic mass with hemorrhage and necrosis. The peripheral solid portions usually enhance with intravenous contrast and can have curvilinear calcifications as well. The lesion is more commonly seen in the tail of the pancreas. The differential diagnosis includes pseudocyst, mucinous cystic neoplasm, or a nonfunctioning islet cell tumor that has undergone cystic degeneration. The lack of history for pancreatitis makes pseudocyst unlikely. Both mucinous cystic neoplasm and a nonfunctioning islet cell tumor can have the same radiographic appearance as the solid and papillary epithelial neoplasm. The treatment, however, is the same and consists of surgical resection.

CASE 6

Clinical History: (A) 57-year-old man presents initially with pancreatitis; (B) the same patient presents 2 years later with a recurrent episode of pancreatitis; (C) 2 weeks later, the patient is readmitted for abdominal pain and hematemesis.

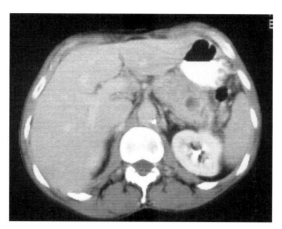

Figure 2.6 A

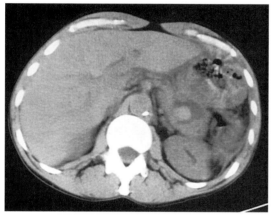

Figure 2.6 B

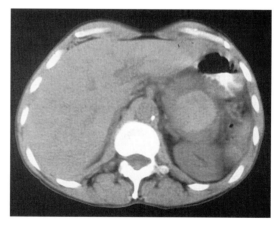

Figure 2.6 C

Findings: (A) CECT demonstrates a small pseudocyst in the tail of the pancreas. (B) NECT 2 years later demonstrates a small hematoma within the pseudocyst in the tail of the pancreas. (C) NECT 2 weeks later shows a large hematoma in the tail of the pancreas.

Differential Diagnosis: None.

Diagnosis: Hematoma secondary to a pseudoaneurysm of the splenic artery from pancreatitis.

Discussion: Pseudoaneurysms can be seen as a complication of pancreatitis secondary to the erosion of a peripancreatic artery by pancreatic enzymes. Commonly involved vessels include the splenic artery, gastroduodenal artery, and pancreaticoduodenal arcades. On NECT the hyperdense hematoma can frequently be seen as noted in this example. With contrast enhancement, the pseudoaneurysm can sometimes be demonstrated as an enhancing cystic structure within or adjacent to a pseudocyst. Diagnosis can be confirmed by angiography. Rupture of a pseudoaneurysm has a high mortality rate of approximately 37%. Embolization of a pseudoaneurysm can be performed during the acute phase of pancreatitis until surgery can be performed at a later date. Embolization by itself has been used therapeutically as well.

CASE 7

Clinical History: 44-year-old man with repeated bouts of pancreatitis.

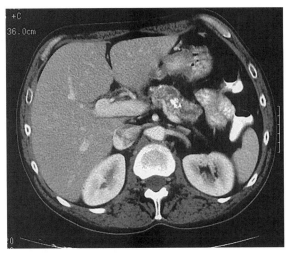

Figure 2.7 A

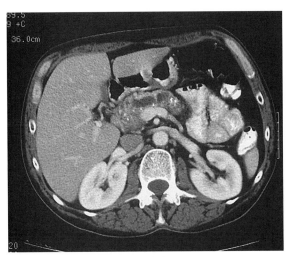

Figure 2.7 B

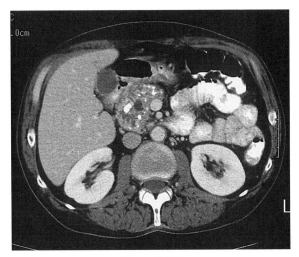

Figure 2.7 C

Findings: CECT demonstrates multiple pancreatic calcifications with an irregularly dilated pancreatic duct.

Differential Diagnosis: None.

Diagnosis: Chronic pancreatitis.

Discussion: Chronic pancreatitis is most commonly secondary to underlying alcohol consumption in the United States. The alcohol alters the function of the acinar cells resulting in concentration of proteins in the ducts. This leads to stone formation, ductal stenosis and dilatation, and acinar atrophy. The ductal dilatation in chronic pancreatitis is most commonly irregular in appearance (73%), followed by smooth (15%), and beaded (12%). Pancreatic ductal dilatation is seen in 68% of patients with chronic pancreatitis, with atrophy in 54%, and calcifications in 50%. This case demonstrates the typical findings of chronic pancreatitis with calcifications and ductal dilatation. There is always a concern for an underlying pancreatic adenocarcinoma in a patient with chronic pancreatitis causing pancreatic ductal dilatation. The head of the pancreas, however, is diffusely calcified with no focal low attenuation mass present. Pancreatic adenocarcinomas rarely calcify. If there is continued concern for a malignancy, then ERCP or biopsy is required. Correlation with serum CA 19-9 levels is also helpful because it is elevated in pancreatic adenocarcinoma.

CASE 8

Clinical History: 69-year-old woman with abdominal pain and weight loss.

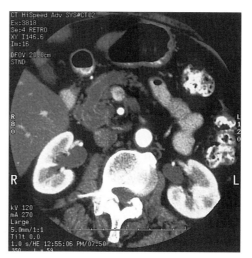

Figure 2.8 A

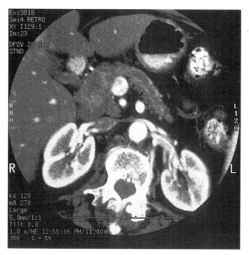

Figure 2.8 B

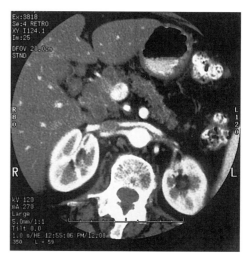

Figure 2.8 C

Findings: CECT demonstrates a markedly dilated pancreatic duct and low attenuation areas within the head of the pancreas and the uncinate process. No pancreatic calcifications are seen.

Differential Diagnosis: Chronic pancreatitis, ampullary carcinoma.

Diagnosis: Ductectatic mucinous cystadenocarcinoma.

Discussion: Ductectatic mucinous cystadenocarcinoma is similar histologically to a mucinous cystic neoplasm but differs in that it involves a side branch of the pancreatic duct and communicates with the pancreatic duct. This lesion produces mucin which fills the pancreatic duct and causes it to dilate. By ERCP, there are multiple cystic cavities, usually in the uncinate process, which communicate with the main pancreatic duct. There is also a large amount of mucin coming from the ampulla as it is cannulated by the endoscopist. The low attenuation lesions seen in the head of the pancreas and uncinate process represent cystic cavities that communicate with the duct. Spread of the cancer outside of the pancreas occurs late in the course of the disease so this neoplasm has a fairly good prognosis after resection.

CASE 9

Clinical History: 26-year-old man with abdominal pain.

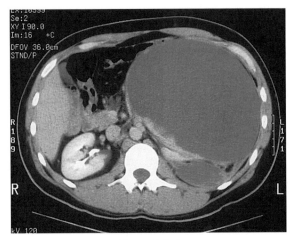

Figure 2.9 A

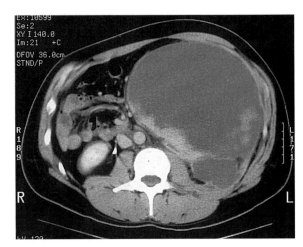

Figure 2.9 B

Findings: CECT demonstrates a 19-cm cystic lesion with peripheral mural nodules in the pancreas.

Differential Diagnosis: Pseudocyst, mucinous cystic neoplasm, nonfunctioning islet cell tumor.

Diagnosis: Solid and papillary epithelial neoplasm of the pancreas.

Discussion: The differential diagnosis for a large cystic mass in the pancreas in a young adult is limited. Excluding an abscess and hematoma, the differential for a large mass in the region of the pancreas would include a mesenchymal tumor such as a leiomyosarcoma and lymphoma, which are both solid in appearance. For a large cystic lesion arising in the pancreas or peripancreatic region, the differential would include a pseudocyst, nonfunctioning islet cell tumor with cystic degeneration, or a solid and papillary neoplasm of the pancreas. The lack of history for pancreatitis would exclude pseudocyst and the age would make a nonfunctioning islet cell tumor and mucinous cystic neoplasm less likely. Prognosis for this patient is excellent with surgical excision.

CASE 10

Clinical History: 73-year-old woman with steatorrhea.

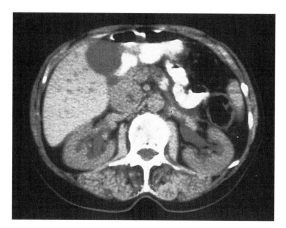

Figure 2.10 A

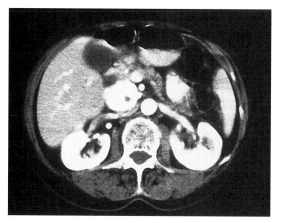

Figure 2.10 B

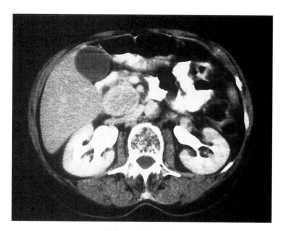

Figure 2.10 C

Findings: (A) NECT demonstrates a 3-cm mass in the head of the pancreas. (B) Arterial phase of a CECT demonstrates intense contrast enhancement of this lesion. (C) Equilibrium-phase CECT demonstrates persistent enhancement in the periphery with the center of the lesion remaining hypodense.

Differential Diagnosis: Pancreatic adenocarcinoma, metastasis, acinar cell neoplasm.

Diagnosis: Islet cell tumor (somatostatinoma).

Discussion: Somatostatinoma is a rare islet cell tumor of the pancreas that inhibits the release of pepsin, secretin, pancreatic exocrine enzymes, and causes intestinal hypomotility. These lesions tend to be very slow growing although greater than 50% are malignant. As with other islet cell tumors, somatostatinomas are hypervascular and demonstrate intense contrast enhancement. Somatostatinomas and other islet cell tumors can be isodense or slightly hyperdense on the equilibrium phase of a CECT and can be difficult to detect. The NECT and arterial phase are often necessary to better identify these lesions as is shown in this case. Pancreatic adenocarcinomas are hypovascular and would not demonstrate intense enhancement as is seen in this case on the arterial phase of the CECT. Metastases are unlikely because the lesion is solitary and there is no known primary.

CASE 11

Clinical History: 23-year-old woman with abdominal discomfort.

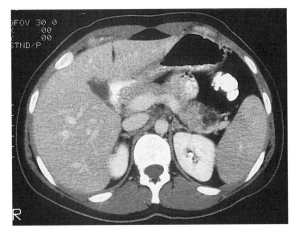

Figure 2.11 A

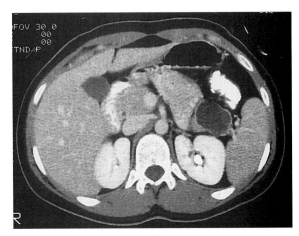

Figure 2.11 B

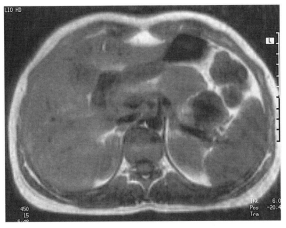

Figure 2.11 C

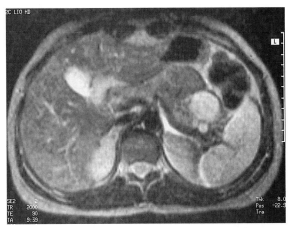

Figure 2.11 D

Findings: (A, B) CECT demonstrates a 3.5-cm septated cystic mass in the tail of the pancreas. (C) T1WI demonstrates this lesion to be of low signal intensity. (D) This same lesion is of marked increased signal intensity (fluid intensity) on the T2WI.

Differential Diagnosis: Pancreatic pseudocyst, solid and papillary neoplasm.

Diagnosis: Mucinous cystic neoplasm.

Discussion: Mucinous cystic neoplasm is a primary cystic neoplasm of the pancreas. All mucinous cystic neoplasms are considered to have malignant potential and complete resection is recommended. Most of these lesions occur in patients between the ages of 40–60 years but the range is from 20–80 years of age. By CT imaging, these lesions are predominantly cystic with the cysts larger than 2 cm, hence the term macrocystic. They can be septated and have eggshell-like peripheral calcifications. On MRI, the lesion varies in appearance depending on the cyst content. They are typically hypointense on the T1WI and hyperintense on the T2WI, as is seen in this case. This case is atypical because the age of the patient would favor a solid and papillary neoplasm or a pseudocyst from pancreatitis. Without a history of pancreatitis, a neoplasm (solid and papillary neoplasm versus mucinous cystic neoplasm) was the top differential diagnosis and surgical resection was performed.

CASE 12

Clinical History: 53-year-old woman with jaundice.

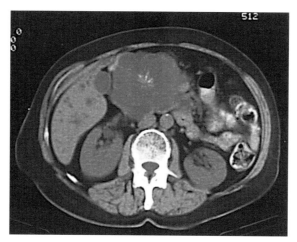

Figure 2.12 A

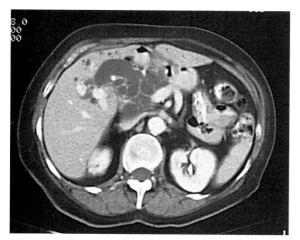

Figure 2.12 B

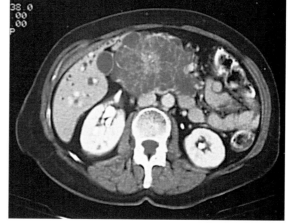

Figure 2.12 C

Findings: (A) NECT demonstrates a low attenuation lesion in the body of the pancreas with central calcifications. (B, C) CECT demonstrates the same lesion to have enhancing septa separating multiple small cysts. Note the dilated CBD and intrahepatic biliary ducts.

Differential Diagnosis: None.

Diagnosis: Microcystic adenoma.

Discussion: Microcystic adenoma is almost always a benign neoplasm of the pancreas arising from the duct cells. They typically occur in older women between the ages of 50–70 years. This lesion has been associated with von Hippel-Lindau disease. This lesion can occur anywhere within the pancreas and is considered to be one of the cystic neoplasms of the pancreas. The cysts tend to be small measuring less than 2 cm in size. The septa forming the cysts can enhance after intravenous contrast administration and if the cysts are very small, the lesion can appear solid. Calcifications within a central stellate fibrotic scar are characteristic of this lesion as is seen in this example. Other cystic neoplasms of the pancreas include a mucinous cystic neoplasm, which tends to have larger cysts and a necrotic islet cell tumor. Neither of these lesions would have the central calcifications and innumerable small cysts.

CASE 13

Clinical History: 45-year-old man with severe abdominal pain and fevers.

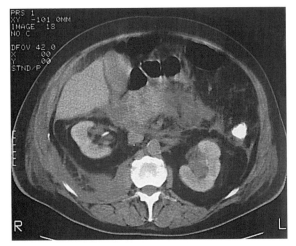

Figure 2.13 A

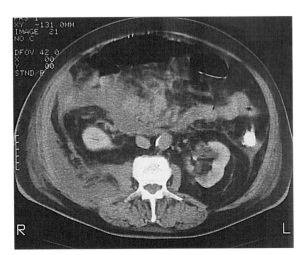

Figure 2.13 B

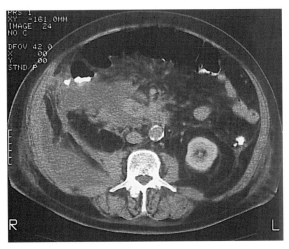

Figure 2.13 C

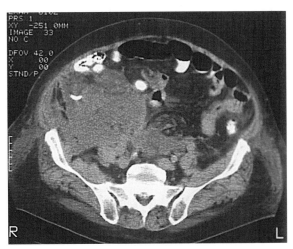

Figure 2.13 D

Findings: CECT demonstrates extensive peripancreatic inflammation and phlegmon predominantly around the head and body of the pancreas. These fluid collections extend down into the pelvis.

Differential Diagnosis: None.

Diagnosis: Pancreatitis.

Discussion: This case demonstrates the spaces in the retroperitoneum. The pancreas is located within the anterior pararenal space just anterior to Gerota's fascia, which separates it from the kidney. Fluid and phlegmon from pancreatitis will pool within the anterior pararenal space and frequently spare the kidney and the perirenal space as is seen in this case. The fluid has also accumulated in the posterior pararenal space, which is not contiguous with the anterior pararenal space at this level. It is separated from it by fat and the lateral conal fascia. The three spaces, anterior and posterior pararenal space and perirenal space, communicate in the infrarenal space. This is well demonstrated in this case in which the fluid in the anterior and posterior pararenal space becomes one fluid collection in the right pelvis. This anatomy is important to understand because it helps define the source of an abnormality in the retroperitoneum.

CASE 14

Clinical History: 75-year-old woman with weight loss.

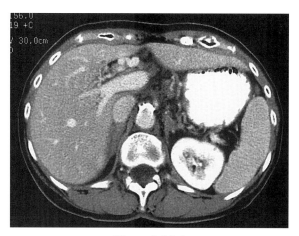

Figure 2.14 A

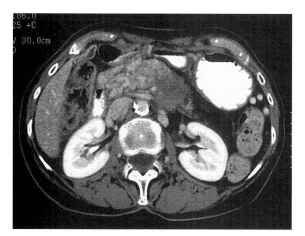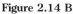

Figure 2.14 B

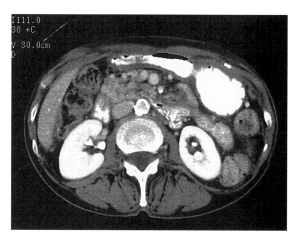

Figure 2.14 C

Findings: CECT demonstrates a low attenuation lesion surrounding the superior mesenteric artery in the body of the pancreas. There is thrombosis of the splenic vein and superior mesenteric vein (SMV). Note the collateral vessels anterior to the pancreas, medial to the stomach, and in the left flank.

Differential Diagnosis: Pancreatitis.

Diagnosis: Pancreatic adenocarcinoma with splenic vein and SMV thrombosis.

Discussion: The key role for CT in the evaluation of pancreatic masses is to determine the resectability particularly of a pancreatic adenocarcinoma. One of the most reliable staging criteria for resectability is the presence of vascular invasion. The fat plane between the pancreas and the SMV can be obliterated normally. This does not necessarily indicate vascular invasion by the malignancy. However, if the SMV is obstructed by the mass then vascular invasion is likely present. In contradistinction, if the perivascular fat around the SMA is obliterated by the mass or there is thickening of the vessel, then vascular invasion is suspected. The presence of mesenteric, gastric, and omental collateral vessels should also suggest SMV or splenic vein thrombosis. These collaterals, typically the gastrocolic trunk entering the SMV, are seen well on CECT, as noted in this example.

CASE 15

Clinical History: 35-year-old woman with episodes of hypoglycemia.

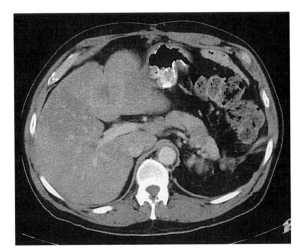

Figure 2.15 A

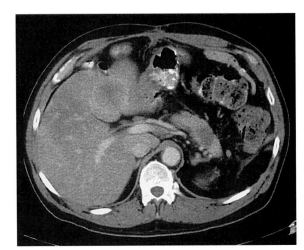

Figure 2.15 B

Findings: CECT demonstrates a 2-cm low attenuation lesion in the tail of the pancreas. A small calcification is seen in the center. A hypervascular metastasis is seen in the left lobe of the liver.

Differential Diagnosis: Pancreatic adenocarcinoma, metastasis.

Diagnosis: Islet cell tumor (insulinoma).

Discussion: Islet cell tumors are endocrine neoplasms of the pancreas that can secrete hormones such as insulin, glucagon, and somatostatin. Because of their hormone secretion, these patients usually present early in the course of the disease when the lesion is still small. Except for insulinomas, the majority of these lesions are malignant but tend to be slow growing. Insulinoma is the most common islet cell tumor and typically presents in the fourth through sixth decade. Insulinomas are small with most being <1.5 cm and solitary. Small calcifications can be present as in this case. Insulinomas are most often hypervascular and can be isodense to hyperdense on CECT. This case is unusual because the lesion is hypodense on the CECT, allowing it to be seen against the enhanced pancreas. The hypervascular metastasis in the liver, the lesion in the pancreas, and the history of hypoglycemia are clues to the diagnosis in this case.

CASE 16

Clinical History: 18-year-old woman with abdominal pain and bloating.

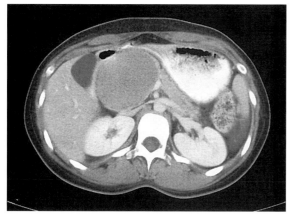

Figure 2.16 A

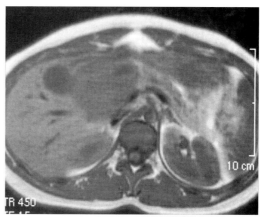

Figure 2.16 B

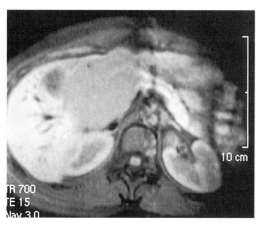

Figure 2.16 C

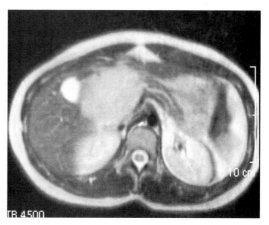

Figure 2.16 D

Findings: (A) CECT demonstrates a 6-cm low attenuation lesion in the head of the pancreas. (B) T1-weighted MRI demonstrates a homogeneous low signal intensity lesion relative to the pancreas. (C) This same lesion enhances with gadolinium. (D) It is hyperintense on the T2WI.

Differential Diagnosis: Islet cell tumor.

Diagnosis: Solid and papillary epithelial neoplasm.

Discussion: In an 18-year-old woman, there are not many diagnostic possibilities for a pancreatic mass. Of the pancreatic neoplasms, the most likely diagnosis is a solid and papillary epithelial neoplasm. Because of its size, a nonfunctioning islet cell tumor is also a possibility. The patient is too young for an adenocarcinoma, microcystic adenoma, and a mucinous cystic neoplasm. Adolescents can get pancreatitis usually from trauma, drugs, or postviral infections but a history of pancreatitis is usually known. The lesion enhances which excludes a pseudocyst, choledochal cyst or duplication cyst. Lymphoma is a possibility but no other evidence for adenopathy is present.

CASE 17

Clinical History: 38-year-old man with history of peptic ulcer disease.

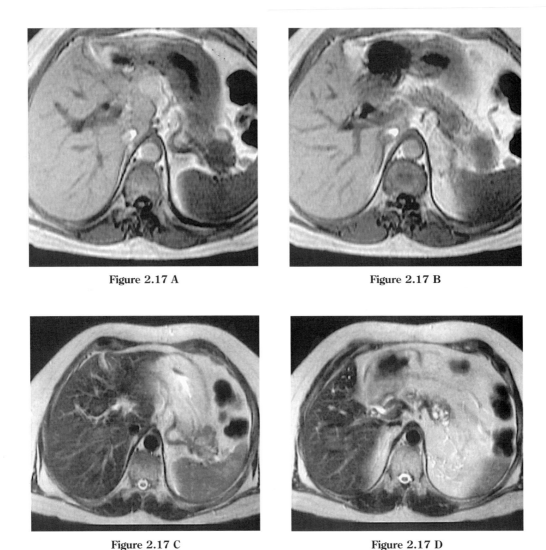

Figure 2.17 A

Figure 2.17 B

Figure 2.17 C

Figure 2.17 D

Findings: (A, B) T1-weighted MR demonstrates two low signal intensity lesions within the body and tail of the pancreas. (C, D) This same lesion is of increased signal intensity on the T2 images. Note the thickened stomach as well.

Differential Diagnosis: Metastases, lymphoma.

Diagnosis: Multiple gastrinomas in a patient with MEN I syndrome.

Discussion: Multiple endocrine neoplasia (MEN) type I syndrome consists of a pituitary adenoma, parathyroid adenoma, and pancreatic islet cell tumor. The islet cell tumors can either be insulinomas, gastrinomas, or VIPomas. This patient had multiple gastrinomas resulting in Zollinger-Ellison syndrome causing a thickened stomach wall. Few diseases will cause multiple lesions in the pancreas. These lesions did not appear cystic excluding pseudocysts. Other lesions include metastases and lymphoma. Gastric cancer with metastases to the pancreas is a possibility but no other metastases are present in the abdomen. Lymphoma can also involve the stomach and pancreas but widespread lymphadenopathy is usually present. Gastrinomas can be multiple in up to 60% of cases, especially if associated with MEN I. The thickened gastric wall is due to the excess acid produced by the stomach secondary to the elevated serum gastrin levels. A careful history of the patient's family revealed that other people in the family had similar problems as well.

CASE 18

Clinical History: 51-year-old man with pancreatic insufficiency and abdominal pain.

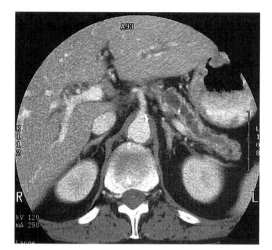

Figure 2.18 A

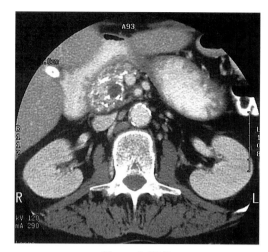

Figure 2.18 B

Findings: CECT demonstrates calcifications throughout the pancreas as well as an irregularly dilated pancreatic duct.

Differential Diagnosis: None.

Diagnosis: Chronic pancreatitis.

Discussion: In the United States, the most common cause for chronic pancreatitis is oral intake of alcohol. Other causes have been implicated including hereditary pancreatitis, cystic fibrosis, hyperlipidemia, and hyperparathyroidism. Pathologically, there is progressive fibrosis and destruction of the pancreas with atrophy of the acini. This leads to stone formation and loss of both endocrine and exocrine function. Radiologically, there are multiple calcifications throughout the pancreas, which are predominantly intraductal in location. There can be atrophy of the pancreas as well as pancreatic and biliary dilatation. The biliary dilatation is thought to be due to stenosis of the common bile duct as it passes through the fibrotic head of the pancreas.

CASE 19

Clinical History: 60-year-old woman with weight loss.

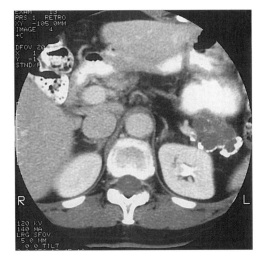

Figure 2.19 A

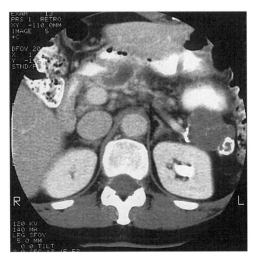

Figure 2.19 B

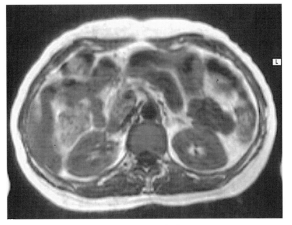

Figure 2.19 C

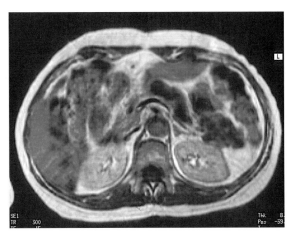

Figure 2.19 D

Findings: (A, B) CECT demonstrates a 4-cm septated cystic mass in the tail of the pancreas. Note the peripheral calcifications. (C) T1WI demonstrates this same lesion to be of low signal intensity. (D) Post-gadolinium T1WI demonstrates enhancement of the multiple septa in the lesion.

Differential Diagnosis: Microcystic adenoma, pseudocyst.

Diagnosis: Mucinous cystic neoplasm.

Discussion: 85–90% of cysts in the pancreas are pseudocysts from pancreatitis. These lesions lack an inner epithelial lining. The other 10–15% of cysts are of duct cell origin. These consist of cysts (either congenital or associated with Von Hippel-Lindau or autosomal dominant polycystic kidney disease), or cystic neoplasms (microcystic adenomas or mucinous cystic neoplasms).

Mucinous cystic neoplasms tend to have cysts greater than 2 cm and are few in number. There is often a thick wall present in the periphery of the tumor, which can calcify as is seen in this case. The septa that form these cysts enhance with contrast administration (gadolinium and iodinated contrast). Approximately 85% of these lesions are found in the tail of the pancreas with a marked female preponderance (9:1). A microcystic adenoma is unlikely because they tend to have tiny cysts with central calcifications rather than peripheral. Pseudocyst is a good differential diagnosis and a thorough history is necessary to exclude it.

CASE 20

Clinical History: 81-year-old woman with abdominal pain and weight loss.

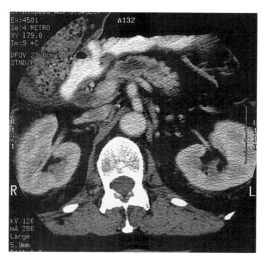

Figure 2.20 A

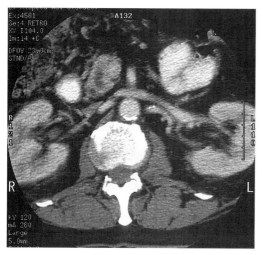

Figure 2.20 B

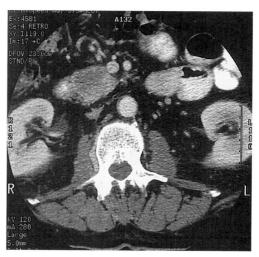

Figure 2.20 C

Findings: CECT demonstrates a 4-cm low-attenuation lesion in the head of the pancreas. Note the dilated common bile and pancreatic ducts.

Differential Diagnosis: Focal pancreatitis, islet cell tumor, metastasis.

Diagnosis: Pancreatic adenocarcinoma.

Discussion: Risk factors for pancreatic adenocarcinomas include smoking, long standing diabetes, and hereditary pancreatitis. Alcohol is a cause for pancreatitis but is not a risk factor for adenocarcinoma. Elevated liver enzymes and laboratory findings of obstructive jaundice are commonly seen because most lesions occur in the head of the pancreas. The importance of CT for pancreatic adenocarcinoma is in both detection and staging. CT findings that exclude resectability include retroperitoneal extension, vascular invasion, adjacent organ involvement except the duodenum, lymphadenopathy, distant metastases, and ascites. In this case, there is no vascular invasion, lymphadenopathy or ascites seen but involvement of the duodenum is questionable. Approximately 50% of patients who are thought to be resectable by CT is found to have local invasion or liver metastases at time of surgery.

CASE 21

Clinical History: 42-year-old man from Argentina presents with abdominal pain and fevers.

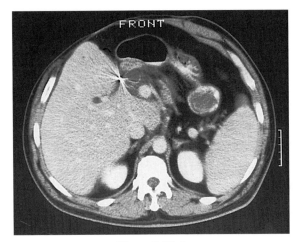

Figure 2.21 A

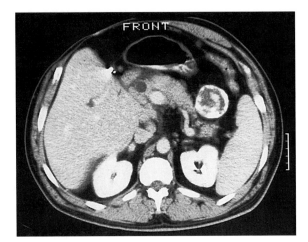

Figure 2.21 B

Findings: CECT demonstrates a 4-cm calcified cystic lesion arising from the body of the pancreas.

Differential Diagnosis: Old hematoma, abscess, pseudocyst, mucinous cystic neoplasm.

Diagnosis: Echinococcal cyst of the pancreas.

Discussion: The liver is the most common organ affected by this parasite (75–80% of cases) but other organs can also be involved such as the brain, lung, and kidney. Infection in humans is from the feces of the dog contaminated by the parasite. The eggs hatch in the GI tract and enter the portal system where access to the rest of the body is obtained. The differential diagnosis for a calcified cystic lesion in the pancreas is similar to that of the rest of the abdomen. It includes an old abscess, hematoma, or in the case of the pancreas a pseudocyst. Cystic neoplasms can also have peripheral eggshell-like calcifications such as a mucinous cystic neoplasm. This patient was found to have similar lesions in the liver which were confirmed as hydatid cysts.

CASE 22

Clinical History: 77-year-old woman with jaundice and weight loss.

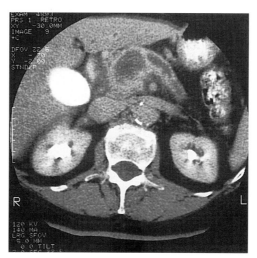

Figure 2.22 A

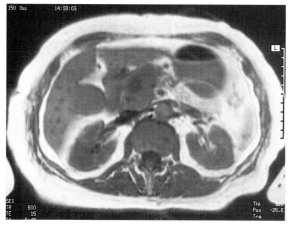

Figure 2.22 B

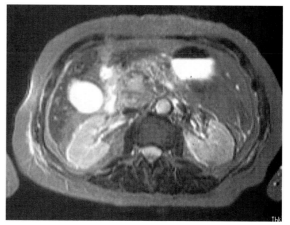

Figure 2.22 C

Findings: (A) CECT demonstrates a necrotic mass in the head of the pancreas with pancreatic ductal dilatation. The mass abuts the SMV. (B) T1WI demonstrates a low signal intensity mass in the head of the pancreas. No flow void is seen in the SMV. (C) T2WI demonstrates an area of high signal intensity corresponding to the necrosis.

Differential Diagnosis: Pancreatitis, metastasis, islet cell tumor.

Diagnosis: Pancreatic adenocarcinoma with SMV thrombosis.

Discussion: One of the critical factors in staging a patient with pancreatic adenocarcinoma is involvement of vascular structures, especially the SMV and SMA. Loss of the fat plane between the pancreas and the SMV can be seen normally. However, SMV thrombosis suggests vascular involvement by the tumor and would render the patient unresectable. This may be difficult to ascertain on CECT as is seen in this example. MRI or helical CT during the arterial phase with 3-D reconstruction are better suited for evaluating for vascular involvement. Typically a flow void is seen in the vessels on T1WI with loss of the flow void and high signal intensity centrally indicative of a thrombosis of the vessel. This is well demonstrated in this case. Gradient echo sequences can also be used to evaluate retroperitoneal vasculature. MRI can also be used to evaluate for peripancreatic extension, lymphadenopathy, liver metastases, and ductal dilatation.

CASE 23

Clinical History: 29-year-old man with abdominal pain and weight loss.

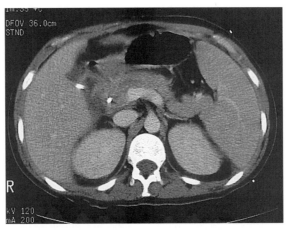

Figure 2.23 A

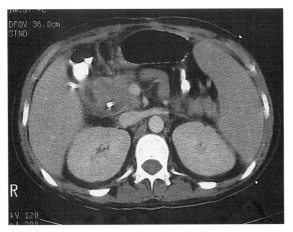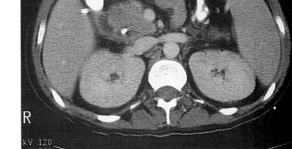

Figure 2.23 B   **Figure 2.23 C**

Findings: CECT demonstrates a low attenuation lesion diffusely infiltrating the head of the pancreas. Note the peripancreatic stranding.

Differential Diagnosis: Pancreatitis, pancreatic adenocarcinoma, metastasis.

Diagnosis: Pancreatic lymphoma.

Discussion: Primary lymphoma of the pancreas is extremely rare, with peripancreatic lymphoma being much more common. Non-Hodgkin's lymphoma is more common than Hodgkin's lymphoma in the pancreas, with histiocytic and Burkitt's lymphoma the most common subtypes.

It is often difficult to distinguish between peripancreatic and pancreatic lymphoma because lymph nodes can often invade the pancreas due to its lack of serosa. Also confusing the picture is the presence of pancreatitis, which can sometimes accompany lymphoma due to obstruction of the duct. Lymphoma of the pancreas can present either as a solitary mass or as multiple solid masses. Alternatively, the pancreas can be diffusely involved simulating pancreatitis. In this case, the age of the patient makes adenocarcinoma unlikely. The lack of other lesions and of a known primary makes metastases unlikely as well. Pancreatitis is a good consideration and often biopsy is necessary to distinguish these two entities.

CASE 24

Clinical History: 79-year-old woman with fever.

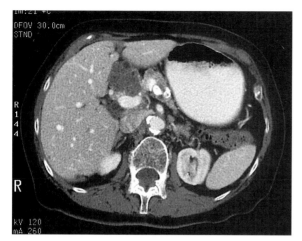

Figure 2.24 A

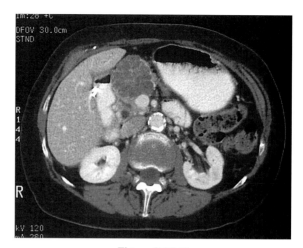

Figure 2.24 B

Findings: CECT demonstrates a 4-cm low attenuation mass with multiple internal small cysts at the junction of the body and head of the pancreas.

Differential Diagnosis: None.

Diagnosis: Microcystic adenoma.

Discussion: Approximately 95% of the non-neoplastic cystic masses of the pancreas are pseudocysts. The remaining others are true cysts either congenital in origin or associated with von Hippel-Lindau or polycystic kidney disease. Cystic neoplasms include microcystic adenoma, mucinous cystic neoplasm, solid and papillary epithelial neoplasm, lymphangioma, teratoma and a necrotic nonfunctioning islet cell tumor. Except for the microcystic adenoma, most of the other neoplasms tend to have one or a few large cysts (>2 cm) and resemble pseudocysts in appearance. The solid portion of these lesion varies depending on the cell type and aggressiveness of the lesion. Microcystic adenoma, on the other hand, will have innumerable small (<2 cm) cysts as is seen in this case. The age, sex, and appearance of this lesion is characteristic for a microcystic adenoma.

CASE 25

Clinical History: 71-year-old woman with left upper quadrant pain.

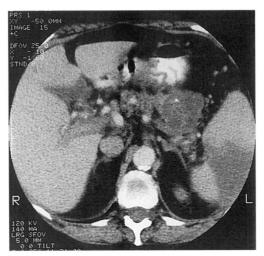

Figure 2.25 A

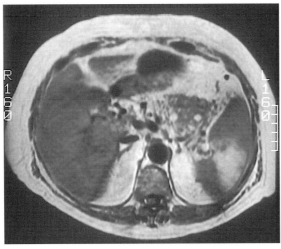

Figure 2.25 B

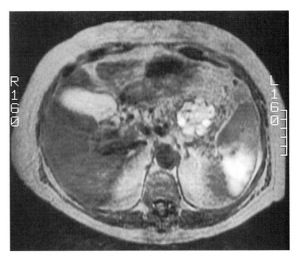

Figure 2.25 C

Findings: (A) CECT demonstrates a 4-cm low attenuation lesion composed of multiple small cysts. A small calcification is seen in the center of the lesion. Note a splenic infarct and nonvisualization of the splenic vein. Multiple small collaterals are present. (B) T1WI demonstrates this lesion to be predominantly low in signal intensity with several hyperintense small cysts. The splenic infarct is again seen. (C) T2WI demonstrates the lesion to be hyperintense.

Differential Diagnosis: Mucinous cystic neoplasm.

Diagnosis: Microcystic adenoma.

Discussion: Microcystic adenoma is a benign neoplasm arising from the duct cells. It is typically composed of innumerable small cysts filled with glycogen. If the cysts are very small, the lesion can appear solid by CT and have central calcifications. Often the cysts will be hyperintense on T1WI secondary to proteinaceous material and hemorrhage as is seen in this case. Mucinous cystic neoplasms usually have larger cysts and appear similar to pseudocysts from pancreatitis. The diagnosis of a microcystic adenoma is crucial for the patient because a partial pancreatectomy carries a high morbidity and mortality rate. Because the patients are typically older (>60 years), they are often poor surgical candidates as well. This case is unusual because there has been thrombosis of the splenic vein by this lesion. Although uncommon, obstruction of the splenic vein as well as the pancreatic and biliary duct can occur. The splenic vein thrombosis led to the splenic infarct, which was the cause of the patient's discomfort.

Clinical History: 49-year-old man with severe abdominal pain and weight loss over the past 6 months.

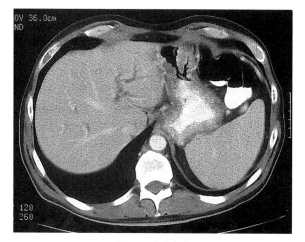

Figure 2.26 A

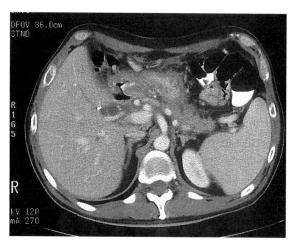

Figure 2.26 B

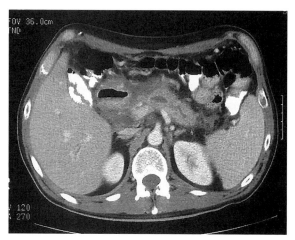

Figure 2.26 C

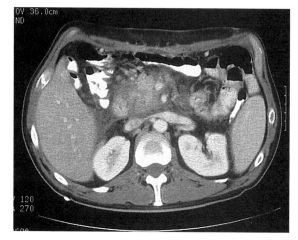

Figure 2.26 D

Findings: CECT demonstrates an edematous swollen pancreas with peripancreatic inflammation and phlegmon formation. Note the dilated intrahepatic and pancreatic ducts.

Differential Diagnosis: None.

Diagnosis: Pancreatitis secondary to a pancreatic adenocarcinoma.

Discussion: Pancreatitis can be due to several causes with alcohol and biliary stones accounting for the majority of cases. Other causes include iatrogenic (post ERCP), trauma, post-infection, hereditary pancreatitis, and drugs. Pancreatic carcinoma is a rare cause of pancreatitis making up less than 5% of the cases of pancreatitis. It is often very difficult to diagnose pancreatic cancer in a patient with pancreatitis. The diagnosis should be suggested in a middle-aged or elderly patient with no identifiable cause for pancreatitis. Biliary dilatation and longstanding elevated bilirubin levels are less common in focal pancreatitis and would suggest the diagnosis of an adenocarcinoma. Pancreatitis also tends to spread anteriorly in the retroperitoneum whereas pancreatic cancer more commonly spreads in a retropancreatic direction. Obliteration of the fat surrounding vessels can be seen in both pancreatitis and cancer but is more typical in pancreatic cancer. Pancreatic cancer in this patient was suggested and the diagnosis confirmed by ERCP.

CASE 27

Clinical History: 52-year-old man with history of recurrent pancreatitis presents with abdominal bloating.

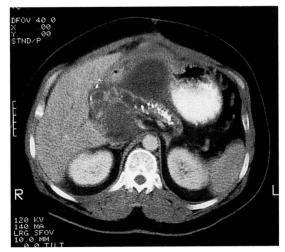

Figure 2.27 A

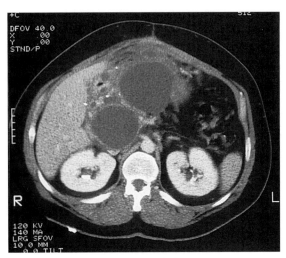

Figure 2.27 B

Findings: CECT demonstrates findings of chronic pancreatitis with a dilated pancreatic duct and pancreatic calcifications. A 5-cm and 7-cm cystic lesion is seen in the region of the head of the pancreas.

Differential Diagnosis: Mucinous cystic neoplasm, necrotic tumor (metastasis, nonfunctioning islet cell tumor).

Diagnosis: Pancreatic pseudocyst.

Discussion: Pancreatic pseudocyst formation is one of the many complications of acute pancreatitis. The majority of peripancreatic fluid collections will resolve spontaneously without drainage. Approximately 10% of patients, however, will form a pseudocyst . These cysts differ from true congenital cysts in that they do not have an inner epithelial lining. A fluid collection is not usually considered a true pseudocyst until it is approximately 6 weeks old and has developed a mature fibrotic wall. At that time it is unlikely to resolve on its own. Drainage of noninfected pseudocysts is usually reserved for those larger than 5 cm, those that are enlarging, or those that are symptomatic for the patient. The main differential diagnosis for a pseudocyst is a mucinous cystic neoplasm. Patients with mucinous cystic neoplasms do not usually have a history of pancreatitis or demonstrate signs of chronic pancreatitis as is seen in this case. If no history of pancreatitis can be elicited, then a mucinous cystic neoplasm must be considered.

CASE 28

Clinical History: 9-year-old boy with epigastric pain and increasing abdominal girth.

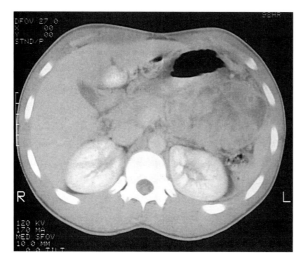

Figure 2.28 A

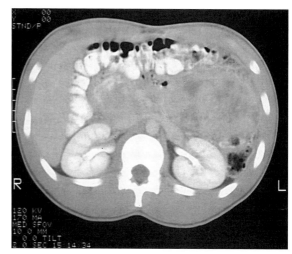

Figure 2.28 B

Findings: CECT demonstrates a large 7-cm heterogeneous enhancing mass arising from the tail of the pancreas.

Differential Diagnosis: Lymphoma, retroperitoneal sarcoma, hematoma, solid and papillary epithelial neoplasm.

Diagnosis: Pancreaticoblastoma.

Discussion: Pancreaticoblastomas are a rare neoplasm of the pancreas composed of epithelial cells sometimes intermixed with mesenchymal tissue. They typically arise in children between the ages of 1–8 years and are usually large at the time of presentation. Hemorrhage and necrosis are commonly present. Prognosis is fairly good if distant metastases have not occurred. The difficulty in diagnosing this lesion is discerning the organ of origin. If it arises from the pancreas then in this age group, the most likely diagnosis would be a pancreaticoblastoma, or less likely, a solid and papillary epithelial neoplasm. Other large masses in the abdomen could be due to a retroperitoneal sarcoma or lymphoma. If there is a history of trauma, then a large hematoma could have this heterogeneous appearance as well. Pancreaticoblastomas can have an elevated alpha fetoprotein as well. If this is inconclusive, then diagnosis can be made by biopsy.

CASE 29

Clinical History: 61-year-old man with weight loss.

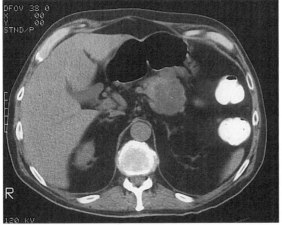

Figure 2.29 A

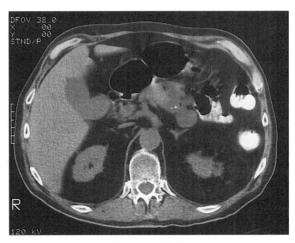

Figure 2.29 B

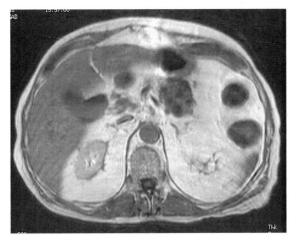

Figure 2.29 C

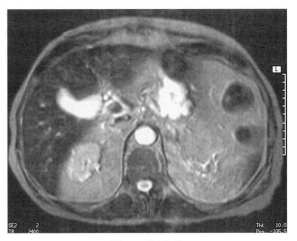

Figure 2.29 D

Findings: (A, B) NECT demonstrates a low attenuation lesion in the body of the pancreas with small calcifications. (C) MRI demonstrates this lesion to be of low signal intensity on the T1-weighted sequence. (D) The same lesion is of high signal intensity on the T2 image. The signal characteristics follow that of water. Note the linear low signal area on the T2 image, which represents a fibrous scar.

Differential Diagnosis: Mucinous cystic neoplasm.

Diagnosis: Microcystic adenoma.

Discussion: Microcystic adenoma is almost always a benign cystic lesion of the pancreas which is often lobulated due to the multiple small cysts. The cysts are filled with glycogen-rich fluid and range in size from 1 mm up to 2 cm. On MRI, the cysts usually follows the signal characteristics of water depending on the amount of protein and glycogen within the fluid. Because they are hypervascular, the cysts can occasionally hemorrhage and be bright on T1WI. The central scar and septa will typically be dark on both the T1- and T2-weighted images, as is seen in this case.

Mucinous cystic neoplasms tend to have a few large cysts rather than multiple small cysts as is seen in this case. They most often resemble a pseudocyst. Necrotic nonfunctioning islet cell tumors can also have a cystic component but are usually much larger in size with more of a solid component than is seen here. Adenocarcinomas are typically solid and found in the head of the pancreas. The multiple small cysts, age of the patient, and calcifications are characteristic for a microcystic adenoma.

CASE 30

Clinical History: 46-year-old man with history of alcoholism.

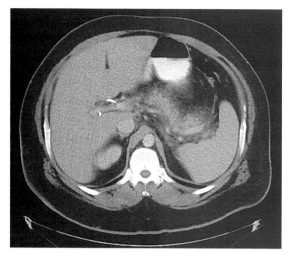

Figure 2.30 A

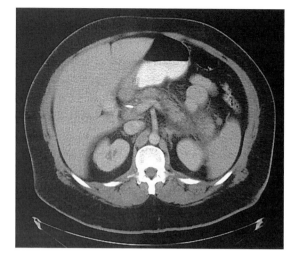

Figure 2.30 B

Findings: CECT demonstrates a swollen pancreas with peripancreatic inflammation. There are no peripancreatic fluid collections or phlegmon formation.

Differential Diagnosis: None.

Diagnosis: Pancreatitis.

Discussion: Complications from pancreatitis can have devastating repercussions for the patient. A grading system for pancreatitis was devised by Balthazar to help predict the outcome of these patients. Grade A: normal pancreas radiographically; Grade B: enlargement of the pancreas with no peripancreatic disease; Grade C: peripancreatic inflammation; Grade D: single peripancreatic fluid collection or phlegmon; Grade E: two or more peripancreatic fluid collections or the presence of gas. Grades A and B carry a better prognosis with a shorter uncomplicated hospital stay than grades D and E. Because no pancreatic fluid collections are present, two of the most worrisome complications, pseudocyst and abscess formation, are unlikely in grades A and B. Deaths from pancreatitis occurred almost exclusively in patients with grades D and E.

Clinical History: 46-year-old woman with abdominal pain and elevated amylase.

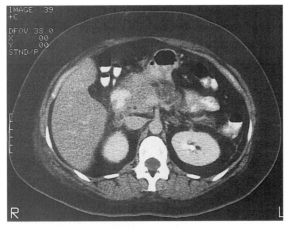

Figure 2.31 A

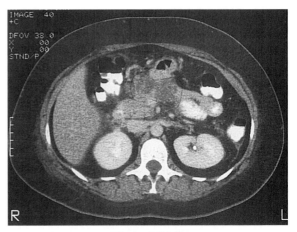

Figure 2.31 B

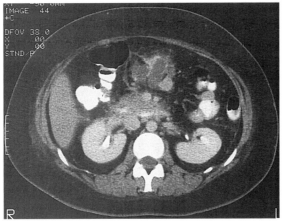

Figure 2.31 C

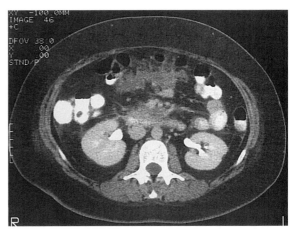

Figure 2.31 D

Findings: CECT demonstrates peripancreatic inflammation and phlegmon spreading anteriorly to the transverse colon.

Differential Diagnosis: None.

Diagnosis: Pancreatitis.

Discussion: This case nicely demonstrates one of the many pathways of spread to and from the pancreas. Although the pancreas resides in the anterior pararenal space of the retroperitoneum, it has access to many parts of the abdomen. Pancreatitis or a pancreatic malignancy can spread by direct extension to other organs in the anterior pararenal space such as the duodenum, ascending and descending colon. A pancreatic process can also reach the transverse colon via the transverse mesocolon. As can be seen in this example, the phlegmon from the pancreatitis tracked anteriorly through the transverse mesocolon to eventually reach the transverse colon. This can produce a thickened mucosa seen by barium enema or CT scan. Note that no loops of small bowel are involved by this process since the small bowel is attached to the retroperitoneum via the small bowel mesentery which is not directly related to the pancreas. A pancreatic malignancy can also spread to the transverse colon in a similar manner.

CASE 32

Clinical History: 62-year-old man with weight loss.

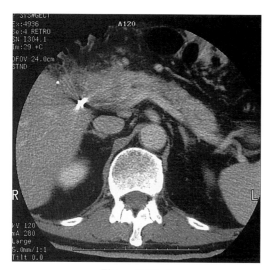

Figure 2.21 A

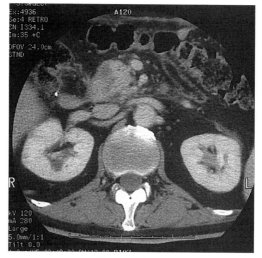

Figure 2.21 B

Findings: CECT demonstrates a low attenuation mass in the head of the pancreas. No dilated ducts are present.

Differential Diagnosis: Focal pancreatitis, metastases, islet cell tumor.

Diagnosis: Pancreatic adenocarcinoma.

Discussion: Pancreatic adenocarcinoma arises from the duct cells of the pancreas and accounts for approximately 80–95% of the nonendocrine malignancies of the pancreas. These tumors occur most commonly in the head of the pancreas and in patients between the ages of 50–70 years. It rarely occurs in patients younger than 40 years of age. Pancreatic adenocarcinomas are hypovascular relative to the normal pancreas therefore, they have low attenuation on a CECT. Because they commonly occur in the head of the pancreas, they can present with symptoms of biliary obstruction even when the tumor is still small due to the desmoplastic reaction. Most lesions range in size between 2–5 cm. Other entities in the differential diagnosis include pancreatitis, islet cell tumors, and metastases. Pancreatitis and functioning islet cell tumors can usually be excluded by history. A nonfunctioning islet cell tumor is usually larger in size when they present clinically. Metastases tend to be multiple and a primary malignancy is typically known by the time a pancreatic metastasis is found.

Clinical History: 57-year-old woman with abdominal pain and a palpable mass.

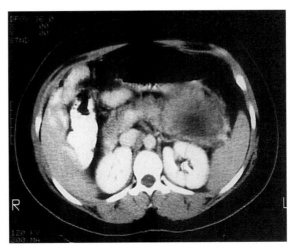

Figure 2.33 A

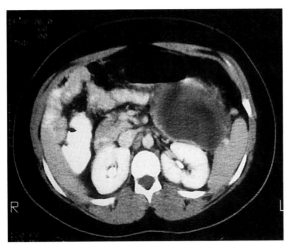

Figure 2.33 B

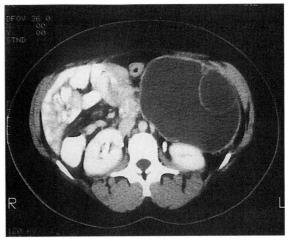

Figure 2.33 C

Findings: CECT demonstrates a large 10-cm cystic lesion with a single septation seen in the tail of the pancreas.

Differential Diagnosis: Pseudocyst.

Diagnosis: Mucinous cystic neoplasm.

Discussion: Mucinous cystic neoplasm is lined by mucin-producing columnar cells and arise from the ductal epithelium. They can fill on ERCP if they communicate with the pancreatic duct. As with most cystic neoplasms, the larger the solid portion of the lesion the worse the prognosis.

A large cystic lesion in an older woman will most likely be a pseudocyst or mucinous cystic neoplasm. These two are often too difficult to distinguish if the history is equivocal. Both can become large and have thick walls and calcifications. Percutaneous biopsy is not helpful since a negative biopsy is not reliable and the entire lesion is often necessary to make the diagnosis.

Clinical History: 44-year-old man with severe abdominal pain, fever, and elevated white blood cell count.

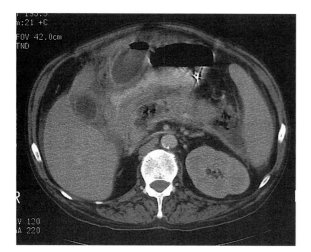 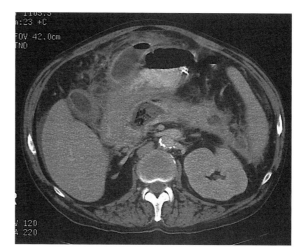

Figure 2.34 A   **Figure 2.34 B**

Findings: CECT demonstrates an edematous and swollen pancreas with peripancreatic inflammation and stranding. Note the two fluid pockets that contain mottled gas in the body and tail of the pancreas.

Differential Diagnosis: None.

Diagnosis: Necrotizing pancreatitis with abscess formation.

Discussion: Many complications can occur in pancreatitis. Necrotizing pancreatitis is one of the most worrisome. In necrotizing pancreatitis, there is destruction of the pancreatic parenchyma due to the pancreatic enzymes. This can lead to infection of the pancreas and adjacent phlegmon by gram-negative bacteria, which carries an extremely high mortality rate. CT findings include lack of enhancement of the normal pancreas post contrast and formation of a low attenuation area in the pancreas region. The presence of gas with an enhancing rim is highly suggestive of an abscess but sterile necrosis cannot be excluded. Often needle aspiration is needed to confirm the presence of an abscess.

Clinical History: 64-year-old man with history of smoking, now with weight loss.

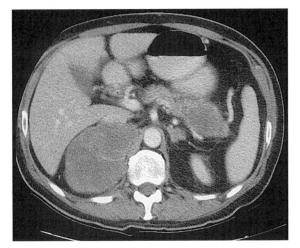

Figure 2.35 A

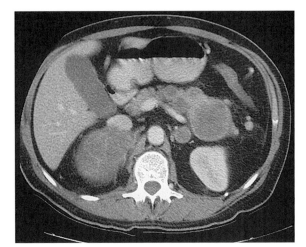

Figure 2.35 B

Findings: CECT demonstrates multiple low attenuation lesions within the pancreas. Note the large right adrenal mass and the smaller left adrenal lesion.

Differential Diagnosis: Islet cell tumor, lymphoma.

Diagnosis: Metastatic bronchogenic carcinoma.

Discussion: Metastatic disease to the pancreas is extremely rare and typically occurs during the advanced stages of a malignancy. Most metastases to the pancreas arise by direct extension from an adjacent organ. Other metastases are hematogenous in nature such as lung cancer, breast cancer, and melanoma. Multiple masses in the pancreas are very rare but when present can be due to metastases, multiple islet cell tumors (usually gastrinomas), and lymphoma. In this case, the finding of bilateral adrenal masses with multiple pancreatic masses is supportive of metastatic lung cancer.

CASE 36

Clinical History: 46-year-old man with weight loss.

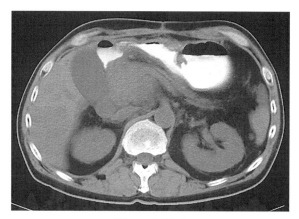

Figure 2.36 A

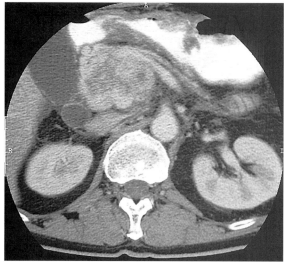

Figure 2.36 B

Figure 2.36 C

Findings: (A) NECT demonstrates a large mass in the head of the pancreas. (B, C) CECT demonstrates a heterogeneous enhancing 6-cm mass with central necrosis in the head of the pancreas.

Differential Diagnosis: Pancreatic adenocarcinoma, metastasis, sarcoma, acinar cell neoplasm.

Diagnosis: Nonfunctioning islet cell tumor.

Discussion: Nonfunctioning islet cell tumor accounts for approximately 15–30% of the islet cell tumors and the vast majority have malignant biological behavior. Nonfunctioning islet cell tumors are similar to other islet cell tumors histologically but they secrete only a small amount of hormones. Therefore, they are not easily detected clinically. These neoplasms are usually slow growing and will typically be large at the time of diagnosis. Because of their slow nature, when discovered liver and regional metastases are frequently present. Nonfunctioning islet cell tumors are isodense to the pancreas on a NECT. They have heterogeneous contrast enhancement on CECT with areas of hemorrhage and necrosis frequently seen due to their large size. Calcifications can be present as well. The differential diagnosis is limited for a large lesion in the pancreas. Pancreatic adenocarcinomas are usually much smaller at the time of presentation and will not typically have hemorrhage and necrosis. Sarcoma and acinar cell neoplasm are frequently large lesions but are rare.

CASE 37

Clinical History: 33-year-old man with long-standing respiratory insufficiency.

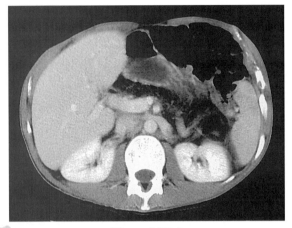

Figure 2.37 A

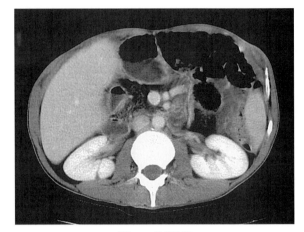

Figure 2.37 B

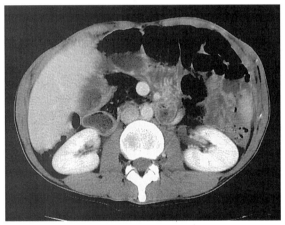

Figure 2.37 C

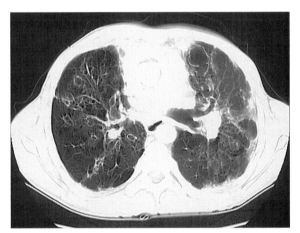

Figure 2.37 D

Findings: CECT of the abdomen demonstrates complete fatty replacement of the pancreas. Image of the chest demonstrates bronchiectasis and pulmonary fibrosis.

Differential Diagnosis: Obesity, normal variant in elderly patients, pancreatic duct obstruction, severe malnutrition, Schwachman syndrome, Cushing's syndrome.

Diagnosis: Cystic fibrosis.

Discussion: Cystic fibrosis is characterized by the formation of thick secretions due to dysfunction of the exocrine glands including pancreatic insufficiency. There is also dysfunction of the mucociliary transport system, which results in recurrent pulmonary infections. A typical finding in cystic fibrosis is complete fatty replacement of the pancreas. The diagnosis is confirmed in this case by the age of the patient and the coexisting lung disease. The fatty replacement seen in elderly patients, obese patients and patients with Cushing's syndrome tends to be marbled in appearance rather than diffuse total replacement as is seen in this case. Pancreatic duct obstruction is associated with pancreatic atrophy rather than fatty transformation. Schwachman syndrome is a rare disorder in the family of metaphyseal dysplasias which has coexisting fatty replaced pancreas.

SUGGESTED READING

Inflammation

Balthazar EJ. CT diagnosis and staging of acute pancreatitis. Radiol Clin North Am 1989;27:19–37.

Balthazar E, Ranson BM, Naidich D, et al. Acute pancreatitis: prognostic value of CT. Radiology 1985;156:767–772.

Balthazar E, Robinson D, Megibow A, et al. Acute pancreatitis: value of CT in establishing prognosis. Radiology 1990;174:331–336.

Beger H, Bittner R, Block S, et al. Bacterial contamination of pancreatic necrosis. Gastroenterology 1986;91:443–438.

Bradley E, Clements JL, Gonzalez AC. The natural history of pancreatic pseudocysts: a unified concept of management. Am J Surg 1979;137:135–141.

Burke JW, Erickson SJ, Kellum CD. Pseudoaneurysms complicating pancreatitis: detection by CT. Radiology 1986;161:447–450.

Freeny PC. Classification of pancreatitis. Radiol Clin North Am 1989;27:1–3.

Friedman AC, Dachman AH. Radiology of the liver, biliary tract and pancreas. St. Louis, Mosby, 1994.

Kalmer JA, Matthews CC, Bishop LA. Computerized tomography in acute and chronic pancreatitis. South Med J 1984;77:1393–1396.

Karasawa E, Goldberg HI, Moss AA, et al. CT pancreatogram in carcinoma of pancreas and chronic pancreatitis. Radiology 1983;148:489–493.

Luetmer PH, Stephens DH, Ward EM. Chronic pancreatitis: reassessment with current CT. Radiology 1989;171:353–357.

Neff CC, Simeone JF, Wittenberg J, et al. Inflammatory pancreatic masses. Radiology 1984;150:35–38.

Stabile BE, Wilson SE, Debas HT. Reduced mortality from bleeding pseudocysts and pseudoaneurysms caused by pancreatitis. Arch Surg 1983;118:45–51.

White AF, Baum S, Buranasiri S. Aneurysms secondary to pancreatitis. Am J Roentgenol 1976;127:393–396.

White EM, Wittenberg J, Mueller PR. Pancreatic necrosis: CT manifestations. Radiology 1986;158:343–346.

Neoplasms

Buetow PC, Parrino TV, Buck JL, et al. Islet cell tumors of the pancreas: pathologic-imaging correlation among size, necrosis and cysts, calcification, malignant behavior and functional status. AJR 1995;165:1175–1179.

Burgener FA, Hamlin DJ. Histiocytic lymphoma of the abdomen. AJR 1981;137:337–342.

Chio BI, Kim KW, Han MC, et al. Solid and papillary eipthelial neoplasms of the pancreas: CT findings. Radiology 1988;166:413–416.

Compagno J, Oertel JE. Mucinous cystic neoplasms of the pancreas with overt and latent malignancy (cystadenocarcinoma and cystadenoma). Am Soc Clin Pathol 1978;69:573–580.

Dunnick NR, Long JA, Krudy A, et al. Localizing insulinomas with combined radiographic methods. AJR 1980;135:747–752.

Frable WJ, Still WJS, Kay S. Carcinoma of the pancreas, infantile type. Cancer 1971;27:667–673.

Freeny PC, Mark, WM, Ryan JA, et al. Pancreatic ductal adenocarcinoma: diagnosis and staging with dynamic CT. Radiology 1988;166:125–133.

Friedman AC, Dachman AH. Radiology of the liver, biliary tract and pancreas. St. Louis, Mosby, 1994.

Friedman AC, Lichtenstein JE, Dachman AH. Cystic neoplasms of the pancreas. Radiology 1983;149:45–50.

Friesen SR. Tumors of the endocrine pancreas. N Engl J Med 1982;306:580–590.

Frucht H, Doppman JL, Norton JA, et al. Gastrinomas: Comparison of MR imaging with CT, angiography, and US. Radiology 1989;171:713–717.

Fugazzola C, Procacci C, Andreis IAB. The contribution of ultrasonography and computed tomography in the diagnosis of nonfunctioning islet cell tumors of the pancreas. Gastrointest Radiol 1990;15:139–144.

Galiber AK, Reading CC, Charboneau JW, et al. Localization of pancreatic insulinoma: comparison of pre- and intraoperative US with CT and angiography. Radiology 1988;166:405–408.

Gold J, Rosenfield AT, Sostman D, et al. Nonfunctioning islet cell tumors of the pancreas: radiographic and ultrasonographic appearances in two cases. Am J Roentgenol 1978;131:715–717.

Gorman B, Charboneau JW, James EM, et al. Benign pancreatic insulinoma: preoperative and intraoperative sonographic localization. AJR 1986;147:929–934.

Gunther RW, Klose JK, Ruckert K, et al. Islet-cell tumors: detection of small lesions with computed tomography and ultrasound. Radiology 1983;148:485–488.

Horie A, Yano Y, Yasunori K, et al. Morphogenesis of pancreatoblastoma, infantile carcinoma or the pancreas. Cancer 1977;39:247–254.

Hosoki T. Dynamic CT of pancreatic tumors. AJR 1983;104:959–965.

Itai Y, Ohhashi K, Furui S, et al. Microcystic adenoma of the pancreas: spectrum of computed tomographic findings. J Comput Assist Tomogr 1988;12:797–803.

Jenson RT. Zollinger-ellison syndrome: current concepts and management. Ann Intern Med 1983;98:59–75.

Johnson CD, Stephens DH, Charboneau JW, et al. Cystic pancreatic tumors: CT and sonographic assessment. AJR 1988;151:1133–1138.

Karasawa E, Goldberg HI, Moss AA, et al. CT pancreatogram in carcinoma of the pancreas and chronic pancreatitis. Radiology 1983;148:489–493.

Kraus BB, Ros PR. Insulinoma: diagnosis with suppressed MR imaging. AJR 1994;162:69–70.

Morohoshi T, Kanda M, Horie A, et al. Immunocytochemical markers of uncommon pancreatic tumors. Cancer 1987;5:739–747.

Radin DR, Colletti PM, Forrester DM. Pancreatic acinar cell carcinoma with subcutaneous and intraosseous fat necrosis. Radiology 1986;158:67–68.

Ros PR, Hamrick-Turner, Chiechi, et al. Cystic masses of the pancreas. Radiographics 1992;12:673–686.

Rossi P, Allison DJ, Bezzi M, et al. Endocrine tumors of the pancreas. Radiol Clin North Am 1989;27:129–161.

Rossi P, Baert A, Passariello R, et al. CT of functioning tumors of the pancreas. AJR 1985;144:57–60.

Stamm B, Burger H, Hollinger A. Acinar cell cystadenocarcinoma of the pancreas. Cancer 1987;60:2542–2547.

Teefey SA, Stephens DH, Sheedy PF, et al. CT appearance of primary pancreatic lymphoma. Gastrointest Radiol 1986;11:41–43.

chapter 3

GASTROINTESTINAL TRACT

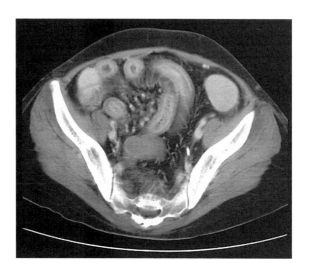

CASE 1

Clinical History: 27-year-old woman with bloody diarrhea and weight loss.

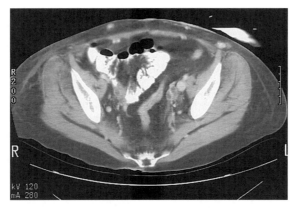

Figure 3.1 A

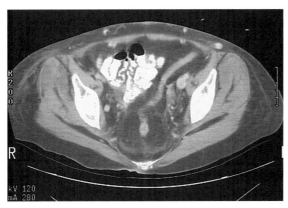

Figure 3.1 B

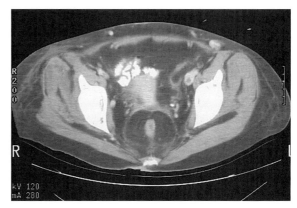

Figure 3.1 C

Findings: CECT of the pelvis demonstrates a narrowed rectosigmoid colon with extensive fat seen surrounding this loop of bowel.

Differential Diagnosis: Ulcerative colitis, radiation colitis.

Diagnosis: Crohn disease with "creeping fat."

Discussion: Crohn disease is a chronic inflammatory process with predilection for the terminal ileum. Involvement of the colon and terminal ileum is seen in approximately 40–45% of patients and colonic involvement alone in 30% of patients. "Creeping fat" represents fibrofatty proliferation typically seen in patients with Crohn disease. It is thought to occur as a response to repeated episodes of inflammation resulting in separation of loops of bowel, most frequently seen in the small bowel mesentery but can occur in the colon as well. The narrowed rectosigmoid colon and fatty proliferation seen in this example could be due to either ulcerative colitis or Crohn disease. Diagnosis could be confirmed by searching for inflammatory bowel disease in other areas of the GI tract. This would suggest the diagnosis Crohn disease, which tends to have skip lesions. Radiation enteritis frequently involves loops of small bowel located within the radiation therapy port. The normal loops of small bowel in the pelvis makes radiation enteritis unlikely.

CASE 2

Clinical History: 46-year-old man with long history of abdominal pain.

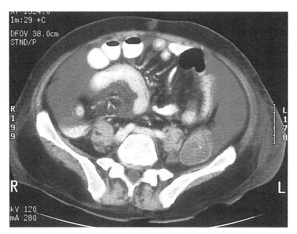

Figure 3.2 A

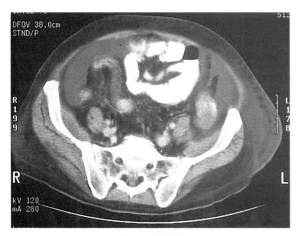

Figure 3.2 B

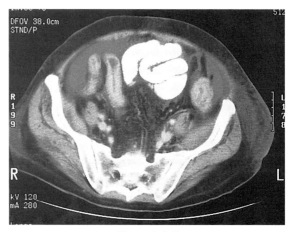

Figure 3.2 C

Findings: CECT demonstrates thickening and irregularity of the wall of the terminal ileum. Inflammatory changes are noted in the adjacent mesentery as well as increased attenuation of the fat. There is thickening and proliferation of the mesenteric fat. Ascites is present.

Differential Diagnosis: Infectious enteritis (tuberculosis, Yersinia), ischemia, lymphoma.

Diagnosis: Crohn disease.

Discussion: Crohn disease is a chronic disease of the GI tract, which is characterized by transmural inflammatory reaction, granulomas, skip lesions, fistula formation, and mesenteric abnormalities. Within the mesentery, there will be inflammatory changes including stranding, phlegmon, and abscess formation. The attenuation of the mesentery is often increased and the sharp definition between the bowel and fat is lost. This fibrofatty change is the cause for the increased separation of the loops of bowel seen in Crohn disease. Almost any segment of the GI tract can be involved by Crohn disease, although the terminal ileum and ascending colon are the most commonly involved areas. Ischemia would most likely involve more loops of small and large bowel rather than just the terminal ileum. Infectious enteritis and lymphoma could both appear similar on CT and would have to be considered. In this case, however, the bowel wall thickening of the terminal ileum as well as increased attenuation of the adjacent fat with bowel loop separation makes Crohn disease the best diagnosis.

CASE 3

Clinical History: 62-year-old man with severe abdominal pain and a palpable mass in the right lower quadrant.

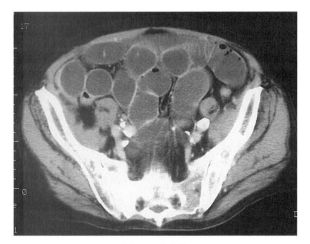

Figure 3.3 A

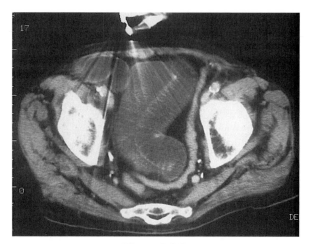

Figure 3.3 B

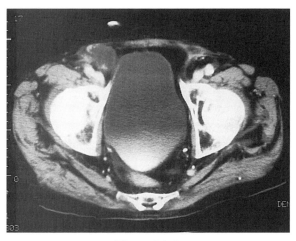

Figure 3.3 C

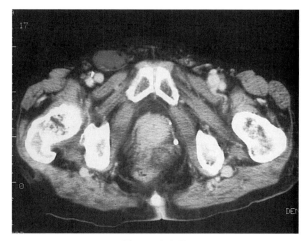

Figure 3.3 D

Findings: CECT demonstrates multiple dilated loops of small bowel, which can be followed into the right groin laying anterior to the femoral vessels.

Differential Diagnosis: None.

Diagnosis: Small bowel obstruction secondary to a right inguinal hernia.

Discussion: Inguinal hernias can be either direct or indirect. Indirect hernias are the most common and occur predominantly in males. The peritoneal sac along with intraabdominal contents enters the inguinal canal and exits at the external ring. In males, a hernial sac follows the spermatic cord and enters into the scrotum. Because of its long course, indirect hernias can become incarcerated leading to bowel infarction. Direct hernias, on the other hand, are less common and occur when the hernia enters medial to the inferior epigastric vessels. The finding of abdominal contents (small bowel, sigmoid colon, cecum, mesenteric fat) in the inguinal canal anterior to the femoral vessels is diagnostic of an inguinal hernia. In males, this is easily seen as asymmetry in the spermatic cord when compared with the other side. Frequently, hernias are asymptomatic and easily reducible. They can, however, lead to small bowel obstruction due to incarceration as in this case.

CASE 4

Clinical History: 65-year-old man with history of multiple myeloma.

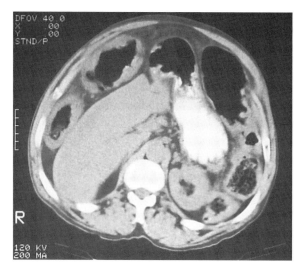

Figure 3.4 A

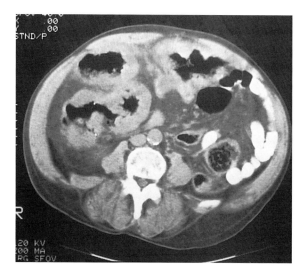

Figure 3.4 B

Findings: CECT demonstrates nodular thickening and dilatation of the ascending and transverse colon. The descending colon appears normal.

Differential Diagnosis: Pseudomembranous colitis, infectious colitis, Crohn colitis, ischemia.

Diagnosis: Amyloidosis of the colon.

Discussion: Amyloidosis is a heterogeneous group of disorders that results in deposition of proteins in various tissues of the body. This leads to tissue hypoxia, mucosal edema, and ulceration. Amyloidosis can be primary or secondary. Primary amyloidosis is probably an inherited disorder of plasma cell function, whereas secondary is a reactive disease to a chronic inflammatory process or illness. CT findings of amyloidosis include loss of haustration with thickening and nodularity of the mucosa and muscular wall. The bowel can be dilated or narrowed by this process. This appearance is often nonspecific. The involvement of the ascending and transverse colon is a good site for ischemia but there is lack of involvement of the small bowel. The diffuse thickening of the colon is also seen in pseudomembranous colitis and infectious colitis, which would be indistinguishable from amyloidosis in this example.

CASE 5

Clinical History: 42-year-old man with abdominal pain, fever, and chronic GI problems.

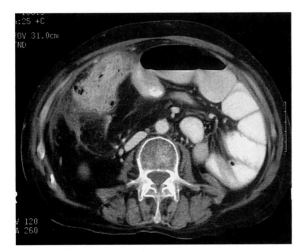

Figure 3.5 A

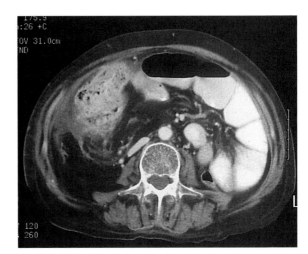

Figure 3.5 B

Findings: CECT demonstrates a large inflammatory mass involving the cecum with mottled air and pericecal inflammation. There is also a small bowel obstruction.

Differential Diagnosis: Cecal diverticulitis, perforated neoplasm, typhlitis, infectious colitis (tuberculosis, amebiasis).

Diagnosis: Crohn colitis with abscess formation.

Discussion: Crohn disease can have many complications including fistulas and occasionally adenocarcinoma. Because the process is transmural, fistulas and abscesses occur more commonly than with ulcerative colitis, which affects primarily the mucosa and submucosa. The mottled gas within the inflammatory mass in the region of the cecum suggests an abscess. Abscesses can occur in the right lower quadrant from several sources. In the younger population, appendicitis is the primary consideration. The presence of an appendicolith would ensure the diagnosis. In the older population, a perforated neoplasm and cecal diverticulitis are common causes. Diverticulitis in the cecum constitutes approximately 5–10% of all diverticulitis and other diverticula are usually present. Typhlitis occurs in patients who are immunocompromised especially with lymphoma or leukemia. Tuberculosis can have this appearance and a search for other evidence of tuberculosis, especially in the lung, should be performed.

CASE 6

Clinical History: 56-year-old woman with history of breast cancer and hysterectomy.

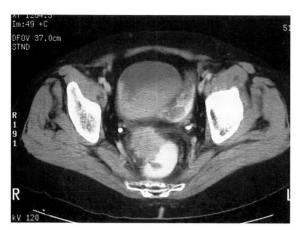

Figure 3.6 A

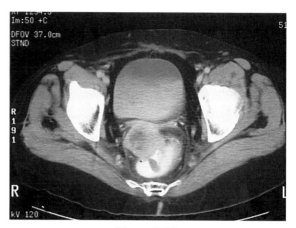

Figure 3.6 B

Findings: CECT demonstrates a 4-cm polypoid lesion with areas of necrosis in the right anterior portion of the rectum.

Differential Diagnosis: Adenocarcinoma, abscess, lymphoma.

Diagnosis: Breast cancer metastasis to the rectum.

Discussion: Metastases to the colon are fairly common but often are asymptomatic and are found incidentally by autopsy. Malignancies can spread to the colon by way of direct extension as is seen in prostate, ovarian, uterine, and cervical carcinomas. Intraperitoneal seeding and hematogenous spread can also occur. The most common malignancies to spread hematogenously include melanoma, breast, and lung cancer. Breast metastases can present as an eccentric mass or as an irregular circumferential stricture (linitis plastica). The stricture appearance can simulate Crohn disease of the colon. An eccentric mass is most often going to be confused with an adenocarcinoma of the colon. A metastasis, however, will appear as an extrinsic mass invading into the lumen whereas a colon cancer will be a mass growing out from the colonic mucosa. Very little perirectal stranding and lack of extraluminal air makes an abscess unlikely in this case. Lymphoma tends to involve the cecum and often are large.

CASE 7

Clinical History: 33-year-old man with severe acute abdominal pain and sepsis.

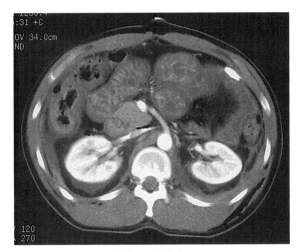

Figure 3.7 A

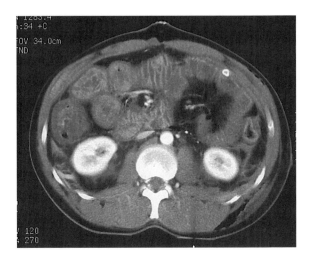

Figure 3.7 B

Findings: CECT demonstrates extensive bowel wall thickening of the small bowel, ascending colon and cecum. A "double halo sign" is seen in the ascending colon

Differential Diagnosis: Diffuse hemorrhage, infectious colitis (yersinia, campylobacter), Crohn disease.

Diagnosis: Ischemic bowel.

Discussion: Acute mesenteric artery ischemia is commonly seen in the elderly due to cardiac problems (arrhythmias, congestive heart failure, myocardial infarction) and atherosclerotic disease. In other age groups, mesenteric ischemia can be due to sepsis, hypotension, and hypovolemia. This leads to decreased blood flow in the SMA, which causes ischemia of the ileum and proximal colon. CT findings include bowel wall thickening of the small bowel and proximal colon and the "double halo" sign. The double halo sign represents enhancement of the mucosa surrounded by edema in the bowel wall. Pneumatosis, portal venous air, or air in the mesenteric veins all signify bowel ischemia and is easily seen on CT. Often air in stool can be mistaken for pneumatosis so careful examination is necessary to ensure the location of the air. Atherosclerotic disease or a clot in the SMA can sometimes be seen on a CT as well. Crohn disease does not usually involve a large amount of small bowel. The characteristic location, double halo sign, and extensive small bowel involvement makes ischemic bowel the best diagnosis.

CASE 8

Clinical History: 57-year-old man with abdominal pain.

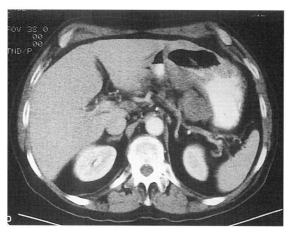

Figure 3.8 A

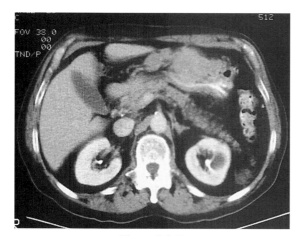

Figure 3.8 B

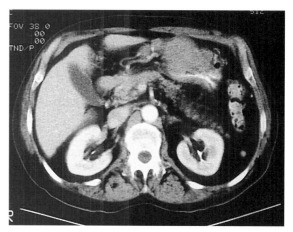

Figure 3.8 C

Findings: CECT demonstrates a 3 x 5 cm mass involving the anterior wall of the antrum. A soft tissue mass is also seen in the gastrohepatic ligament.

Differential Diagnosis: Adenocarcinoma, metastasis.

Diagnosis: NonHodgkin lymphoma of the stomach.

Discussion: Lymphoma of the stomach accounts for approximately 3–5% of gastric neoplasms with NHL making up the majority of these cases. Radiographically, lymphoma can present as a solitary submucosal mass as in this case. Gastric lymphoma can become large and present as a necrotic, ulcerating exophytic mass in the gastric wall. Lymphoma can also be an infiltrating process, presenting as thickened gastric folds that are difficult to distinguish from gastritis. Hodgkin's disease rarely involves the stomach but when present may mimic linitis plastica. In any mass arising from the gastric wall, the differential diagnosis includes gastric adenocarcinoma. In favor of lymphoma, there is adenopathy and the preserved pliability of the gastric wall. In most cases, biopsy is necessary to confirm the diagnosis.

CASE 9

Clinical History: 40-year-old man status post endoscopy currently with abdominal pain.

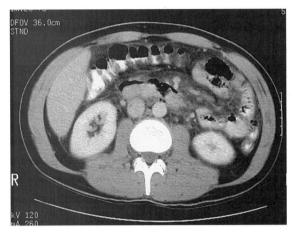

Figure 3.9 A

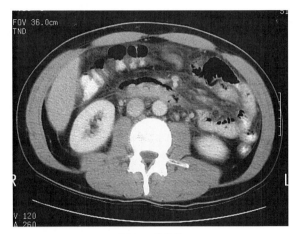

Figure 3.9 B

Findings: CECT demonstrates extraluminal air in the retroperitoneum just anterior to the duodenum. Stranding and inflammation is also present in the mesentery as well as small lymph nodes.

Differential Diagnosis: None.

Diagnosis: Duodenal perforation with pneumoperitoneum.

Discussion: Pneumoretroperitoneum can be caused by perforation of a retroperitoneal loop of bowel such as the duodenum, ascending, and descending colon. This could be secondary to blunt or penetrating trauma, perforated ulcer or neoplasm, or iatrogenic bowel injury, such as in this case. Retroperitoneal abscesses can also cause gas in the retroperitoneum, but the gas tends to be mottled in an inflammatory mass. Retroperitoneal gas is often difficult to diagnose on plain films because it does not tend to collect under the diaphragm as in pneumoperitoneum. CT is much better suited for diagnosing pneumoretroperitoneum because the air will collect along fascial planes. Air can be seen as linear gas collections in the anterior pararenal space and along the margins of the psoas muscles. The gas can sometimes cross Gerota's fascia and enter into the perirenal space outlining the kidney. In this example, extraluminal air is seen anterior to the duodenum collecting on the underside of the peritoneal reflection. The location of the air and history of an EGD makes a duodenal perforation the best diagnosis.

CASE 10

Clinical History: 27-year-old man with 10-day history of left lower quadrant pain, fevers, and chills.

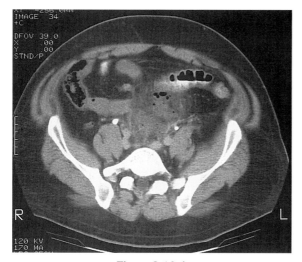

Figure 3.10 A

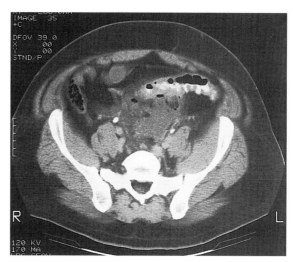

Figure 3.10 B

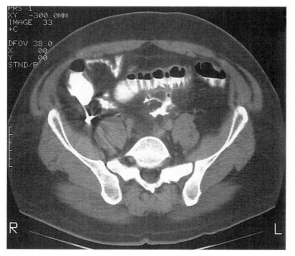

Figure 3.10 C

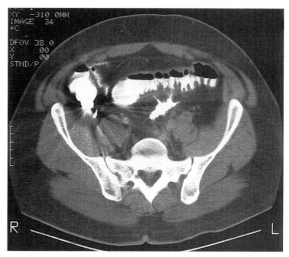

Figure 3.10 D

Findings: (A, B) CECT demonstrates an inflammatory mass that contains air posterior to the sigmoid colon. (C, D) A second CECT performed 9 days later demonstrates extraluminal contrast and air posterior to the sigmoid colon.

Differential Diagnosis: Crohn colitis, traumatic perforation, perforated neoplasm.

Diagnosis: Diverticular abscess.

Discussion: Diverticulitis most commonly occurs in the elderly patient population in whom diverticulosis is more prevalent. Often in debilitated elderly patients, the diagnosis is delayed because many of the symptoms are less pronounced and masked by underlying medical problems such as diabetes, renal failure, and medications. When diverticulitis occurs in the younger patient (<40 years of age), it is often more severe and may require emergent surgery. In this case, there is both extraluminal air and contrast from the adjacent sigmoid colon. Notice how the contrast appears to be spiculated and is surrounded by inflammation indicating perforation or fistula from the bowel. Although this can be due to fistula or abscess formation from Crohn colitis, no findings suggestive of Crohn disease is present. Prior trauma or a perforated neoplasm can also have this appearance and although unlikely in this age group, an underlying neoplasm must be excluded.

CASE 11

Clinical History: 16-year-old boy with severe abdominal pain after a bicycle accident.

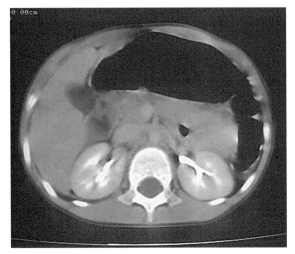

Figure 3.11 A

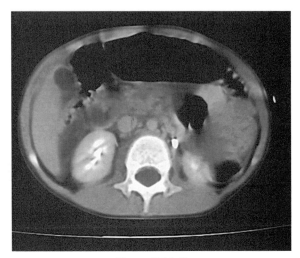

Figure 3.11 B

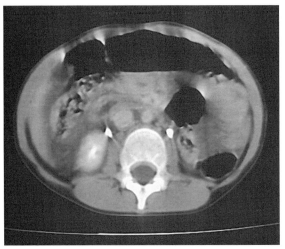

Figure 3.11 C

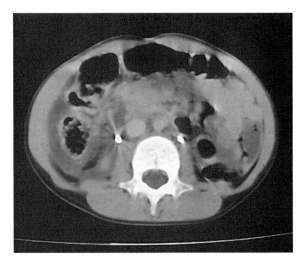

Figure 3.11 D

Findings: CECT demonstrates a fluid-filled proximal duodenum with wall thickening as it passes over the vertebral column. Note the free fluid surrounding the ascending colon.

Differential Diagnosis: None.

Diagnosis: Duodenal rupture.

Discussion: Common locations for injured organs after blunt abdominal trauma are the duodenum and pancreas because they pass over the spine. The pancreas and duodenum, which are fixed, can be crushed against the spine due to the force of the injury. This can lead to either a hematoma or rupture of the duodenum. Because the duodenum is located in the anterior pararenal space, hemorrhage and fluid from the injury will not be seen typically in the peritoneal cavity but in the retroperitoneum. In this case, the fluid is seen surrounding the ascending colon rather than in the paracolic gutter. The partially obstructed proximal duodenum due to the hemorrhage and edema in its fourth portion is another clue to the origin of the injury. These findings suggest injury to the duodenum. Duodenal rupture was found at surgery.

Clinical History: 45-year-old man with abdominal pain and known aneurysm of the aorta.

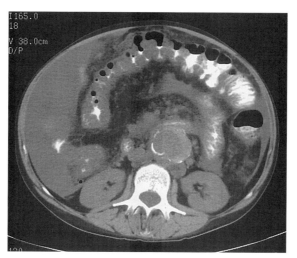

Figure 3.12 A

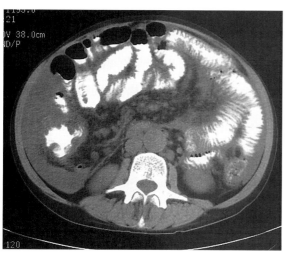
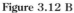

Figure 3.12 B

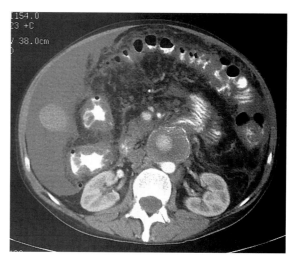

Figure 3.12 C

Findings: NECT demonstrates thickening of multiple loops of small bowel and ascending colon. An abdominal aortic aneurysm and ascites is present as well. CECT demonstrates mural thrombus within the aneurysm.

Differential Diagnosis: Diffuse hemorrhage, infectious colitis, Crohn disease.

Diagnosis: Ischemic bowel.

Discussion: Acute mesenteric ischemia can be caused by a variety of etiologies all of which lead to decreased blood flow in the SMA. This will lead to ischemia of the right colon to the level of the splenic flexure and most of the small bowel. In this patient, there is an aneurysm of the abdominal aorta with a large mural thrombus. This can lead to either occlusion of the origin of the SMA or emboli formation, resulting in mesenteric ischemia. Diffuse hemorrhage can have this appearance as well. This could be due to anticoagulant therapy or blood dyscrasias such as Henoch-Schonlein purpura. The extensive amount of bowel involved would make Crohn disease less likely. The presence of the aneurysm and the involvement of most of the small bowel and proximal colon make ischemia the most likely diagnosis.

CASE 13

Clinical History: 56-year-old man with weight loss and bloody diarrhea.

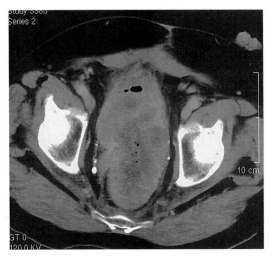

Figure 3.13 A

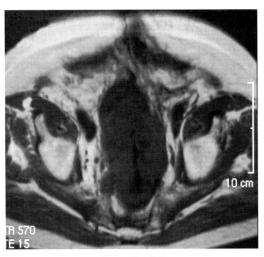

Figure 3.13 B

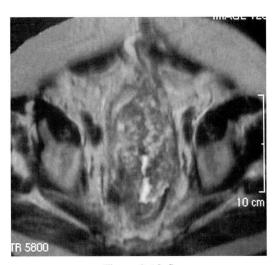

Figure 3.13 C

Findings: (A) CECT demonstrates a large circumferential mass in the rectum. (B) T1-weighted image demonstrates a large mass involving the rectum, which is isointense to muscle. The lumen is markedly narrowed. (C) T2-weighted image demonstrates this mass to be hyperintense. The lumen, which contains fluid, is very bright and is almost obliterated by the tumor.

Differential Diagnosis: Lymphoma, metastases.

Diagnosis: Large adenocarcinoma of the rectum.

Discussion: There are many different malignant neoplasms found in the rectum including adenocarcinoma, lymphoma, carcinoid, squamous cell carcinoma, leiomyosarcomas, and metastases. Adenocarcinoma is by far the most common. These lesions can present as annular constricting, polypoid or infiltrating. The most common is the annular constricting lesion. On MRI, these lesions are isointense to muscle on the T1-weighted images. Because the surrounding fat is of high signal intensity, perirectal extension is well seen. In this example, the outer margin is not well defined. This likely represents extension of tumor through the rectal wall. On the T2-weighted image, the tumor is hyperintense relative to muscle but is now of similar signal to that of fat, making it difficult to see the margins of the lesion. The lumen is almost obliterated by the tumor and accounts for the patient's symptoms. Both lymphoma and metastases could have this appearance although they are less common than adenocarcinomas. Ulcerative colitis does not produce localized bowel wall thickening seen in this case.

CASE 14

Clinical History: 58-year-old man with diarrhea and crampy abdominal pain.

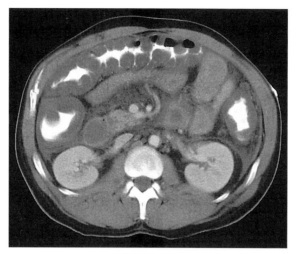

Figure 3.14 A

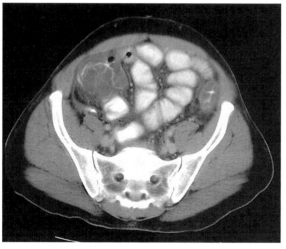

Figure 3.14 B

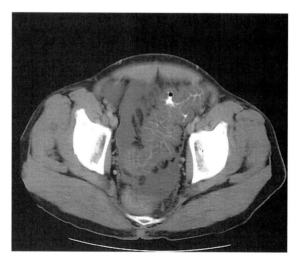

Figure 3.14 C

Findings: CECT demonstrates marked thickening of the ascending, transverse and descending colon. Fluid is also seen in the paracolic gutters. An image in the pelvis demonstrates thickening of the sigmoid colon and rectum. Free fluid is again noted.

Differential Diagnosis: Ulcerative colitis, infectious colitis.

Diagnosis: Pseudomembranous colitis (PMC).

Discussion: The classic findings of PMC are seen in this example. There is thickening of the entire colon (average greater than 15 mm), without small bowel involvement, minimal pericolonic stranding, and ascites. In the transverse colon, slips of contrast can be seen between the thickened pseudomembranes. This "accordion sign" is thought to be specific for advanced stages of PMC. Ulcerative colitis usually has only mild to moderate bowel wall thickening. Involvement of the entire colon without small bowel involvement is unusual for ischemia. Infectious colitis can present in this manner but pericolonic inflammation is typically extensive.

CASE 15

Clinical History: 55-year-old woman with history of cervical cancer.

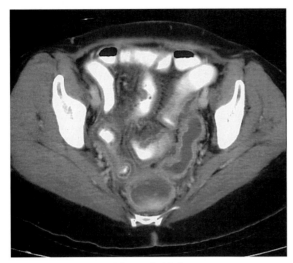

Figure 3.15 A

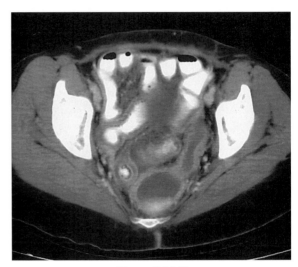

Figure 3.15 B

Findings: CECT demonstrates thickening of both small bowel and rectosigmoid colon in the pelvis. There is also extensive stranding seen in the mesentery.

Differential Diagnosis: Ischemia, Crohn disease, lymphoma.

Diagnosis: Radiation enteritis.

Discussion: Radiation enteritis and colitis can occur several years after radiation therapy. Most commonly this is seen in women with cervical cancer who present with crampy abdominal pain and diarrhea. Because of the mesenteric edema and narrowing of the lumen, the loops of bowel are often separated in the pelvis. Few entities will involve both the rectosigmoid colon and small bowel, such as ischemia (involving multiple branch vessels), Crohn disease, and lymphoma. The key to the diagnosis is the presence of these findings only in the bowel loops localized to one area corresponding to the radiation port (the pelvis in cases of cervical cancer).

CASE 16

Clinical History: 77-year-old man with history of diarrhea and abdominal pain.

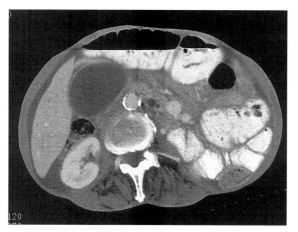

Figure 3.16 A

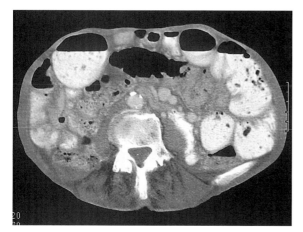

Figure 3.16 B

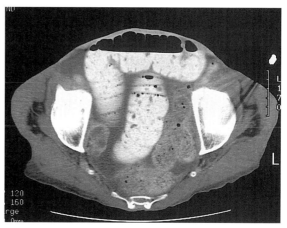

Figure 3.16 C

Findings: CECT demonstrates markedly dilated fluid-filled loops of small bowel. The involved loops of bowel appear effaced, and free fluid and edema are present in the mesentery.

Differential Diagnosis: Scleroderma, small bowel obstruction, ileus.

Diagnosis: Non-tropical Sprue (Celiac disease).

Discussion: Sprue is related to dietary gluten, which causes an immunologic reaction with resultant atrophy of the small bowel villi leading to malabsorption. Genetic factors have been noted in this disease. This malabsorption results in diarrhea, steatorrhea, and abdominal pain possibly related to intermittent intussusception. Diagnosis of sprue is usually made by mucosal biopsy by EGD. The CT findings of sprue are similar to those seen on a small bowel series. There is marked small bowel dilatation usually involving the duodenum and jejunum with loss of normal small bowel folds. The folds present are thickened probably from the associated hypoalbuminemia. There are fluid-filled bowel loops, mesenteric lymphadenopathy, and edema. Other entities to consider in patients with dilated small bowel include scleroderma, small bowel obstruction, and ileus. The small bowel folds in scleroderma and obstruction tend to be normal. Scleroderma does not tend to have excess fluid as is seen in sprue and obstruction. The dilated small bowel with effaced featureless mucosa makes sprue the best diagnosis.

CASE 17

Clinical History: 68-year-old nursing home resident with acute abdominal pain.

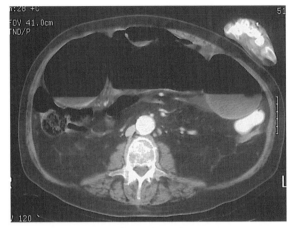

Figure 3.17 A

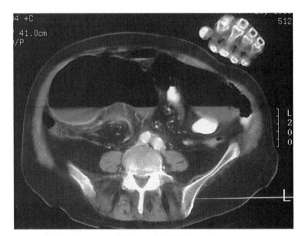

Figure 3.17 B

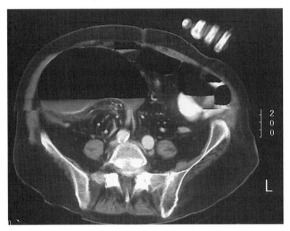

Figure 3.17 C

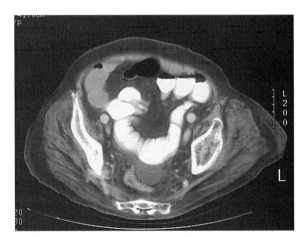

Figure 3.17 D

Findings: CECT demonstrates a markedly dilated transverse colon. A loop of bowel is seen in the right lower quadrant, which tapers to a point with vessels coursing into it. Note the decompressed rectum.

Differential Diagnosis: Obstructed sigmoid colon from other etiologies (neoplasm, adhesions, hernia), ileus.

Diagnosis: Sigmoid volvulus.

Discussion: Any loop of bowel can volvulate at its mesenteric attachment. The majority of colonic volvulus occur in the sigmoid colon. In the United States, the typical patient is from a nursing home and mental institution. These patients typically have chronic constipation and paralytic ileus due to a combination of medications, immobility and handicapped mental status, leading to dilated loops of colon, which volvulate. Radiographically on plain films, there is a dilated loop of sigmoid colon, which is "bean" shaped with its long axis pointing toward the right upper quadrant. The same finding can be seen on a CT scan as well. The dilated colon can be followed to the point of obstruction in the pelvis, with a swirling of vessels to the point of volvulus. CT also excludes other causes of a colonic obstruction such as a neoplasm or hernia. An ileus is unlikely because the distal rectum is decompressed. In this case, the volvulus was reduced by sigmoidoscopy.

CASE 18

Clinical History: 57-year-old man status post gastrojejunostomy with crampy abdominal pain.

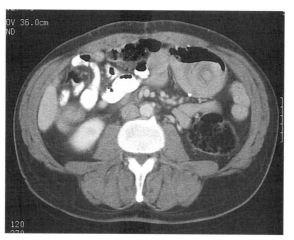

Figure 3.18 A

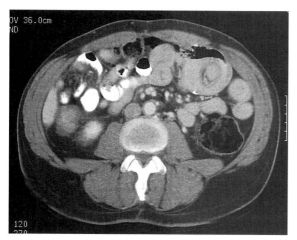

Figure 3.18 B

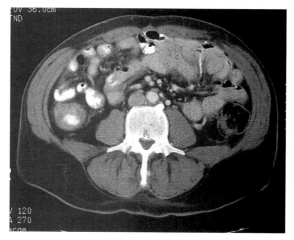

Figure 3.18 C

Findings: CECT demonstrates a circular mass adjacent to the suture line of the gastrojejunostomy. This mass appears to be intraluminal and contains fat.

Differential Diagnosis: None.

Diagnosis: Jejunogastric intussusception.

Discussion: Jejunogastric intussusception can occur after a simple gastrojejunostomy. This usually occurs several years after surgery but can occur early on as well. The jejunal limb invaginates into the stomach secondary to retrograde peristalsis. The efferent limb is involved in about 75% of the cases rather than the afferent limb. Intussusception is recognized easily by CT because typically there is a round soft tissue mass with concentric rings made up of the walls of the jejunum and stomach. The central fat attenuation layer represents herniated mesenteric fat, which has traveled with the loop of jejunum. The other low attenuation ring represents edema in the bowel wall. Diagnosis is crucial because ischemia can occur if the intussusception should persist.

CASE 19

Clinical History: 59-year-old woman with diarrhea, abdominal distension, and crampy abdominal pain.

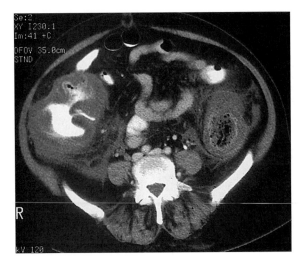

Figure 3.19 A

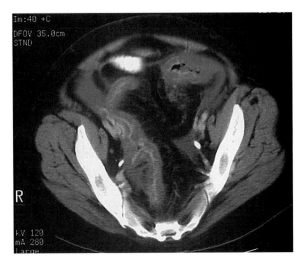

Figure 3.19 B

Findings: CECT demonstrates marked thickening of the ascending, descending, and sigmoid colon. Fluid is also seen in both paracolic gutters. Note the small sliver of contrast between the thickened mucosa.

Differential Diagnosis: Ulcerative colitis, Crohn colitis, infectious colitis.

Diagnosis: Pseudomembranous colitis (PMC).

Discussion: Pseudomembranous colitis is a toxin-mediated disease with no evidence of microbial invasion into the bowel wall mucosa. Diagnosis is made by isolating the toxin in the stool of the affected patient. The causative organism is *Clostridium difficile* and occurs typically after antibiotic use. In PMC, there is usually marked bowel wall thickening with an average of 15 mm. The thickening is homogeneously low in attenuation and is thought to be due to edema in the bowel wall. In this case, the bowel wall measures greater than 2 cm in some areas and is low in density. Ascites is also present in a majority of cases as is seen in this case. This example also demonstrates the "accordion sign." This represents contrast material insinuating between the large pseudomembranes of PMC. This finding is considered specific for pseudomembranous colitis.

CASE 20

Clinical History: 65-year-old woman with epigastric pain and weight loss.

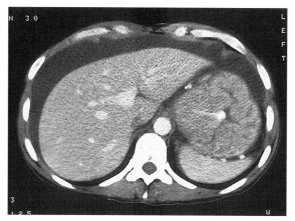

Figure 3.20 A

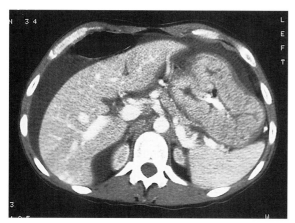

Figure 3.20 B

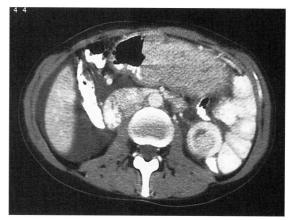

Figure 3.20 C

Findings: CECT demonstrates marked thickening of the stomach with sparing of the antrum.

Differential Diagnosis: Lymphoma, adenocarcinoma, peptic ulcer disease, eosinophilic gastritis, tuberculosis.

Diagnosis: Menetrier disease.

Discussion: Menetrier disease is a protein-losing enteropathy of unknown etiology characterized by massive mucosal hypertrophy, hypoproteinemia, and hypochlorhydria. There is a slight male predominance. Patients present with abdominal pain, weight loss, diarrhea, and peripheral edema from the protein loss. Radiographically, there is marked thickening of the gastric folds with sparing of the antrum in the majority of the cases. Frequently there is abrupt change from abnormal to normal gastric mucosa as in this case. The greatest degree of thickening of the gastric mucosa is commonly seen along the greater curvature. Often the folds become so enlarged that they can appear as a polypoid mass on both CT and upper GI studies. Biopsy is necessary to exclude a malignancy such as lymphoma or adenocarcinoma.

Clinical History: 44-year-old man with a history of pneumonia that did not respond to typical antibiotics now presents with abdominal pain and diarrhea.

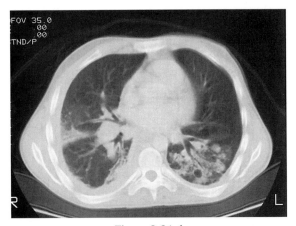

Figure 3.21 A

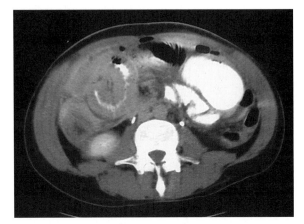

Figure 3.21 B

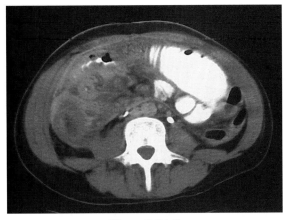

Figure 3.21 C

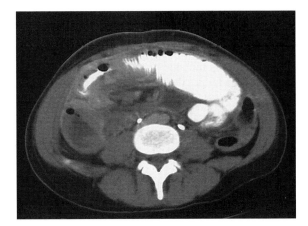

Figure 3.21 D

Findings: CECT demonstrates a LLL pneumonia. CECT of the abdomen demonstrates thickening of the terminal ileum, cecum, and ascending colon.

Differential Diagnosis: Crohn colitis, lymphoma, amebiasis, yersinia, ischemic colitis.

Diagnosis: Tuberculosis.

Discussion: Intestinal tuberculosis is thought to be due to either hematogenous spread, swallowing of infected sputum, or from infected cow's milk. Typically, GI tuberculosis is associated with pulmonary tuberculosis and diagnosis can be suggested by an abnormal radiograph or positive sputum stains and cultures. However, positive chest film findings are present in only 50% of cases of GI tuberculosis.

Findings of tuberculosis are similar to those seen in Crohn disease and should be considered where Crohn disease is a potential diagnosis. Early in the disease, there is thickening and nodularity of the mucosa which involves the cecum more than the terminal ileum. Ulcers form that can heal and form strictures. The cecum can become rigid from the inflammation and scarring and appear cone shaped. This can simulate a carcinoma. Several pathologic processes involve both the terminal ileum and the cecum. Crohn colitis is the most common but other entities such as yersinia colitis, amebiasis, and ischemia can have this appearance as well.

Clinical History: 44-year-old man after brain surgery presents with an acute abdomen requiring emergent exploratory laparotomy.

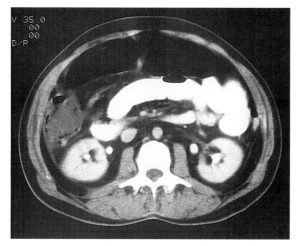 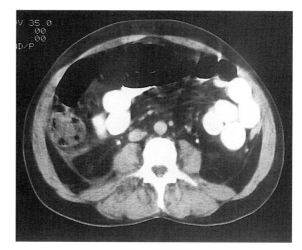

Figure 3.22 A   Figure 3.22 B

Findings: CECT demonstrates thickening of the cecum with inflammatory changes in the pericecal fat. Pneumatosis is present.

Differential Diagnosis: Diverticulitis, perforated cecum.

Diagnosis: Bowel infarction.

Discussion: Colonic ischemia is most commonly seen in the elderly and can be due to a variety of etiologies including cardiac problems (CHF, arrhythmias), trauma, vasculitis, diabetes, and hypotension. Most often a definitive cause is not found. Colonic ischemia can lead to reversible (transient) ischemia, chronic ischemic colitis, strictures, and bowel infarction. Bowel infarction is the most devastating of the possible outcomes and can quickly lead to death if surgery is not performed. CT findings of bowel infarction include bowel wall thickening, inflammatory changes in the pericolonic fat, pneumatosis, and portal venous air. Although pneumatosis can be caused by a variety of benign processes, in the setting of an acute abdomen and bowel wall thickening, ischemia and infarction must be considered as likely etiologies. Infectious colitis and Crohn colitis will rarely produce pneumatosis unless ischemia/infarction is present. Diverticulitis and a perforated cecum from trauma or neoplasm can have associated pneumatosis but an inflammatory mass would most likely be present.

CASE 23

Clinical History: 65-year-old woman with weight loss and guaiac positive stools.

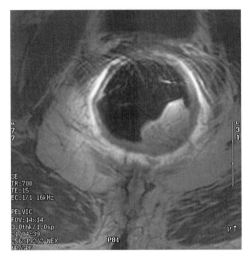

Figure 3.23 A

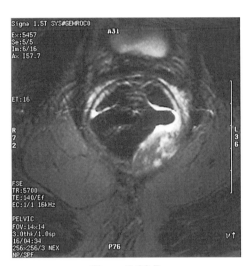

Figure 3.23 B

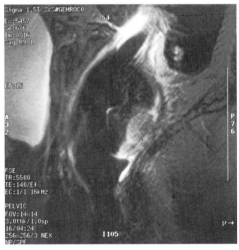

Figure 3.23 C

Findings: (A) T1-weighted endorectal MRI demonstrates an isointense polypoid mass in the left posterior rectum. (B, C) T2-weighted axial and sagittal image demonstrates this lesion to be of increased signal intensity relative to muscle. On all three images, the muscular wall of the bowel is obliterated suggesting invasion through to the perirectal fat.

Differential Diagnosis: Lymphoma, metastases.

Diagnosis: Adenocarcinoma of the rectum with wall invasion.

Discussion: Endorectal MRI is performed by placing an endorectal coil into the rectum. The coil is directional so the probe must be directed toward the region of interest. This allows superb detail of structures adjacent to the rectum such as the uterus, cervix, prostate, and particularly the rectal wall. MRI is also advantageous over CT because multiple planes can be performed. This case demonstrates a typical adenocarcinoma of the rectum. The lesion is isointense to muscle on the T1-weighted image and hyperintense on the T2-weighted images. This lesion is not limited to the mucosa because the bowel wall layers are effaced suggesting invasion of the perirectal fat. A screening MR of the pelvis without the endorectal coil is also performed to rule out adenopathy. The ability to see the lesion in multiple planes is important to delineate crucial anatomy such as the levator ani. All these findings are important in the preoperative staging to determine the best approach.

CASE 24

Clinical History: 57-year-old man with severe abdominal pain.

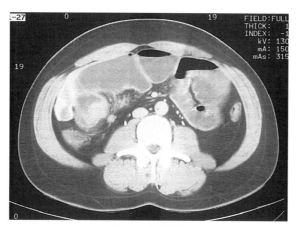

Figure 3.24 A

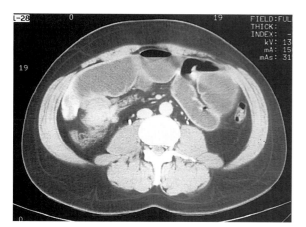

Figure 3.24 B

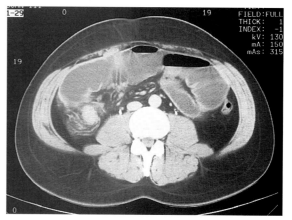

Figure 3.24 C

Findings: CECT demonstrates dilated loops of fluid-filled small bowel and an enhancing mass in the right lower quadrant. Note the large amount of stranding within the mesentery adjacent to the mass.

Differential Diagnosis: Adenocarcinoma, lymphoma, Crohn disease, tuberculosis, focal hemorrhage.

Diagnosis: Carcinoid of the small bowel.

Discussion: Carcinoid is a slow-growing tumor with malignant potential that arises from the enterochromaffin cells in the small bowel. The most common location for a carcinoid tumor in the gastrointestinal tract is the appendix followed by the distal small bowel. Hormonally active substances are secreted by this tumor such as serotonin, histamine, and bradykinin. Carcinoid in the small bowel can be mucosal or submucosal in location. As the tumor grows, an exophytic component is seen which grows out from the tumor into the mesentery. The serotonin causes an intense desmoplastic reaction, which can lead to kinking of the bowel and obstruction. In this example, there is a relatively small mass, but extensive stranding is seen in the mesentery surrounding the mass. This represents the desmoplastic reaction and spread of the tumor. Adenocarcinoma, lymphoma, and hemorrhage will not invoke as much desmoplastic reaction as is seen in this case. Crohn disease can have inflammatory changes around the involved bowel but will typically present as segmental thickening or stricture of the bowel.

CASE 25

Clinical History: 42-year-old man presents with fever, hypotension, and abdominal pain.

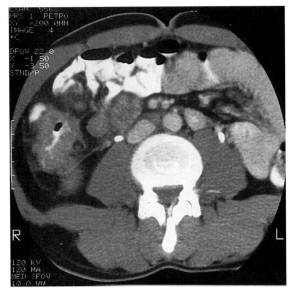

Figure 3.25 A

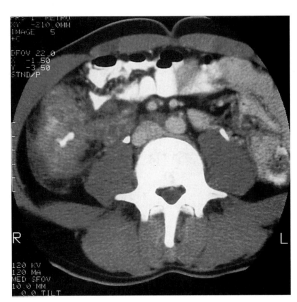

Figure 3.25 B

Findings: CECT demonstrates marked thickening of the cecum with pericecal stranding and inflammation.

Differential Diagnosis: Crohn disease, infectious colitis, typhlitis, perforated neoplasm, diverticulitis.

Diagnosis: Appendicitis.

Discussion: Appendicitis is typically a clinical diagnosis based on laboratory findings and physical exam. Like diverticulitis, the prevalence is higher in Western countries due to the low fiber diet resulting in impaction of the appendix. Appendicitis is more commonly seen in children and adolescents but can be seen in the elderly as well. In the elderly, the diagnosis can be difficult due to the milder symptoms. The CT findings of appendicitis include an inflamed appendix, cecal and pericecal inflammation, an appendicolith, and pericecal fluid collections. CT is excellent for differentiating between mild inflammation versus abscess or extensive phlegmon formation. If there is a periappendiceal abscess present, CT can also be used to guide a percutaneous drainage. Because of the patient's age, appendicitis was not the first diagnosis suggested. The CT appearance of a thickened cecum and pericecal inflammation is nonspecific and could be due to diverticulitis, infectious colitis, or a perforated neoplasm. Appendicitis was found at surgery.

CASE 26

Clinical History: 35-year-old man with rectal pain and weight loss.

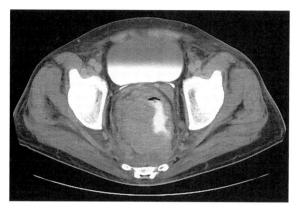

Figure 3.26 A

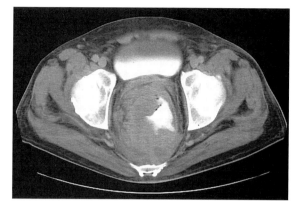

Figure 3.26 B

Findings: CECT demonstrates a large circumferential mass involving the rectum with narrowing and displacement of the lumen to the left.

Differential Diagnosis: Adenocarcinoma, rectal abscess, hemorrhage.

Diagnosis: Lymphoma.

Discussion: Primary rectal involvement by lymphoma is rare but should be considered in a patient with preexisting disease. Primary lymphoma is more commonly seen in the rectum and cecum but secondary lymphoma can occur anywhere in the colon. Lymphoma can present as a large exophytic mass or as an infiltrating mass causing an annular stricture. Typically, only a short segment of bowel is involved and the mass at presentation can be large measuring up to 12 cm in size. These large lesions can necrose, ulcerate, and fistulize to adjacent structures. In this example, the large circumferential bulky mass should suggest a malignancy such as adenocarcinoma or lymphoma. Hemorrhage and an abscess could also appear as a bulky mass but low attenuation fluid is normally present in or around the mass. Ulcerative colitis, ischemia, and pseudomembranous colitis usually involve a longer segment of bowel with diffuse bowel wall thickening rather than a large bulky mass.

CASE 27

Clinical History: 66-year-old man post cardiac arrest and a prolonged period of hypotension.

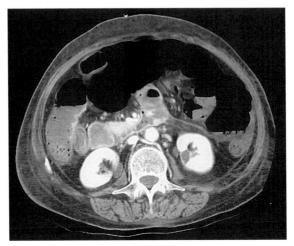

Figure 3.27 A

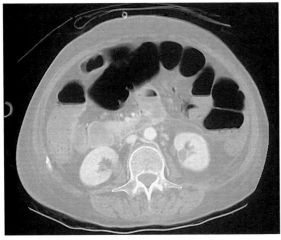

Figure 3.27 B

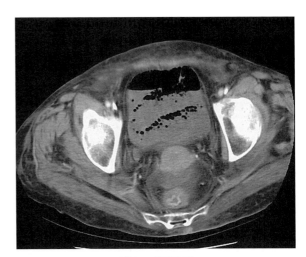

Figure 3.27 C

Findings: CECT demonstrates dilated loops of large bowel and a small pocket of air in a mesenteric vein. This is better seen when the same image is displayed in lung windows. Images through the pelvis demonstrate fluid-filled loops of small bowel adjacent to each other with pneumatosis.

Differential Diagnosis: None.

Diagnosis: Ischemic bowel with pneumatosis and venous air.

Discussion: Ischemic bowel can be due to a variety of causes including prolonged hypotension as in this case. The CT findings are often nonspecific including thickened bowel within a vascular territory or watershed zone, stranding and inflammation around the affected bowel, and pneumatosis and venous air in the abdomen. Although pneumatosis can be due to benign causes including COPD, infection, and prior abdominal intervention, with the appropriate history, ischemic bowel must be considered. In addition to pneumatosis, venous air in the mesentery and portal vein air can be present as well in an ischemic bowel. This is often difficult to see on standard soft tissue windows and is often better seen in either lung or bone windows as demonstrated in this example.

CASE 28

Clinical History: 46-year-old man with diarrhea and abdominal pain.

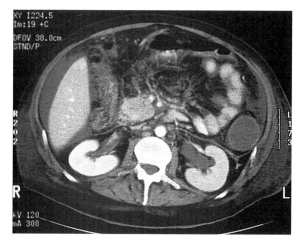

Figure 3.28 A

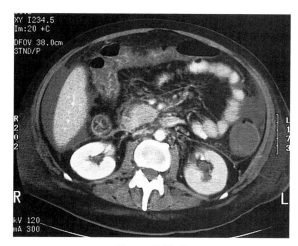

Figure 3.28 B

Findings: CECT demonstrates thickening of the ascending and transverse colon. There is also ascites and edema of the mesentery.

Differential Diagnosis: Ischemia, infectious colitis (tuberculosis, amebiasis), lymphoma.

Diagnosis: Crohn colitis.

Discussion: Crohn colitis is a disease of unknown etiology that is characterized by transmural inflammation of the GI tract in a discontinuous fashion (skip lesions) usually involving the terminal ileum and proximal colon. Complications include fistulas, abscess formation, and adenocarcinoma. The earliest changes of Crohn colitis includes aphthous ulcers and thickening of the bowel wall. This is followed by deeper ulcers, rigidity of the bowel wall, and a "cobblestone appearance" of the mucosa. The cobblestone appearance is due to ulcers separated by areas of edematous mucosa. Finally, there is stricture formation of the bowel. The involvement of the proximal colon in this case leads to a narrow differential. When ischemia involves the proximal colon it will also involve the distal small bowel because this is the vascular supply of the SMA. Pseudomembranous colitis typically involves the entire colon and there is a greater degree of bowel wall thickening. Ulcerative colitis begins in the rectum and progresses proximally and does not involve the terminal ileum. Infectious colitides usually involve a smaller segment of bowel rather than a long segment as is seen in this example. Crohn colitis would be the best diagnosis.

CASE 29

Clinical History: 50-year-old man with abdominal pain and weight loss.

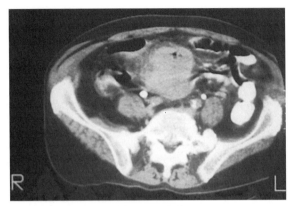

Figure 3.29 A

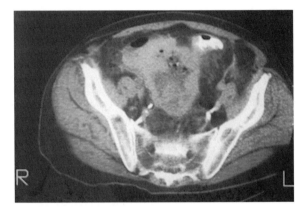

Figure 3.29 B

Findings: CECT demonstrates an 8-cm necrotic mass in the mid pelvis that appears to be in close association with a loop of small bowel. Air is seen within the lesion.

Differential Diagnosis: Adenocarcinoma, metastasis, sarcoma, abscess, lymphoma.

Diagnosis: Carcinoid tumor.

Discussion: Carcinoid tumor is the most common neoplasm of the small bowel and appendix. Within the small bowel, the majority are found in the ileum followed by the jejunum and duodenum. When the lesions are small (<1 cm), they will present as a submucosal lesion. As the tumor grows, it can penetrate the mucosa and cause ulceration and obstruction. The lesion will frequently grow through the serosa and present primarily as a mesenteric mass as in this example. Because of the secretion of serotonin, there is marked desmoplastic reaction leading to kinking of the bowel and tethering of the folds. The large mass seen in this case is unusual because carcinoid tumors will usually present as a smaller mass with an intense desmoplastic reaction. This necrotic mass is more typical of a large adenocarcinoma or sarcoma. An abscess from diverticulitis can also have this appearance and clinical correlation is necessary.

CASE 30

Clinical History: 79-year-old man with weight loss and bloody stools.

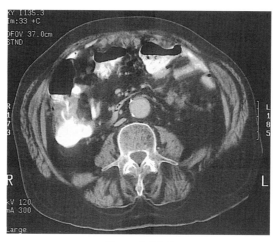

Figure 3.30 A

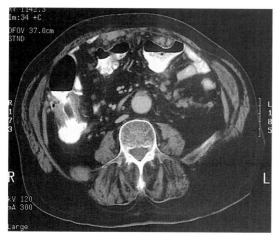

Figure 3.30 B

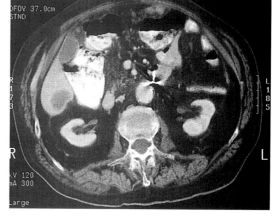

Figure 3.30 C

Findings: CECT of the upper abdomen demonstrates a low attenuation mass in the right lobe of the liver. CECT of the cecum reveals a constricting lesion of the cecum. Note the lymphadenopathy in the omentum and mesentery.

Differential Diagnosis: Lymphoma.

Diagnosis: Metastatic colon cancer.

Discussion: A constricting lesion in the cecum can be due to a variety of etiologies. Tuberculosis can have this appearance (tuberculoma) and is more common in the right colon. A stricture from ischemia is also a possibility although no other signs of ischemia in the remaining bowel are seen. Crohn colitis without terminal ileum involvement is rare. The presence of a liver lesion, adenopathy in the omentum, and an "applecore" lesion in the cecum suggest a malignancy. Both lymphoma and adenocarcinoma would be a good possibility in this case.

CASE 31

Clinical History: 71-year-old woman with abdominal pain and fever.

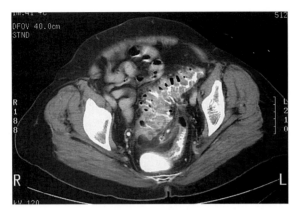

Figure 3.31 A

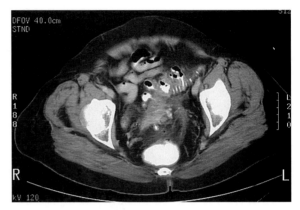

Figure 3.31 B

Findings: CECT demonstrates multiple diverticula in the sigmoid colon with stranding and inflammatory changes seen around the sigmoid colon.

Differential Diagnosis: Infectious colitis, inflammatory bowel disease.

Diagnosis: Diverticulitis.

Discussion: Diverticula of the colon are thought to be due to two main factors: increased pressure within the colonic lumen and relative weakness of the bowel wall. The increased pressure and the higher incidence in the sigmoid colon are thought to be secondary to several factors. When stool reaches the sigmoid colon, most of the water has been removed. This plus a low fiber diet causes the need for higher pressures to move the stool through the sigmoid colon. In the colon, the sigmoid has the smallest lumen requiring the highest pressures. The colonic wall is weakest where the blood vessels penetrate the wall to reach the submucosa, around the taenia mesocolica, and on the mesenteric side of the taenia libera and taenia omentalis, where diverticula are found. This case demonstrates a subtle case of diverticulitis. There is inflammation seen in and around the wall of the sigmoid colon with extension into the pericolonic fat. This in conjunction with the presence of multiple diverticula, makes diverticulitis the most likely diagnosis. Other CT findings include fistula formation to adjacent structures like the bladder, abscess formation, and extraluminal contrast or air.

CASE 32

Clinical History: 71-year-old woman with severe epigastric pain and weight loss.

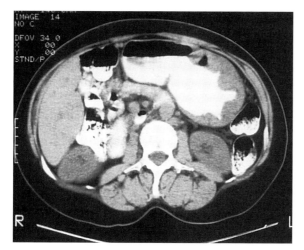
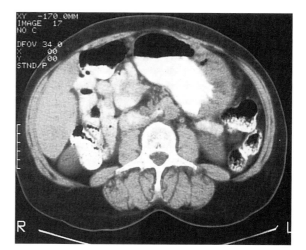

Figure 3.32 A   **Figure 3.32 B**

Findings: NECT demonstrates marked thickening of the body and fundus of the stomach with sparing of the antrum.

Differential Diagnosis: Lymphoma, adenocarcinoma, peptic ulcer disease, eosinophilic gastritis, tuberculosis, Crohn disease.

Diagnosis: Menetrier disease.

Discussion: Menetrier disease is characterized by hyperplasia of the gastric mucous glands causing increased secretions of mucus and protein. Patients also have decreased acid production, resulting in thickened gastric folds, hypochlorhydria, and hypoproteinemia. Menetrier disease typically involves the body and fundus of the stomach, sparing the antrum. The mucosa is markedly thickened as in this case. The main differential diagnoses are lymphoma and adenocarcinoma of the stomach. Biopsy is necessary to exclude a malignancy. Peptic ulcer disease and gastritis do not usually cause gastric thickening to this extent. Other entities such as Crohn disease, eosinophilic gastritis, and tuberculosis are rare but could be considered as well.

Clinical History: 25-year-old man with severe right lower quadrant pain, fever, and leukocytosis.

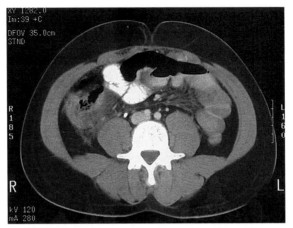

Figure 3.33 A

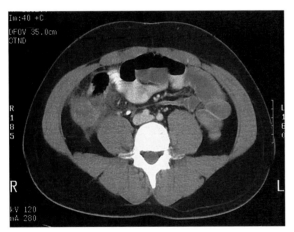

Figure 3.33 B

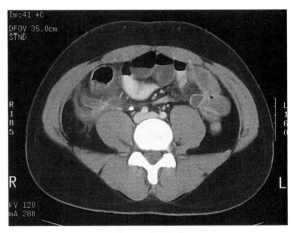

Figure 3.33 C

Findings: CECT demonstrates an inflammatory mass adjacent to the cecum with stranding and phlegmon surrounding it.

Differential Diagnosis: Crohn colitis, typhlitis, infectious colitis (tuberculosis, amebiasis), perforated neoplasm, diverticulitis.

Diagnosis: Perforated appendix with periappendiceal abscess.

Discussion: Appendicitis is the most common abdominal surgical emergency in the United States. It occurs most commonly in the late teens and twenties but has been shown in the elderly as well. Obstruction of the appendix leading to appendicitis can be due to an appendicolith, foreign body, adhesion, neoplasm, or Crohn colitis. CT findings of appendicitis include appendicolith, wall thickening, periappendiceal/pericecal abscess or phlegmon, and cecal and ascending colon wall thickening. It is often difficult to identify an abnormal appendix or to find an appendicolith to diagnose appendicitis. More commonly a periappendiceal abscess/phlegmon is seen, which is similar in appearance to a perforated neoplasm or diverticulitis. In this patient's age group, the most likely choices include Crohn colitis with an abscess, typhlitis if the patient had lymphoma or leukemia, or appendicitis.

CASE 34

Clinical History: Chronically ill 69-year-old man with diabetes and congestive heart failure presents with 30-lb weight loss and abdominal pain.

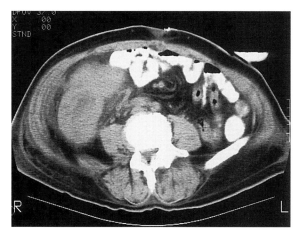

Figure 3.34 A

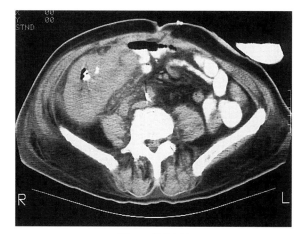

Figure 3.34 B

Findings: NECT demonstrates marked thickening of the cecum and ascending colon. Inflammation is seen in the pericolonic fat.

Differential Diagnosis: Crohn disease, ischemia, typhlitis, diverticulitis, infectious colitis.

Diagnosis: Mucormycosis of the colon.

Discussion: Mucormycosis or colonic zygomycosis is an extremely rare cause of colonic thickening. It is found typically in debilitated patients such as those with dehydration, immunosuppression, burns, systemic illnesses, and malnourished children. Zygomycetes are ubiquitous and are found in molding breads, fruits, and vegetables. The most common presentations for mucormycosis are rhinocerebral, pulmonary, and cutaneous. Colonic involvement is rare and most commonly is in the right colon. It usually presents as a focal expanding mass that can ulcerate and demonstrate necrosis. Inflammatory changes are often present in the surrounding tissues. Most right-sided colitides could have this appearance. Terminal ileum disease is not seen in this case, making Crohn disease and ischemia less likely. The patient is not immunocompromised to suggest typhlitis. Other infectious etiologies that have a predilection for the right colon would be tuberculosis and amebiasis.

CASE 35

Clinical History: 27-year-old man with severe epigastric pain.

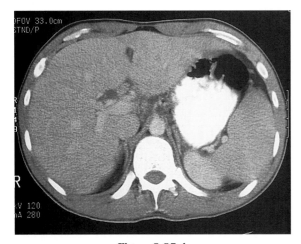

Figure 3.35 A

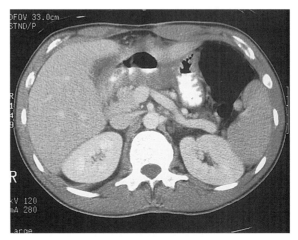

Figure 3.35 B

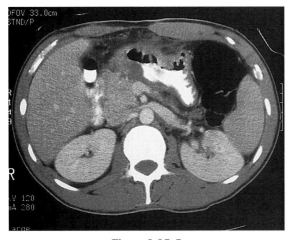

Figure 3.35 C

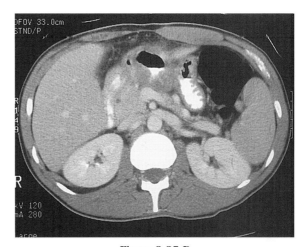

Figure 3.35 D

Findings: CECT demonstrates thickening of the distal antrum of the stomach. The remainder of the stomach is normal.

Differential Diagnosis: Gastric carcinoma, lymphoma, eosinophilic gastritis, antral gastritis.

Diagnosis: Peptic ulcer disease.

Discussion: Peptic ulcers can occur in the stomach or the duodenum. Patients present with symptoms of epigastric pain often precipitated by food. Almost all duodenal ulcers are benign, whereas a small percentage of gastric ulcers can be malignant (ulcerated gastric adenocarcinomas). Careful examination of gastric ulcers must be performed either with follow-up exams or endoscopy with biopsy. Radiographically, besides ulcerations there can be associated thickened folds in the region of the ulcer, which will often radiate to the ulcer crater on a barium exam. On CECT, this will appear as thickening of the gastric wall. In this case, the thickening is limited to the antrum, with the remainder of the stomach being normal. This can represent simple gastritis limited to the mucosal layer or eosinophilic gastritis. Other inflammatory processes are less common such as tuberculosis, sarcoidosis, and Crohn disease. A malignancy must also be excluded. Both lymphoma and adenocarcinoma could have this CT appearance so an endoscopic biopsy is necessary to exclude this possibility.

CASE 36

Clinical History: 35-year-old man with leukemia post a bone marrow transplant.

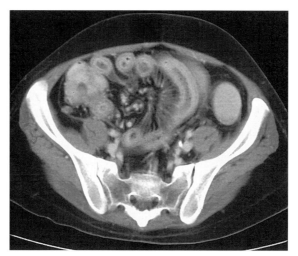

Figure 3.36 A

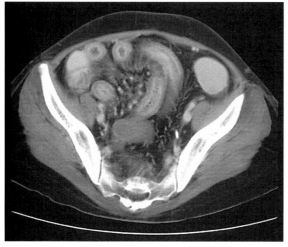

Figure 3.36 B

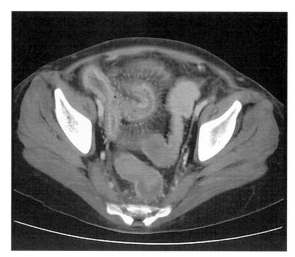

Figure 3.36 C

Findings: Marked thickening of multiple loops of small bowel with mesenteric edema and inflammation

Differential Diagnosis: Viral enteritis, ischemia, radiation, allergic states.

Diagnosis: Graft-versus-host disease (GVHD).

Discussion: Graft-versus-host disease is due to immunocompetent cells in the donor marrow reacting with cells in the recipient. Acute GVHD can occur up to 100 days after transplantation. It commonly affects the skin, liver, and GI tract. In the GI tract, the small bowel is most commonly involved but the stomach, duodenum, and colon can also demonstrate changes as well. There is prolonged coating of the small bowel which can appear as circular collections of barium in cross section or parallel tracks in longitudinal sections. Bowel thickening, mesenteric edema, and adenopathy can also be seen. This appearance can be indistinguishable from viral enteritis, which can also be a complication of bone marrow transplants. Ischemia would typically involve the proximal portion of the colon and clinical history would be necessary to rule out radiation and allergic states.

CASE 37

Clinical History: 76-year-old man with rectal bleeding.

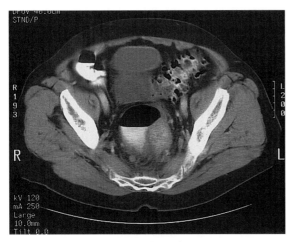

Figure 3.37 A

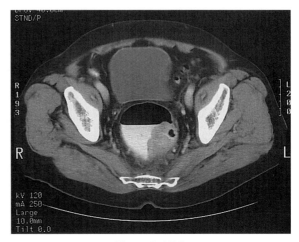

Figure 3.37 B

Findings: CECT demonstrates a 3 × 4 cm polypoid lesion involving the left lateral and posterior wall of the rectum. There is extension of the tumor into the perirectal fat. Note the small lymph node at the 7 o'clock and 5 o'clock position.

Differential Diagnosis: Lymphoma, metastasis, villous adenoma.

Diagnosis: Adenocarcinoma of the rectum.

Discussion: Colon cancer is the most common malignancy of the GI tract. More than 50% of the cases occur in the rectosigmoid. Tumor spreads to adjacent structures and lymph nodes. Metastasis to the liver via the portal venous system occurs in lesions located in the proximal two thirds of the rectum. The lesions in the distal one third of the rectum metastasize to the lung via the hemorrhoidal plexus and IVC. Rectosigmoid lesions demonstrate spread to lymph nodes in the external iliac chain, para-aortic chain, and inguinal region. CT is good at detecting gross extension of the tumor outside the colonic wall but microscopic invasion is often missed. The polypoid lesion in this example is typical for an adenocarcinoma. The size of the lesion (>1 cm), extension outside the wall into the perirectal fat, and presence of small lymph nodes all suggest malignancy. Lymphoma of the colon is typically large in size and usually involves the cecum. The size of this lesion would make a villous adenoma unlikely. No fluid within the lesion is seen to suggest an abscess or hemorrhage. An adenocarcinoma is the best diagnosis.

CASE 38

Clinical History: 39-year-old woman with history of cervical cancer.

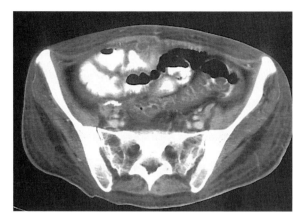

Figure 3.38 A

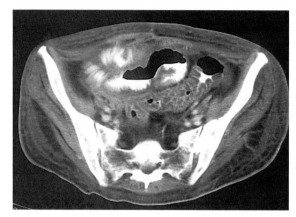

Figure 3.38 B

Findings: CECT demonstrates thickening of the sigmoid colon and adjacent loops of small bowel. The mesentery also appears thickened and inflamed.

Differential Diagnosis: Crohn disease, lymphoma, ischemia.

Diagnosis: Radiation enteritis.

Discussion: Radiation changes in the GI tract for radiation are commonly seen in the rectum, sigmoid, and small bowel with the use of external beam therapy for many pelvic malignancies (i.e., cervical, bladder). A good clinical history will suggest the diagnosis and often eliminate the need for a lengthy workup. CT findings suggestive of radiation enteritis include bowel wall thickening of loops of bowel within the radiation port. It is unusual to have involvement of both the sigmoid colon and small bowel at the same time by the same disease process. This can occur in Crohn disease with skip lesions and ischemia with involvement of multiple branch vessels from vasculitis or emboli. Lymphoma, which is considered a systemic disease, can also affect various loops of bowel. Other CT findings in radiation disease include increased attenuation of the mesenteric fat, mass-like adhesion of the bowel loops, and bowel wall thickening with an average thickness of less than 8 mm.

Clinical History: 35-year-old man with diarrhea and rectal bleeding.

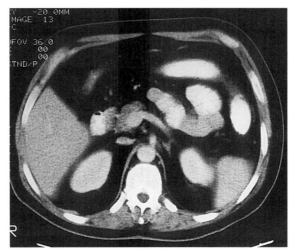

Figure 3.39 A

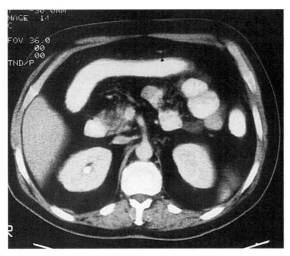

Figure 3.39 B

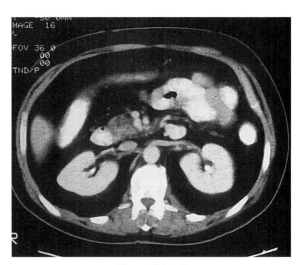

Figure 3.39 C

Findings: CECT demonstrates a smooth, featureless ascending, transverse and descending colon. The entire colon is involved by this process (not shown).

Differential Diagnosis: Crohn disease, cathartic abuse, radiation colitis, treated bacterial and viral colitides.

Diagnosis: Ulcerative colitis.

Discussion: Ulcerative colitis is predominantly a mucosal disease that begins in the rectum and progresses proximally to involve the entire colon. Early in the course of the disease, the mucosa is edematous and hyperemic with areas of ulceration. Thumbprinting can often be seen during this stage as well. Eventually the mucosa becomes friable and denuded with islands of edematous mucosa-forming "pseudopolyps." With further episodes of inflammation and healing, there is distortion of the haustral pattern with eventual loss of haustration and shortening of the colon, leading to a "leadpipe" colon in the chronic phases of ulcerative colitis. This case demonstrates loss of haustration and shortening of the colon typical of ulcerative colitis. Other entities can also cause loss of haustration including cathartic abuse, which predominantly involves the right side of the colon. Any chronic or healed process involving the colon can also lead to loss of haustration including Crohn disease, radiation, and infectious colitides. Both Crohn disease and radiation will rarely involve the entire colon as in this case. Loss of haustration, shortened colon, and pancolonic involvement makes ulcerative colitis the most likely diagnosis.

CASE 40

Clinical History: 76-year-old man with bloody stools and weight loss.

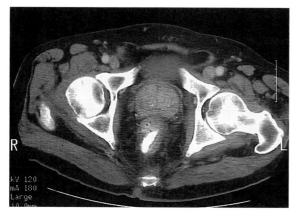

Figure 3.40 A

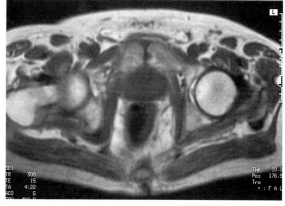

Figure 3.40 B

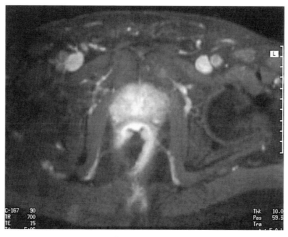

Figure 3.40 C

Findings: (A) CECT demonstrates irregular thickening of the anterior and left lateral rectum. (B) T1-weighted MRI demonstrates the same thickening of the rectum to be isointense to muscle. (C) This lesion is hyperintense on the T1 post gadolinium fat saturation image, and there appears to be extension through the rectal wall.

Differential Diagnosis: Lymphoma, metastases.

Diagnosis: Adenocarcinoma of the rectum.

Discussion: Mild thickening of the bowel, especially of the colon, on a CT scan can often be misleading because it could be due to a neoplasm, adherent fecal material, or a nondistended bowel loop. To avoid overcalling bowel wall thickening, rectal contrast should be administered. MRI, however, is even better suited to evaluate for a colon carcinoma. The T1-weighted images are useful to delineate anatomy, for involvement of adjacent structures by tumor, or searching for lymphadenopathy. The post gadolinium fat saturation T1 images are excellent for seeing the tumor because it will be hyperintense relative to muscle and well delineated from the suppressed perirectal fat. The subtle extension of the tumor through the wall is easily seen. There is no concern on the MRI that this lesion could represent undistended bowel or fecal material.

CASE 41

Clinical History: 40-year-old man with history of rectal pain and diarrhea.

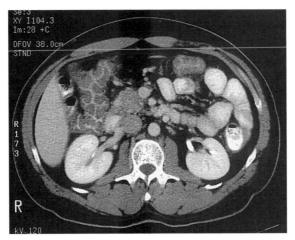

Figure 3.41 A

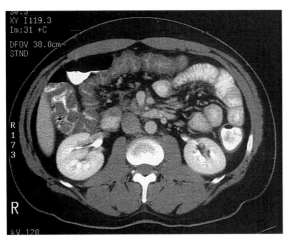

Figure 3.41 B

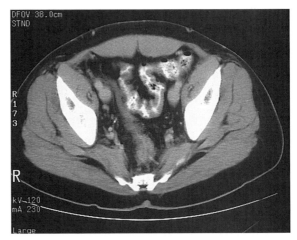

Figure 3.41 C

Findings: CECT of the pelvis demonstrates mild to moderate thickening of the rectum and sigmoid colon. A second image demonstrates thickening of the ascending and transverse colon.

Differential Diagnosis: Pseudomembranous colitis, infectious colitis (CMV, salmonella).

Diagnosis: Ulcerative colitis.

Discussion: Ulcerative colitis is an inflammatory process that involves primarily the colonic mucosa. It begins in the rectum and spreads proximally toward the cecum in a continuous fashion. The terminal ileum can be involved with backwash ileitis but in contrast to Crohn disease, the lumen is usually enlarged rather than strictured. The age of onset is typically in the twenties but ulcerative colitis can be seen at almost any age. On CT, the bowel wall thickening is less pronounced than with other colitides with the average thickening of approximately 8 mm. In addition, the thickening is of heterogeneous density, often with submucosal fat being present. In other colitides, the low attenuation areas in the wall represent edema rather than fat. In this case, the entire colon appears to be involved. Ischemia would be unlikely because this would involve both the SMA and IMA vascular distributions. Pseudomembranous colitis typically has a much thicker wall and there is no history of antibiotic use. Infectious colitis is a good consideration.

CT AND MRI OF THE ABDOMEN AND PELVIS

CASE 42

Clinical History: 39-year-old man with left lower quadrant pain, fever, and leukocytosis.

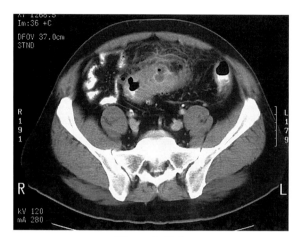

Figure 3.42 A

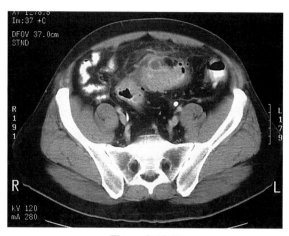

Figure 3.42 B

Findings: CECT demonstrates a large inflammatory mass involving the sigmoid colon. Two small fluid filled pockets are present in this mass as well as marked stranding in the pericolonic fat.

Differential Diagnosis: Infectious colitis, adenocarcinoma, lymphoma.

Diagnosis: Diverticulitis.

Discussion: Diverticula of the colon are acquired herniations of mucosa and submucosa through the muscular layers of the bowel wall. They are found most commonly in the sigmoid colon and are thought to be related to the low fiber diet found in western countries. Diverticulitis occurs secondary to perforation of a diverticulum. This can lead to bowel wall inflammation and spasm, a localized ileus, and abscess formation. Because the perforation usually walls itself off quickly, there is rarely free air present on plain films. On CT, however, extraluminal air can be seen as well as an inflammatory mass, which represents phlegmon or focal abscess. This example demonstrates the characteristic findings of diverticulitis with an inflammatory mass, stranding in the pericolonic fat, and small pus-filled pockets. An underlying malignancy that has perforated could give a similar appearance and should be excluded.

CASE 43

Clinical History: 75-year-old man with diarrhea, abdominal pain, and leukocytosis. The patient is taking antibiotics for a pneumonia.

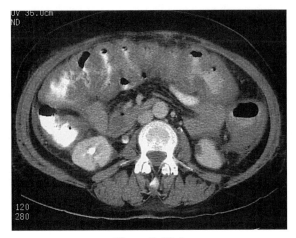

Figure 3.43 A

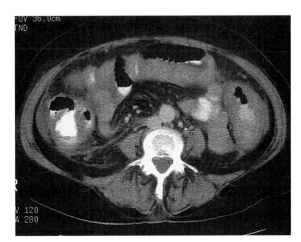

Figure 3.43 B

Findings: CECT demonstrates marked thickening of the ascending, transverse and descending colon with minimal pericolonic stranding. A small amount of ascites is present.

Differential Diagnosis: Ischemic colitis, inflammatory bowel disease, infectious colitis (i.e., Salmonella, Campylobacter).

Diagnosis: Pseudomembranous colitis (PMC).

Discussion: Pseudomembranous colitis forms characteristic yellow or creamy white plaques related to the overgrowth of *Clostridium difficile*. This occurs after the use of almost any antibiotic, but is most closely associated with clindamycin and lincomycin. The patients typically have watery diarrhea, crampy abdominal pain, and occasionally fever. The characteristic CT features include diffuse pancolitis with marked mural thickening, with minimal pericolonic inflammatory changes. The pericolonic stranding that is present is out of proportion to the degree of bowel wall thickening. Ascites is seen in up to 77% of patients with PMC and suggests the acute nature of this disease. Ischemic colitis and Crohn colitis would typically involve the terminal ileum, which was spared in this case. Infectious colitis could have this appearance but pericolonic stranding is usually extensive in those cases. Pseudomembranous colitis is the best choice taking into account the CT findings and clinical history.

CASE 44

Clinical History: 62-year-old man with history of heartburn.

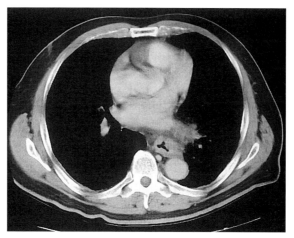

Figure 3.44 A

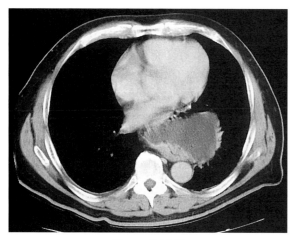

Figure 3.44 B

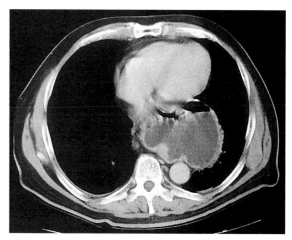

Figure 3.44 C

Findings: CECT demonstrates a fluid-filled structure located anterior and to the left of the aorta and esophagus in the thoracic cavity.

Differential Diagnosis: Sliding hiatal hernia, foregut malformation, pseudocyst.

Diagnosis: Paraesophageal hernia.

Discussion: Paraesophageal hernias occur when a portion of the stomach herniates through the esophageal hiatus to lie anterior to the distal esophagus. The cardia and gastroesophageal junction lie in their normal position below the diaphragm while a variable amount of stomach herniates into the chest. These patients are typically asymptomatic until the hernia becomes large enough to lead to incarceration and gastric infarction. The finding of a portion of the stomach anterior to the distal esophagus with a normally positioned gastroesophageal junction is diagnostic of a paraesophageal hernia. With a sliding hernia, the gastroesophageal junction is above the diaphragm. Because the fluid collection is continuous with the stomach, a pancreatic pseudocyst is excluded. Foregut malformations (esophageal duplication and bronchogenic cysts) usually have a thin wall rather than the thick gastric wall seen in paraesophageal hernias.

CASE 45

Clinical History: 65-year-old man with a long history of smoking presents with abdominal pain.

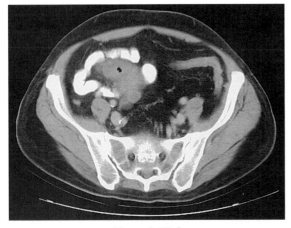

Figure 3.45 A

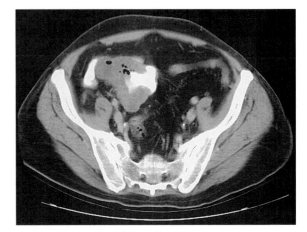

Figure 3.45 B

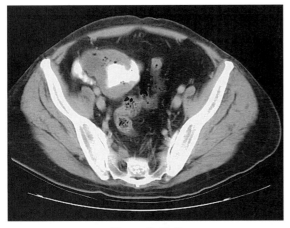

Figure 3.45 C

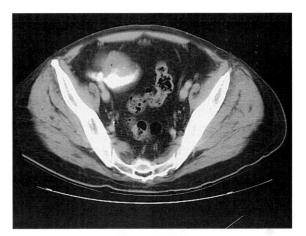

Figure 3.45 D

Findings: CECT demonstrates a soft tissue mass involving the serosal surface of a small bowel loop in the pelvis. There is an area of ulceration present with pockets of air seen within the mass. No bowel obstruction is seen.

Differential Diagnosis: Lymphoma, adenocarcinoma.

Diagnosis: Small bowel metastasis from lung cancer.

Discussion: Metastases to the small bowel can occur by direct extension, peritoneal seeding or as in this case hematogenous spread. The most common hematogenous metastases to the small intestine are melanoma and lung cancer. Radiographically, metastases typically present as multiple nodules or masses on the antimesenteric side. There can be extensive desmoplastic reaction, which causes kinking and tethering of the bowel. In this example, no other loops of bowel were involved, making an inflammatory etiology less likely. Other malignancies such as adenocarcinoma and carcinoid tumor are a possibility but they usually cause luminal narrowing. Lymphoma, however, will not cause obstruction but aneurysmal dilatation. In this case, the lesion appears to grow away from the bowel into the mesentery as typically seen in metastases.

CASE 46

Clinical History: 37-year-old woman with abdominal pain, diarrhea, and new onset of asthma. The patient had an elevated eosinophil count.

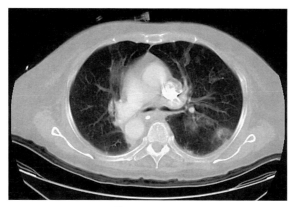

Figure 3.46 A

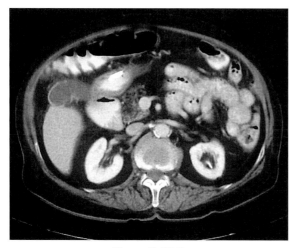

Figure 3.46 B

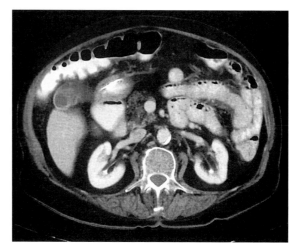

Figure 3.46 C

Findings: (A) CECT of the chest demonstrates bilateral infiltrates. (B, C) CECT of the abdomen demonstrates thickening and distension of the proximal duodenum.

Differential Diagnosis: peptic ulcer disease, eosinophilic gastroenteritis, tuberculosis, Crohn disease, lymphoma.

Diagnosis: Strongyloidiasis.

Discussion: *Strongyloides stercoralis* is a parasite endemic in Africa, Asia, and South America. Cases in the United States are usually from patients who have migrated from these areas or in the AIDS population as an opportunistic infection. The larvae enter the skin reaching the lungs via the venous system. Patients frequently present with new-onset reactive airway disease due to the pneumonitis from the parasite. As with other parasitic infections, peripheral eosinophilia is commonly seen. From the lung, the larvae then migrate to the proximal small bowel, predominantly the proximal duodenum. Radiographically, there are edematous folds, ulcerations, and spasm of the proximal duodenum. As the process progresses, there can be narrowing of the third and fourth portions of the duodenum resulting in proximal dilatation. Thickening of the wall of the proximal duodenum is nonspecific but with pulmonary infiltrates, the differential diagnosis is limited to Strongyloides and tuberculosis. With new onset of asthma and peripheral eosinophilia, the diagnosis of Strongyloides is most likely.

CASE 47

Clinical History: 31-year-old woman with a history of abdominal pain and diarrhea.

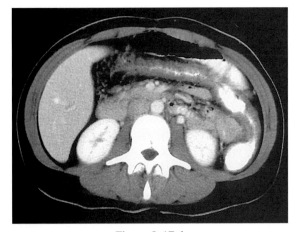

Figure 3.47 A

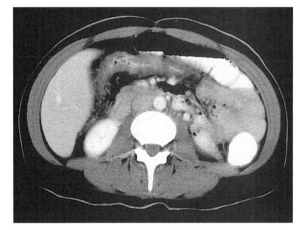

Figure 3.47 B

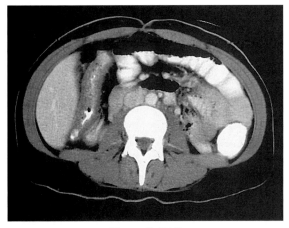

Figure 3.47 C

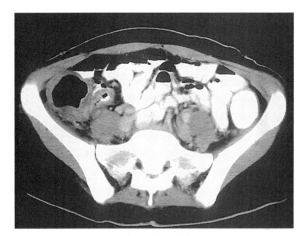

Figure 3.47 D

Findings: CECT demonstrates mild thickening of the terminal ileum, ascending, transverse and descending colon.

Differential Diagnosis: Infectious colitis.

Diagnosis: Crohn disease.

Discussion: This case is unusual because there is involvement of most of the colon and terminal ileum although the rectum and sigmoid colon are spared. This distribution is helpful in narrowing the differential diagnosis. Ischemia would be unlikely because this would represent both SMA and IMA vascular distributions. Ulcerative colitis with backwash ileitis is unlikely due to the lack of rectosigmoid involvement. Pseudomembranous colitis tends to involve most of the colon and there is marked thickening (average 15 mm) not seen in this case. Infectious colitides will rarely involve this extent of colon and terminal ileum as is seen in this case.

CASE 48

Clinical History: 32-year-old woman with abdominal pain.

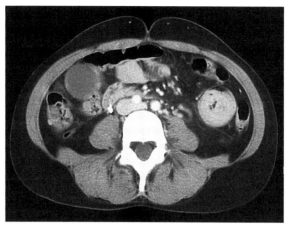

Figure 3.48 A

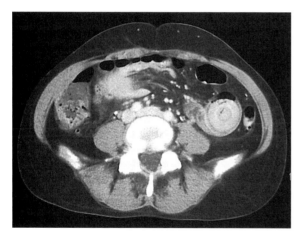

Figure 3.48 B

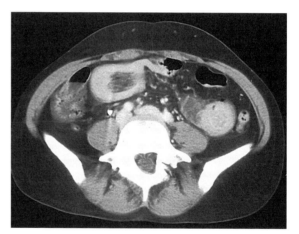

Figure 3.48 C

Findings: CECT demonstrates a round soft tissue mass in the left abdomen with a focal area of fat in its center. There is also an elongated mass in the anterior right abdomen which has mesenteric vessels and fat in it.

Differential Diagnosis: None.

Diagnosis: Two enteroenteric intussusceptions.

Discussion: This case demonstrates the classic CT appearance of an intussusception. An intussusception represents the invagination of one loop of bowel (intussusceptum) into another loop of bowel (intussuscipiens) by peristalsis. The mass in the left abdomen corresponds to the first intussusception scanned in the short axis. In this mass, mesenteric fat can be seen in the center of the intussusception. Three distinct layers of bowel wall can be distinguished. The outer most layer represents the outer wall of the intussuscipiens surrounding air in the bowel lumen. The next two layers are the herniated intussusceptum and are separated in this case by the mesenteric fat. The mass in the anterior abdomen represents a second intussusception but this one is seen longitudinally. Again the mesenteric vessels and fat are seen herniating into the intussuscipiens. This can lead to bowel ischemia. These represent a fairly early stage of intussusception since three distinct layers of bowel wall can still be identified. As the intussusception progresses, there will be loss of the layers secondary to edema in the bowel wall eventually leading to bowel wall ischemia and necrosis.

SUGGESTED READINGS

Neoplasm

Balthazar EJ, Megibow AJ, Hulnick D, et al. Carcinoma of the colon: detection and preoperative staging by CT. AJR 1988;150:301–306.

Bartram CI. Radiology in the current assessment of ulcerative colitis. Gastrointest Radiol 1997;1:383–392.

Buck JL, Sobin LH. Carcinoids of the gastrointestinal tract. Radiographics 1990;10:1081–1095.

Butch RJ, Stark DD, Wittenberg J, et al. Staging rectal cancer by MR and CT. AJR 1986;146:1155–1160.

de Lange, EE, Fechner RE, Edge SB, et al. Preoperative staging of rectal carcinoma with MR imaging: surgical and histopathologic correlation. Radiology 1990;176:623–628.

Ehrlich AN, Stalder G, Geller W, et al. Gastrointestinal manifestations of malignant lymphoma. Gastroenterology 1968;54:1115–1121.

Fiscback W, Kestel W, Kirchner T, et al. Malignant lymphomas of the upper gastrointestinal tract. Cancer 1992;70:1075–1080.

Freeny PC, Marks, WM, Ryan JA, et al. Colorectal carcinoma evaluation with CT: preoperative staging and detection of postoperative recurrence. Radiology 1986;158:347–353.

Gore RM, Levine MS, Laufer I. Textbook of gastrointestinal radiology. Philadelphia: WB Saunders, 1994.

Gould M, Johnson RJ. Computed tomography of abdominal carcinoid tumor. Br J Radiol 1986;59:881–885.

Guinet C, Buy JN, Sezeur A, et al. Preoperative assessment of the extension of rectal carcinoma: correlation of MR, surgical, and histopathologic findings. J Comput Assist Tomogr 1988;12:209–214.

Megibow AJ, Balthazar EJ, Naidich DP, et al. Computed tomography of gastrointestinal lymphoma. AJR 1983;141:541–547.

Picus D, Glazer HS, Levitt RG, et al. Computed tomography of abdominal carcinoid tumors. AJR 1984;143:581–584.

Thompson WM, Halvorsen RA, Foster WL, et al. Preoperative and postoperative CT staging of rectosigmoid carcinoma. AJR 1986;146:703–710.

Weingrad DN, Decosse JJ, Sherlock P, et al. Primary gastrointestinal lymphoma: a 30-year review. Cancer 1982;49:1258–1265.

Williams SM, Berk RN, Harned RK. Radiologic features of multinodular lymphoma of the colon. AJR 1984;143:87–91.

Inflammation

Balthazar EJ, Megibow AJ, Hulnick D, et al. CT of appendicitis. AJR 1986;147:705–710.

Balthazar EJ, Megibow AJ, Schinella RA, et al. Limitations in the CT diagnosis of acute diverticulitis: comparison of CT, contrast enema, and pathologic findings of 16 patients. AJR 1990;154:281–285.

Bartlett JG. Clostridium difficile: clinical considerations. Rev Infect Dis 1990;12:S243–251.

Berkmen YM, Rabinowitz J. Gastrointestinal manifestations of the strongyloidiasis. 1972;115:306–311.

Desai RK, Tagliabue JR, Wegryn SA, et al. CT evaluation of wall thickening in the alimentary tract. Radiographics 1991;11:771–783.

Frager DH, Goldman M, Beneventano TC. Computed tomography in Crohn disease. J Comput Assist Tomogr 1983;7:819–824.

Fishman EK, Kavuru BS, Jones B, et al. Pseudomembranous colitis: CT evaluation of 26 cases. Radiology 1991;180:57–60.

Fultz PJ, Skucas J, Weiss SL. CT in upper gastrointestinal tract perforations secondary to peptic ulcer disease. Gastrointest Radiol 1992;17:5–8.

Gale ME, Birnbaum SG, Gerzof SG, et al. CT appearance of appendicitis and its local complications. J Comput Assist Tomogr 1985;9:34–37.

Gore RM, Marn CS, Kirby DF, et al. CT findings in ulcerative, granulomatous, and indeterminate colitis. AJR 1984;143:279–284.

Hoshino M, Shibata M, Goto N, et al. A clinical study of tuberculous colitis. Jpn Soc Gastroenterol 1979;14:299–305.

Hulnick DH, Megibow AJ, Balthazar EJ, et al. Computed tomography in the evaluation of diverticulitis. Radiology 1984;152:491–495.

Laufer I, Costoppulos L. Early lesions of Crohn's disease. AJR 1978;130:307–311.

Law D, Law R, Eiseman B. The continuing challenge of acute and perforated appendicitis. Am J Surg 1976;131:533–535.

Liberman JM, Haaga JR. Computed tomography of diverticulitis. J Comput Assist Tomogr 1983;7:431–433.

Louisy CL, Barton CJ. The radiological diagnosis of strongyloides stercoralis enteritis. Radiology 1971;98:535–541.

Merine D, Fishman EK, Jones B. Pseudomembranous colitis: CT evaluation. J Comput Assist Tomogr 1987;6:1017–1020.

Michalak DM, Cooney DR, Rhodes KH et al. Gastrointestinal mucromycoses in infants and children: a cause of gangrenous intestinal cellulitis and perforation. J Pediatr Surg 1980;15:320–324.

Philpotts LE, Heiken JP, Westcott MA, et al. Colitis: use of CT findings in differential diagnosis. Radiology 1994;190:445–449.

Ros PR, Buetow PC, Pantograg-Brown L. Pseudomembranous colitis. Radiology 1996;198:1–9.

Scatarige JC, Fishman EK, Crist DW, et al. Diverticulitis of the right colon: CT observations. AJR 1987;148:737–739.

Trinh T, Jones B, Fishman EK. Amyloidosis of the colon presenting as ischemic colitis: a case report and review of the literature. Gastrointest Radiol 1991;16:133–136.

Wank SA, Doffman DL, Miller MJ, et al. Prospective study of the ability of computed axial tomography to localize gastrinomas in patients with Zollinger-Ellison syndrome. Gastroenterology 1987;92:905–912.

Wolfe MM, Jenson RT. Zollinger-Ellison syndrome. N Engl J Med 1987;317:1200–1209.

Zollinger RW. The prognosis in diverticulitis of the colon. Arch Surg 1968;97:418–421.

Miscellaneous

Ballantyne GH, Brandner MD, Beart RW, et al. Volvulus of the colon. Ann Surg 1985;202:83–92.

Bova JC, Friedman AC, Weser E, et al. Adaptation of the ileum in nontropical sprue: reversal of the jejunoileal fold pattern. AJR 1985;144:299–302.

Clark RA. Computed tomography of bowel infarction. J Comp Assist Tomogr 1987;11:757–763.

Doubleday LC, Bernardino ME. CT findings in the perirectal area following radiation therapy. J Comp Assist Tomogr 1980;4:634–638.

Federle MP, Chun G, Jeffrey RB, et al. Computed tomographic findings in bowel infarction. AJR 1984;142:91–95.

Fishman EK, Zinreich ES, Jones B, et al. Computed tomographic diagnosis of radiation ileitis. Gastrointest Radiol 1984;9:149–152.

Fisk JD, Shulman HM, Greening RR, et al. Gastrointestinal radiographic features of human graft-vs-host disease. AJR 1981;136:329–336.

Hill LD. Incarcerated paraesophageal hernia. Am J Surg 1973;126:286–291.

Hillyard RW, El-Mahdi M, Schellhammer PF. Intestinal strictures complicating preoperative radiation therapy followed by radical cystectomy. J Urol 1986;136:98–101.

Iko BO, Teal JS, Siram SM, et al. Computed tomography of adult colonic intussusception: clinical and experimental studies. AJR 1984;143:769–772.

Jeffrey RB, Federle MP, Wall S. Value of computed tomography in detecting occult gastrointestinal perforation. J Comput Assist Tomogr 1983;7:825–827.

Jones B, Bayless T, Fishman EK. Lymphadenopathy in celiac disease: computed tomographic observations. AJR 1984;141:1127–1132.

Jones B, Kramer SS, Saral R, et al. Gastrointestinal inflammation after bone marrow transplantation: graft versus-host disease or opportunistic infection? AJR 1988;150:277–281.

Mathis JM, Zelenik ME, Staab EV. CT detection of bowel infarction. Comput Radiol 1985;9:177–179.

O'Connell DJ, Thompson AJ. Lymphoma of the colon: the spectrum of radiologic changes. Gastrointest Radiol 1978;2:377–385.

Olmsted WW, Cooper PH, Madewell JE. Involvement of the gastric antrum in Menetrier's disease. AJR 1976;126:524–529.

Pandolfo I, Blandio A, Gaeta M, et al. CT findings in palpable lesions of the anterior abdominal wall. J Comput Assist Tomogr 1986;10:629–633.

Perez C, Llauger J, Puig J, et al. Computed tomographic findings in bowel ischemia. Gastrointest Radiol 1989;14:241–245.

Reese DF, Hodgson JR, Dockerty MB. Giant hypertrophy of the gastric mucosa (Menetrier's disease): a correlation of the roentgenographic pathologic, and clinical findings. AJR 1962;88:619–626.

Rosen A, Korobkin M, Silverman PM, et al. Mesenteric vein thrombosis: CT identification. AJR 1984;143:83–86.

Rosenberg HK, Seola FT, Koch P, et al. Radiographic features of gastrointestinal graft-vs-host disease. Radiology 1981;138:371–374.

Salmonowiz E, Frick MP, Sommer G, et al. Symptomatic inguinal hernia: association with intraabdominal mass lesions. Gastrointest Radiol 1983;8:371–374.

Styles RA, Larsen CR. CT appearance of adult intussusception. J Comp Assist Tomogr 1983;7:331–333.

Williams SM, Harned RK, Settles RH. Adenocarcinoma of the stomach in association with Menetrier's disease. Gastrointest Radiol 1978;3:387–390.

Scott JR, Miller WT, Urso M, et al. Acute mesenteric infarction. AJR 1971;113:269–278.

Searcy RM, Malagelada JR. Menetrier's disease and idiopathic hypertrophic gastropathy. Ann Intern Med 1984;100:555–570.

Skaane P, Schindler G. Computed tomography of adult ileocolic intussusception. Gastrointest Radiol 1985;10:355–357.

Smerud MJ, Johnson CD, Stephens DH. Diagnosis of bowel infarction: a comparison of plain films and CT scans in 23 cases. AJR 1990;154:99–103.

Trier JS. Celiac sprue. N Engl J Med 1991;325:1709–1719.

Uflacker R, Goldany MA, Constant S. Resolution of mesenteric angina with percutaneous transluminal angioplasty of a superior mesenteric artery stenosis using a balloon catheter. Gastrointest Radiol 1980;5:367–369.

chapter 4

SPLEEN

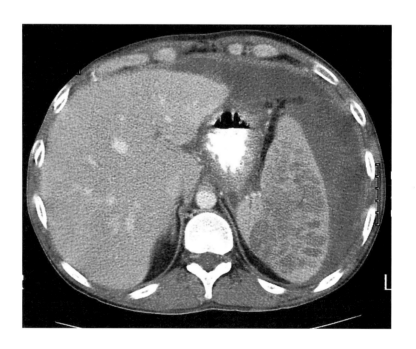

CASE 1

Clinical History: 49-year-old woman with weight loss and left upper quadrant pain.

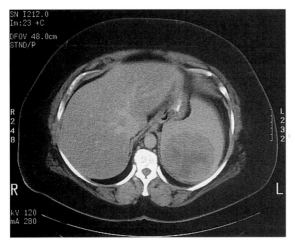

Figure 4.1 A

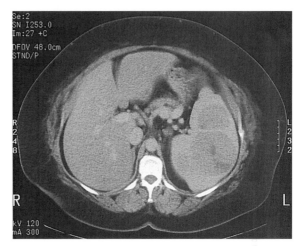

Figure 4.1 B

Findings: CECT demonstrates multiple large hypodense lesions within the spleen. No lesions are seen in the liver.

Differential Diagnosis: Abscess, lymphoma.

Diagnosis: Melanoma metastases.

Discussion: Metastatic disease to the spleen is uncommon and typically occurs in patients with widespread metastatic disease. Most metastases spread hematogenously via the splenic artery. Less common pathways include the splenic vein in patients with portal hypertension, lymphatics, and intraperitoneal seeding (such as in ovarian cancer). The most common primaries include melanoma, breast, lung, and ovary. Enhancement is seen in the periphery of these lesions with central areas of necrosis. This excludes predominantly cystic lesions such as hydatid cysts and pancreatic pseudocysts. The multiplicity and large size make hemangiomas less likely. This case is unusual because liver metastases are typically present in melanoma when splenic metastases of this size occur. Both abscess and lymphoma can present with large, hypodense lesions in the spleen without hepatic involvement. They would be excellent diagnostic considerations.

CASE 2

Clinical History: 73-year-old woman with weight loss.

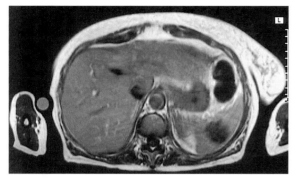

Figure 4.2 A

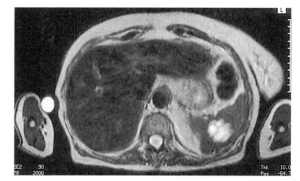

Figure 4.2 B

Findings: (A) T1WI shows a focal irregular low intensity lesion in the spleen. (B) This same lesion is hyperintense on the T2WI. The lesion has signal characteristics similar to water.

Differential Diagnosis: Hemangioma, lymphangioma, infarct, abscess, hematoma.

Diagnosis: Metastasis from ovarian cancer.

Discussion: Excluding lymphoma, metastases to the spleen are uncommon occurring in approximately 7% of patients with widespread malignancy. The most common metastases to the spleen are melanoma followed by breast, lung, ovary, and GI tract malignancies. The majority of metastases from these primaries are multiple but they can be solitary and diffusely infiltrating as well. The MR signal characteristics of splenic metastases are nonspecific being hypointense on the T1WI and hyperintense on the T2WI. The signal characteristic of this lesion is similar to CSF and is due to the high water content. Hemangiomas are hyperintense on T2WI but are not typically as hypointense on the T1WI, as is seen in this case. The exception is the cystic hemangiomas, which also follow the signal characteristic of water. Other cystic lesions such as infarct, lymphangioma, abscess, and hematoma can all have a similar appearance due to the high fluid content. Often biopsy is necessary to make the diagnosis.

CASE 3

Clinical History: 31-year-old man with left upper quadrant and splenomegaly.

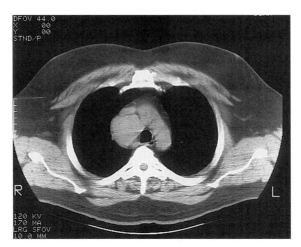

Figure 4.3 A

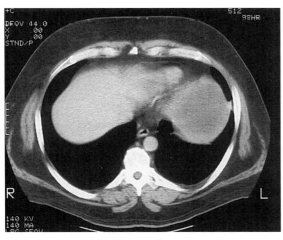

Figure 4.3 B

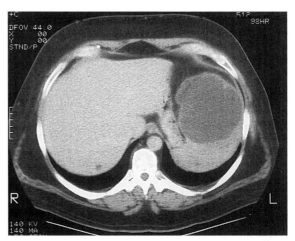

Figure 4.3 C

Findings: (A) CECT of the chest demonstrates large paratracheal adenopathy. (B, C) CECT of the abdomen demostrates a large 8-cm cystic lesion in spleen.

Differential Diagnosis: Abscess, infarct, metastasis, hemangioma, lymphangioma.

Diagnosis: Lymphoma.

Discussion: A single large mass in the spleen from lymphoma is unusual and is more commonly seen in high grade lymphoma in its advanced stages. Splenic lymphoma can become large and extend through the splenic capsule and involve adjacent organs such as the stomach or pancreas. Lymphoma does not enhance on CECT and the cystic necrosis seen in this case is rare. The large cystic mass seen in this example is indistinguishable from an abscess or infarct. The presence of the mediastinal adenopathy is the only clue to the diagnosis. The accuracy of detecting splenic lymphoma ranges from 50–65%. The presence of splenomegaly is nonspecific and ⅓ of these patients do not have splenic lymphoma. Diffuse lymphomatous involvement of the spleen (<5 mm) is also difficult to detect by CT as well. The presence of abdominal lymphadenopathy with splenic enlargement or lesions is highly suggestive of splenic lymphoma and may obviate the need for splenectomy.

CASE 4

Clinical History: 43-year-old woman who was kicked in the abdomen by a horse.

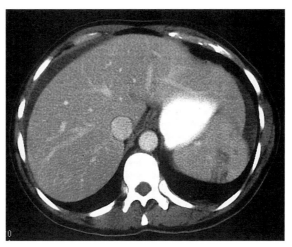

Figure 4.4 A

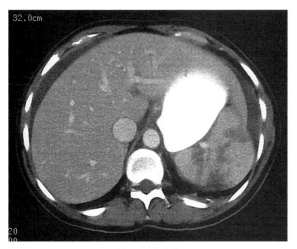

Figure 4.4 B

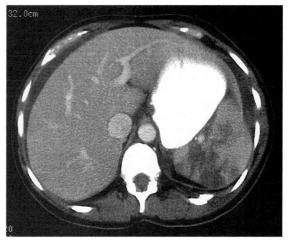

Figure 4.4 C

Findings: CECT demonstrates a stellate area of low attenuation in the spleen with extension to the splenic hilum.

Differential Diagnosis: None.

Diagnosis: Splenic fracture.

Discussion: Injury to the spleen can be demonstrated on a CT scan in several ways. There can be an intrasplenic or sub-capsular hematoma that typically appear as focal areas of low attenuation. Areas of high attenuation can also be present representing acute to subacute hemorrhage. A laceration can occur which will appear as a linear area of low attenuation which does not extend completely across the spleen. This is in contradiction to a fracture that will extend across the spleen, commonly to the splenic hilum. A shattered spleen involves multiple areas of fracture and hematoma, which results in a fragmented spleen. This case demonstrates a fracture of the spleen that extends completely across the spleen to involve the splenic hilum. In addition, larger focal areas of low attenuation are present, representing intrasplenic hematomas. Luckily for this patient, the hilar vessels were not injured and the hematocrit remained stable, thus requiring only conservative management.

CASE 5

Clinical History: 25-year-old man with diffuse joint pain.

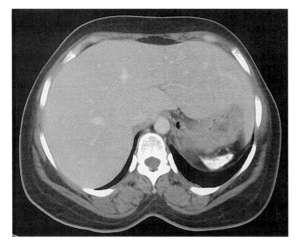

Figure 4.5 A

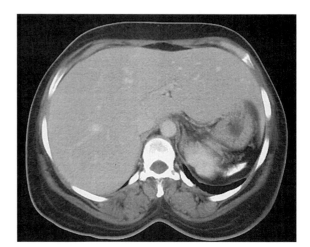

Figure 4.5 B

Findings: CECT demonstrates a densely calcified small spleen.

Differential Diagnosis: Hemochromatosis, Thorotrast.

Diagnosis: Autosplenectomy from sickle cell disease.

Discussion: Autosplenectomy or end-stage spleen is typically seen in patients who have homozygous sickle cell disease. During the first year of life, microinfarctions of the spleen occur secondary to the veno-occlusive disease. This leads to perivascular fibrosis with subsequent decrease in function and size of the spleen. In addition, there is hemosiderin and calcium deposition. Occasionally, the splenic calcifications can be seen on plain film, but they are much better detected on CT. The typical CT finding in sickle cell's autosplenectomy is a small calcified nonfunctioning spleen. Other causes for a dense spleen include secondary hemochromatosis and Thorotrast administration. In these processes, however, the liver is also frequently involved and will demonstrate increased attenuation on a NECT. Also, the small size of the spleen is more commonly seen in sickle cell disease rather than hemochromatosis due to the microinfarcts and fibrosis. The spleen in Thorotrast is also small but Thorotrast is also seen in the liver and abdominal lymph nodes.

CASE 6

Clinical History: 36-year-old asymptomatic woman.

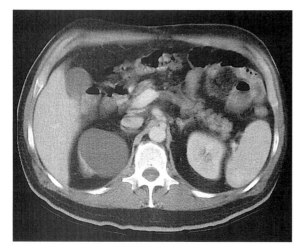

Figure 4.6 A

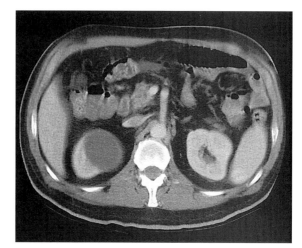

Figure 4.6 B

Findings: CECT demonstrates a 2-cm hyperdense lesion in the posterior portion of the spleen. A right renal cyst is present.

Differential Diagnosis: Angiosarcoma.

Diagnosis: Hemangioma.

Discussion: Hemangiomas are the most common benign primary tumor of the spleen. They can appear solid or cystic with central or peripheral calcifications. Typically, hemangiomas are asymptomatic but can rupture in up to 20% of cases when they become large. Hemangiomas can also be multiple and associated with a generalized angiomatosis (Klippel-Trenaunay-Weber syndrome). A hyperdense lesion in the spleen on a CECT is typical of a hemangioma. Most other lesions in the spleen are hypodense with variable contrast enhancement. Angiosarcomas can be hyperdense by CECT but are extremely rare and are secondary to Thorotrast (Thorium dioxide) administration. No other evidence of Thorotrast use is present such as a hyperdense liver and spleen. The age of the patient would also make it unlikely because Thorotrast use was discontinued in the 1950s.

CASE 7

Clinical History: 1-year-old girl with multiple congenital abnormalities status post a Kasai procedure for biliary atresia.

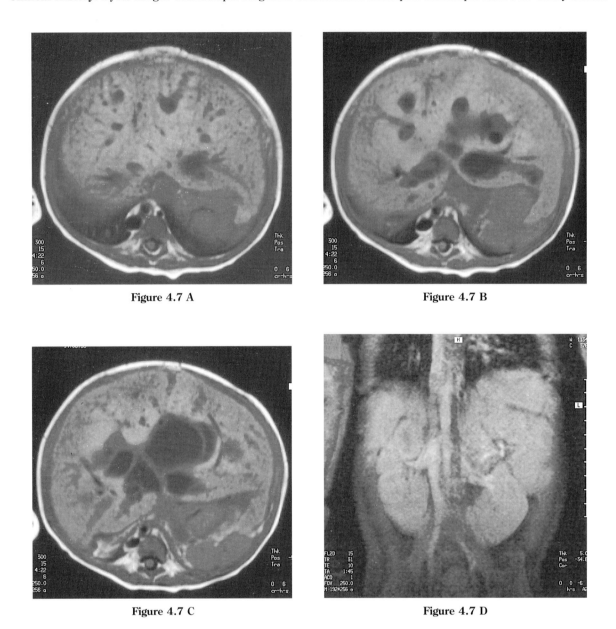

Figure 4.7 A

Figure 4.7 B

Figure 4.7 C

Figure 4.7 D

Findings: (A, B, C) T1WI axial images demonstrate a large midline liver with a loop of bowel seen in the porta hepatis sequela from the Kasai procedure. There is intrahepatic biliary dilatation. Note the multiple soft tissue masses in the left upper quadrant. A right-sided arch and azygous continuation is present on these images and the coronal gradient echo image (D).

Differential Diagnosis: None.

Diagnosis: Polysplenia.

Discussion: Polysplenia syndrome is a congenital abnormality involving multiple organ systems characterized by bilateral left-sidedness. These patients have bilateral morphologic left lungs, multiple spleens, azygous continuation of the inferior vena cava, and abdominal situs ambiguous. Other congenital abnormalities include cardiac anomalies (ventricular septal defects, transposition of the great vessels) and gastrointestinal anomalies (esophageal atresia, biliary atresia). The key findings in this case to make the diagnosis of polysplenia is the presence of a midline liver, right-sided aortic arch, azygous continuation of the inferior vena cava, and the history of a Kasai procedure for biliary atresia. With these findings and the multiple soft tissue masses in the left upper quadrant, the diagnosis of polysplenia is made. A nuclear medicine scan could be performed to confirm that the upper quadrant masses are multiple spleens.

CASE 8

Clinical History: 36-year-old woman involved in a motor vehicle accident.

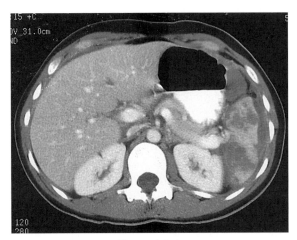

Figure 4.8 A

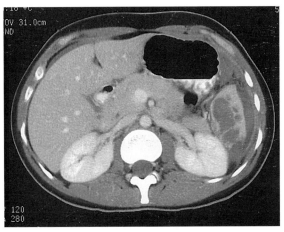

Figure 4.8 B

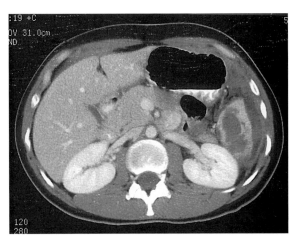

Figure 4.8 C

Findings: CECT demonstrates multiple focal areas of low attenuation throughout the spleen with subcapsular and extracapsular fluid.

Differential Diagnosis: None.

Diagnosis: Splenic rupture.

Discussion: The spleen is the most commonly injured organ after blunt trauma to the abdomen. This can be due to motor vehicle accidents, falls, or direct blows. Other injuries to the spleen include penetrating trauma and iatrogenous causes.

CT is excellent in detecting splenic injury with a sensitivity of approximately 90–95%. Typically splenic hematoma and laceration will appear as a low-density fluid collection on a CECT. On rare occasions, however, the hematoma can be isodense to the spleen on a CECT and hyperdense on a NECT. Therefore, some authors have advocated the use of both NECT and CECT for the evaluation of blunt abdominal trauma. The small subtle lesions missed by a CECT are frequently not surgical injuries so in most institutions, CECT only is performed.

This example is worrisome by CT criteria due to the presence of intraparenchymal, subcapsular, and extracapsular hemorrhage. The extracapsular extension can lead to massive intra-abdominal hemorrhage, which may not be clinically suspected until the CT is performed.

CASE 9

Clinical History: 58-year-old woman receiving chemotherapy.

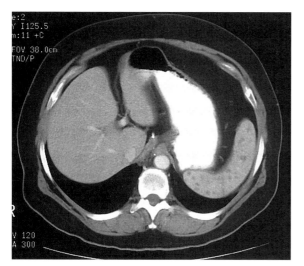

Figure 4.9 A

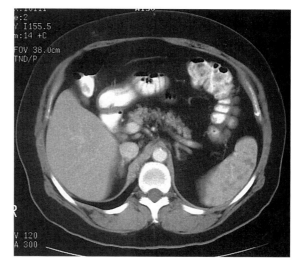

Figure 4.9 B

Findings: CECT demonstrates multiple small low attenuation lesions in the spleen.

Differential Diagnosis: Metastases, peliosis, lymphoma.

Diagnosis: Splenic candidiasis.

Discussion: Splenic fungal infections occur in patients who are immunocompromised from chemotherapy, leukemia, lymphoproliferative disorders, and HIV. The most common fungal organism is Candida followed by Aspergillus and Cryptococccus. Infection of the spleen is thought to be due to colonization of the gastrointestinal tract with widespread dissemination once the patient becomes neutropenic. Diagnosis is often difficult because blood cultures are negative in up to 50% of cases and the symptoms are nonspecific (fever, abdominal pain). The CT appearance is nonspecific with metastases and lymphoma having similar imaging findings. CT, however, is helpful in guiding biopsies and assessing response to treatment.

CASE 10

Clinical History: 41-year-old woman with weight loss and night sweats.

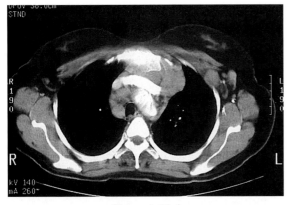

Figure 4.10 A

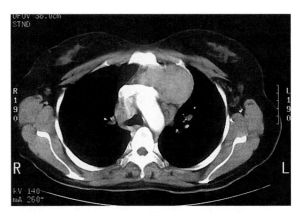

Figure 4.10 B

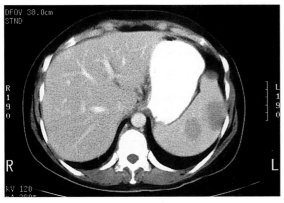

Figure 4.10 C

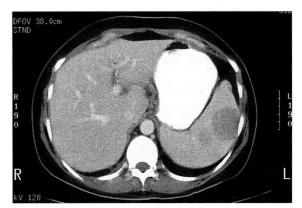

Figure 4.10 D

Findings: (A, B) CECT demonstrates adenopathy involving the anterior mediastinum, paratracheal, and pretracheal regions. (C, D) CECT of the abdomen demonstrates three low attenuation lesions within the spleen.

Differential Diagnosis: None.

Diagnosis: Lymphoma.

Discussion: Lymphomatous involvement of the spleen associated with nodal disease and systemic involvement is much more common than primary splenic lymphoma without nodal disease. Involvement of the spleen can be seen in both Hodgkin and nonHodgkin's lymphoma. CECT is accurate in detecting splenic lymphoma in its late stages but is less accurate in early stages where the lesions are small or diffusely infiltrating the spleen. In these cases, splenectomy is often necessary to confirm the diagnosis. Splenic lymphoma can present by CT imaging as diffuse splenic enlargement, multiple small masses (<2 cm), and one or multiple large masses. The presence of multiple hypodense lesions in the spleen is nonspecific and can be seen in metastases and abscesses. In this case, the presence of mediastinal involvement with multiple splenic lesions is almost diagnostic of lymphoma.

CASE 11

Clinical History: 68-year-old asymptomatic man with a remote history of trauma to the abdomen.

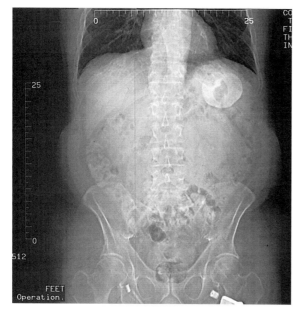

Figure 4.11 A

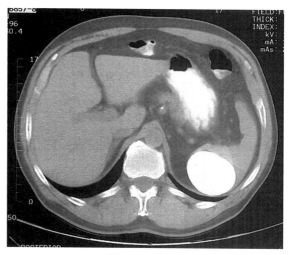

Figure 4.11 B

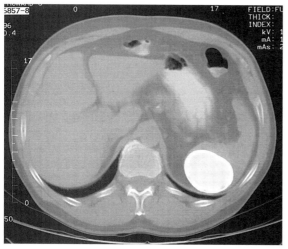

Figure 4.11 C

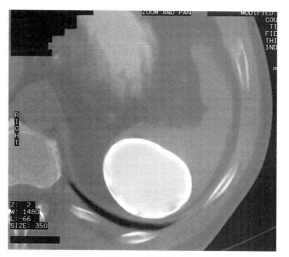

Figure 4.11 D

Findings: (A) CT scout image demonstrates a round calcified lesion in the left upper quadrant. (B) NECT demonstrates a 6-cm densely calcified lesion in the spleen. (C, D) Bone windows demonstrate that the center of this lesion is of water density.

Differential Diagnosis: Epidermoid cyst, postinfectious cyst, hydatid cyst, infarct, pancreatic pseudocyst.

Diagnosis: Posttraumatic cyst.

Discussion: Cysts in the spleen can be divided into true cysts (primary or epidermoid) and false cysts (secondary or posttraumatic). True cysts possess an endothelial lining. Secondary cysts do not possess an endothelial lining but have a fibrous capsule. They are a result of prior infections, infarctions, or hematoma within the spleen. False cysts tend to be subcapsular in location and can calcify in the periphery in up to 50% of the cases as in this example. Other lesions that can present with eggshell calcifications include epidermoid cysts, hydatid cysts, and pancreatic pseudocysts. Clinical history is helpful in these situations to help narrow the differential diagnosis. The remote history of trauma, lack of clinical symptoms, and calcified rim is suggestive of the diagnosis of posttraumatic (false) cyst.

CASE 12

Clinical History: 38-year-old woman with abdominal pain and a known hematological disorder.

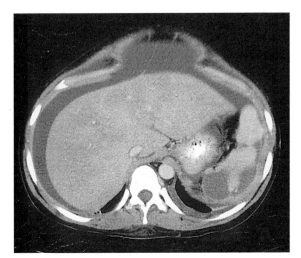

Figure 4.12 A

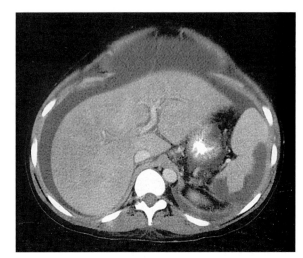

Figure 4.12 B

Findings: CECT demonstrates multiple peripheral low density defects in the spleen. Also note the patchy enhancement of the liver and nonvisualization of the hepatic veins. An abdominal wall defect is also present.

Differential Diagnosis: Subcapsular hematoma, metastases.

Diagnosis: Splenic infarcts and Budd-Chiari syndrome in polycythemia vera.

Discussion: The classic appearance for splenic infarcts is multiple peripheral low attenuation defects in the spleen. A subcapsular hematoma typically causes compression of the splenic parenchyma in a crescentic manner rather than scalloping the surface as is seen in this case. Hematogenous metastases can present with multiple peripheral defects but they typically involve the spleen diffusely. Serosal metastases such as from ovarian cancer, however, will typically scallop the surface of the spleen but will often demonstrate mass effect and bulge out beyond the expected contour of the spleen. Infarcts tend to preserve the splenic contour unless there is an associated subcapsular bleed. The finding of both Budd-Chiari syndrome and splenic infarcts is very suggestive of an underlying hypercoaguable state such as from a hematologic disorder. This patient was hypercoaguable due to polycythemia vera, which led to the splenic infarcts and thrombosis of the hepatic veins.

CASE 13

Clinical History: 74-year-old asymptomatic woman noted to have splenomegaly by physical examination.

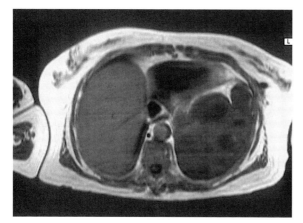

Figure 4.13 A

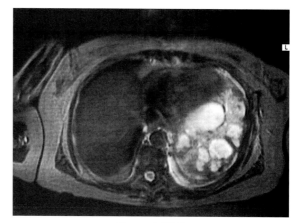

Figure 4.13 B

Findings: (A) T1-weighted image demonstrates multiple hypointense round lesions within the spleen. Some of the lesions have areas of high intensity. (B) These same lesions are hyperintense on the T2-weighted image.

Differential Diagnosis: Hemangioma, metastases, infarcts, abscess, hydatid cysts.

Diagnosis: Lymphangiomatosis.

Discussion: Lymphangiomas are benign vascular lesions comprised of cystic spaces filled with proteinaccous and fatty matcrial (lymph) rather than blood. These vascular spaces are lined by endothelium and can be single or multiple (lymphangiomatosis). Most lymphangiomas occur at a young age but can present later in life secondary to pain from hemorrhage into the vascular spaces. The MR characteristics of these lesions are similar to that of other cystic lesions. They will be hypointense on the T1WI and hyperintense on the T2WI. Because they contain proteinaceous/fatty material and can hemorrhage, these cystic spaces can have areas of high signal intensity on the T1WI as in this case. Lymphangiomas can be indistinguishable from infarcts, metastases, abscesses, and hydatid cysts. Clinical history is often helpful in narrowing the differential diagnoses.

CASE 14

Clinical History: 51-year-old man from Argentina presents with fever.*

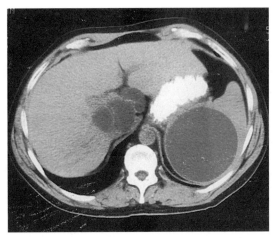

Figure 4.14 A

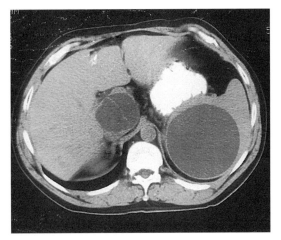

Figure 4.14 B

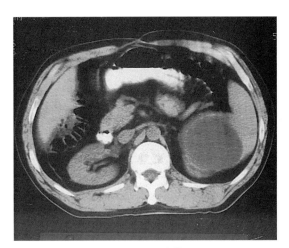

Figure 4.14 C

Findings: NECT demonstrates an 8-cm cyst in the posterior portion of the spleen. There is also a septated cystic lesion in the caudate lobe of the liver.

Differential Diagnosis: Epidermoid cyst, posttraumatic cyst, pancreatic pseudocyst, pyogenic abscess, infarct, neoplasm (hemangioma, lymphoma, lymphangioma, metastases).

Diagnosis: Echinococcal cyst.

Discussion: A cystic lesion in the spleen is a nonspecific finding. Cystic lesions can be congenital (epidermoid cyst), inflammatory (abscess, hydatid cyst), vascular (infarct, peliosis), posttraumatic (hematoma, false cyst), or neoplastic (hemangioma, lymphangioma, lymphoma, metastases). The finding of a second cystic lesion in the liver narrows the differential diagnosis considerably. The finding of simultaneous hepatosplenic cystic lesions can be seen in metastases, abscesses, and hydatid cysts. The other lesions are much less likely. *Echinococcus granulosus* is the most common organism and typically involves the liver, lung, bone, and brain. Involvement of the spleen can occur by either hematogenous spread or peritoneal seeding from a ruptured liver cyst. The lesion is typically water density with a thin wall that can occasionally calcify. Complications of hydatid cyst include cyst infection and anaphylaxis from rupture.

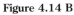

*Case courtesy of Luis Ros, MD, Zaragoza, Spain.

CT AND MRI OF THE ABDOMEN AND PELVIS

Clinical History: 64-year-old man with weight loss.

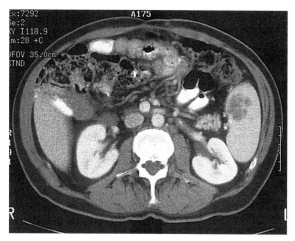

Figure 4.15 A

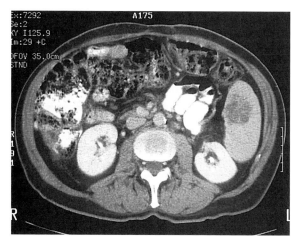

Figure 4.15 B

Figure 4.15 C

Findings: CECT demonstrates a 3-cm heterogeneously enhancing lesion in the spleen.

Differential Diagnosis: Lymphoma, metastasis, hamartoma, angiosarcoma.

Diagnosis: Hemangioma.

Discussion: Hemangioma can be divided histologically into three types: capillary, cavernous, and mixed. Cavernous hemangiomas typically have a combination of both solid and cystic components. The solid components enhance with intravenous contrast giving the lesion a heterogeneous appearance. Cavernous hemangiomas when solid can have the centripetal enhancement seen in hepatic hemangiomas. Capillary hemangiomas have homogeneous enhancement. A heterogenous hypodense lesion in the spleen is nonspecific. Most primary lesions of the spleen such as a hamartoma, angiosarcoma, and lymphoma can all have this appearance. Metastases are hypodense but will typically be multiple. Both abscesses and infarcts will not have enhancement of the central areas as is seen in this example.

CASE 16

Clinical History: 66-year-old woman with abdominal bloating and weight loss.

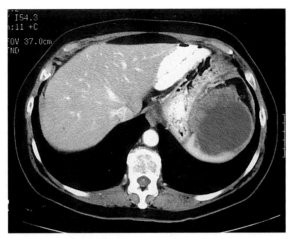

Figure 4.16 A

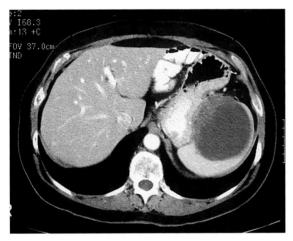

Figure 4.16 B

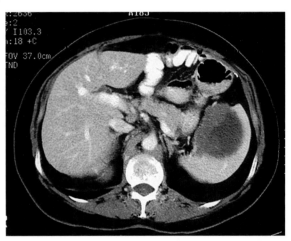

Figure 4.16 C

Findings: CECT demonstrates a large cystic mass involving the anterior surface of the spleen. Note the solid peripheral component to the cystic lesion.

Differential Diagnosis: Hydatid cyst, pancreatic pseudocyst, abscess, hematoma, infarct.

Diagnosis: Ovarian metastasis.

Discussion: A cystic lesion within the spleen is a nonspecific finding. Note, however, that a large portion of the lesion extends outside the expected confines of the spleen. This is the key to the diagnosis in this case. It is crucial to recognize this lesion is not an intraparenchymal lesion but is a serosal metastasis compressing on the splenic parenchyma. Serosal implants are commonly seen in malignancies that spread by intraperitoneal seeding such as ovarian and gastric carcinomas. The presence of a soft tissue component in the periphery of the cystic lesion makes a hydatid cyst and pancreatic pseudocyst unlikely. Hematomas and infarcts tend to be predominantly intraparenchymal. A large abscess would be difficult to exclude in this case and correlation with clinical history would be necessary.

Clinical History: 42-year-old woman with protein C deficiency presents with left upper quadrant pain.

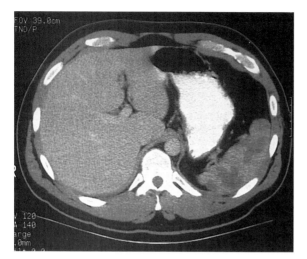

Figure 4.17 A

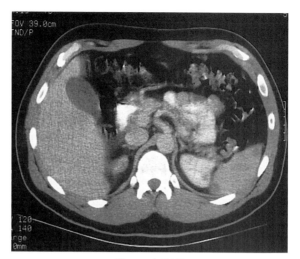

Figure 4.17 B

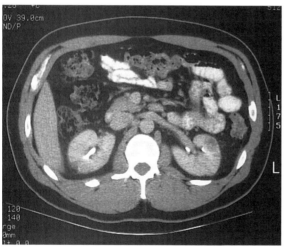

Figure 4.17 C

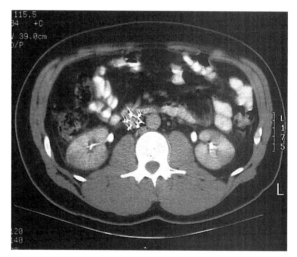

Figure 4.17 D

Findings: CECT demonstrates irregular areas of low attenuation in the spleen. Several wedge-shaped defects are also seen in the spleen and both kidneys. An IVC filter is in place as well.

Differential Diagnosis: Metastases, disseminated infection (Candidiasis).

Diagnosis: Multiple splenic and renal infarcts.

Discussion: There are multiple causes for splenic infarcts including emboli and hematologic diseases. Protein C deficiency results in a hypercoaguable state that can lead to emboli formation. The IVC filter was placed due to repeated pulmonary emboli despite anticoagulation. Infarcts can have a variety of CT appearances ranging from the classic peripheral wedge-shaped defect to focal round lesions and ill-defined areas of low attenuation. These lesions are best demonstrated on a CECT. During the acute stage, infarcts are ill-defined and heterogeneous due to areas of hemorrhage within them. As an infarct begins to fibrose, it will appear better demarcated and may cause contraction of the surrounding normal spleen. The appearance of the spleen in this example is nonspecific, and the lesions could represent metastases or fungal abscess. However, the clinical history and the finding of multiple wedge-shaped defects in the kidneys makes infarcts from multiple emboli the most likely diagnosis. The lack of findings in the liver supports the diagnosis of infarcts in the spleen and kidney since the liver has a dual blood supply making infarcts less common.

CASE 18

Clinical History: 76-year-old woman with right upper quadrant pain.

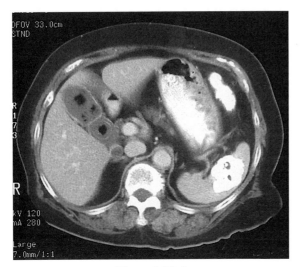

Figure 4.18 A

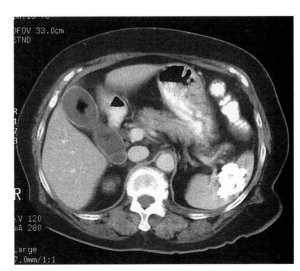

Figure 4.18 B

Findings: CECT demonstrates a heavily calcified lesion within the spleen. Incidentally, there are cholesterol stones within the gallbladder.

Differential Diagnosis: Posttraumatic cyst, postinfectious cyst.

Diagnosis: Calcified hemangioma.

Discussion: Hemangioma is the most common benign primary tumor of the spleen. It is most frequently seen in adults in their 4th through 6th decades of life. Unlike hemangiomas of the liver that are almost always a solid lesion in the spleen, hemangioma frequently has cystic areas (not filled with blood but with clear serous fluid) that can range from small (solid predominance) to very large (cyst predominance). Therefore, splenic hemangioma can present with both cystic and solid components with the solid component enhancing after contrast administration. Coarse thick calcifications can occur in the solid portions. These calcifications to appear in areas of fibrosis corresponding to previously thrombosed zones. Occasionally, like in this case, the entire hemangioma calcifies. The differential diagnoses for a densely calcified splenic mass includes posttraumatic and postinfectious lesions (sequelae of hematoma and abscess). These three entities can be indistinguishable by CT imaging.

CASE 19

Clinical History: 68-year-old man with abdominal discomfort.

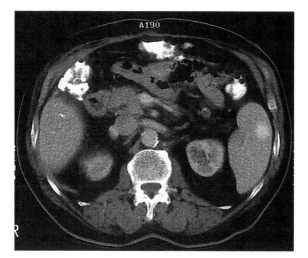

Figure 4.19 A

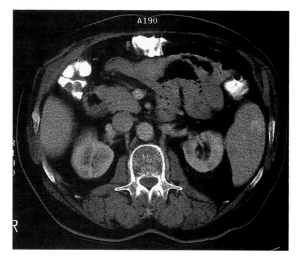

Figure 4.19 B

Findings: CECT demonstrates a 1.5-cm hyperdense lesion in the anterior portion of the spleen.

Differential Diagnosis: Angiosarcoma.

Diagnosis: Hemangioma.

Discussion: Hemangiomas are a benign nonencapsulated neoplasm of the spleen. They are typically less than 2 cm in size and are frequently found incidentally on CT scans. Patients are usually asymptomatic unless the lesion is very large. Large hemangiomas can lead to anemia, thrombocytopenia, and coagulopathy. The CT findings of hemangiomas depend on the histologic type. Hemangiomas can be capillary, cavernous, or mixed. This case is an example of a capillary hemangioma. Capillary hemangiomas have homogeneous contrast enhancement on CECT. They can be isodense or slightly hypodense on a NECT. Punctate or curvilinear calcifications can occur in these lesions. Another lesion that can appear as a hyperdense lesion on a CECT is an angiosarcoma, which may be secondary to Thorotrast administration.

CASE 20

Clinical History: 61-year-old man with left upper quadrant pain.

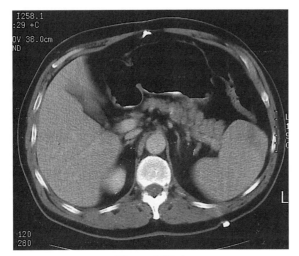

Figure 4.20 A

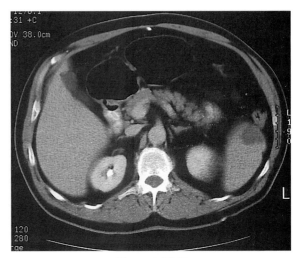

Figure 4.20 B

Findings: CECT demonstrates a 2.5-cm peripheral low attenuation lesion in the anterior portion of the spleen.

Differential Diagnosis: Lymphoma, abscess, primary or metastatic neoplasm.

Diagnosis: Splenic infarct.

Discussion: The appearance of a solitary low density lesion within the spleen is nonspecific. Hodgkins and non-Hodgkin's lymphoma can involve the spleen and appear as a solitary low attenuation lesion. No other evidence of adenopathy is present to support this diagnosis. A solitary metastasis is unusual especially without a history of a primary malignancy. Primary neoplasms of the spleen, although extremely rare, can also have this appearance including hemangiomas, lymphangiomas, and angiosarcomas. Bulging of the splenic contour, which is not present on this examination, would suggest a neoplasm or abscess. A splenic abscess frequently presents as a focal ill-defined low-density lesion in the spleen. The lack of fever and corroborating clinical history makes this diagnosis unlikely. The presence of a single peripheral low density lesion without significant clinical history for abscess or neoplasm makes an infarct the most likely diagnosis.

CASE 21

Clinical History: 30-year-old man presents with hypotension after minor trauma.

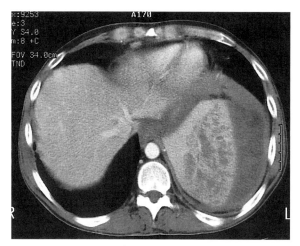

Figure 4.21 A

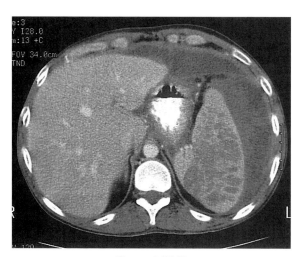

Figure 4.21 B

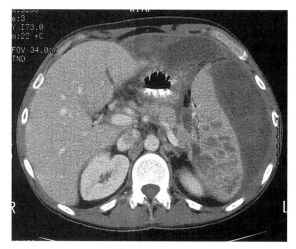

Figure 4.21 C

Findings: CECT demonstrates multiple low attenuation rounded lesions of varying sizes throughout the spleen. Note a large perisplenic hematoma.

Differential Diagnosis: Metastases, abscesses, splenic hematomas.

Diagnosis: Splenic peliosis.

Discussion: Peliosis is a rare disorder that can occur in the liver, spleen, bone marrow, and lungs. It is characterized by diffuse blood-filled cystic spaces of varying sizes ranging from less than 1 cm to up to 3 cm. The exact etiology is unknown, but peliosis is associated with various disorders including malignancies, hematologic diseases (Hodgkin disease, myeloma), steroids, and Thorotrast. Peliosis is usually found incidentally or at autopsy, but can present with hemoperitoneum due to rupture of a blood-filled cystic space. CT findings of peliosis are nonspecific with multiple low attenuation lesions in the spleen. The cystic spaces can occasionally demonstrate enhancement similar to a hemangioma with slow centripetal enhancement. The CT appearance can be similar to metastases, abscesses, and intrasplenic hematomas especially if there is an associated hemoperitoneum. The large amount of hemorrhage out of proportion to the trauma as well as the multiple lesions in the spleen suggested an underlying disorder. Peliosis was discovered at surgery.

CASE 22

Clinical History: 45-year-old man post splenectomy secondary to a motor vehicle accident.

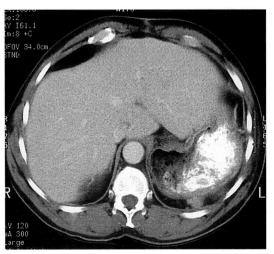

Figure 4.22 A

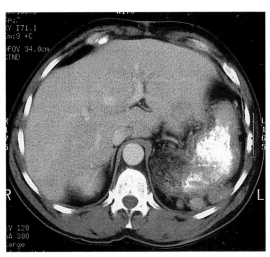

Figure 4.22 B

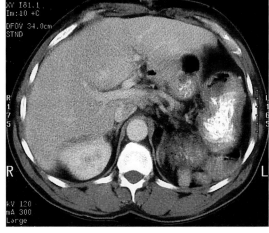

Figure 4.22 C

Findings: CECT demonstrates three small round soft tissue masses posterior to the stomach in the region of the splenic bed.

Differential Diagnosis: Lymph nodes, metastases.

Diagnosis: Splenosis.

Discussion: Splenosis results from autotransplantation of splenic tissue from a prior trauma that required splenectomy, which leads to implantation of splenic tissue anywhere in the peritoneal cavity. The blood supply to these implants is typically from small perforating vessels and will demonstrate enhancement similar to that of the normal spleen. Splenosis can develop several years after an injury and will be discovered incidentally because patients are asymptomatic. The CT appearance of splenosis involves numerous small round enhancing nodules of varying sizes. Without a history of splenic trauma, it would be difficult to distinguish splenosis from peritoneal metastases and lymph nodes. Nuclear medicine with the use of technetium-labeled heat-damaged erythrocytes or sulfur colloid is very sensitive and specific for detecting splenosis.

CASE 23

Clinical History: 60-year-old pedestrian struck by a car.

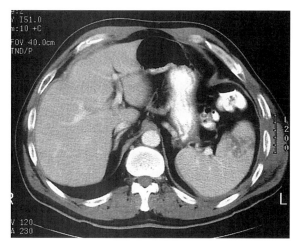

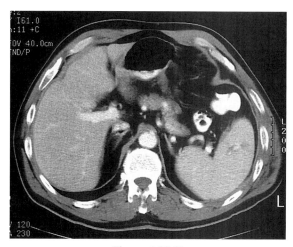

Figure 4.23 A   Figure 4.23 B

Findings: CECT demonstrates a linear low attenuation lesion through the anterior portion of the spleen. Note the small amount of fluid posteriorly.

Differential Diagnosis: None.

Diagnosis: Splenic laceration.

Discussion: The sensitivity of CT for detecting splenic trauma exceeds 90%, but the utility of CT for predicting outcome has been poor. Several CT grading systems for splenic trauma have been devised but the accuracy of these systems is questionable. Ranging from best to worst prognosis, most systems incorporate the findings of a subcapsular hematoma, extracapsular fluid, laceration with or without involvement of major vessels, and a shattered spleen. Despite the discrepancy in the accuracy of predicting outcome, two common factors indicate poor prognosis: hemodynamic instability and injuries to other organs. A shattered spleen with involvement of major vessels is usually suggestive of a large hemoperitoneum, which can lead to hypotension, cardiac decompensation, and shock. A subcapsular hematoma or a splenic fracture not involving the hilum will typically have a small amount of hemorrhage and be clinically stable. In this example, the fracture involved only a small portion of the spleen without major vessel injuries. This patient was hemodynamically stable and treated successfully with conservative management.

CASE 24

Clinical History: 73-year-old woman with left upper quadrant pain and fever.

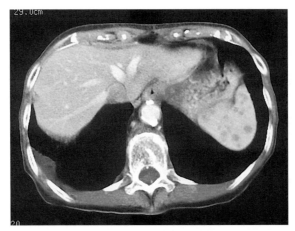

Figure 4.24 A

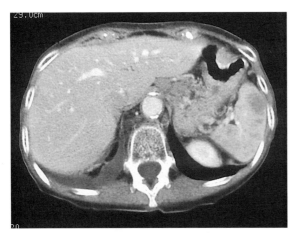

Figure 4.24 B

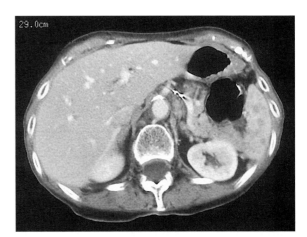

Figure 4.24 C

Findings: CECT demonstrates multiple small hypodense lesions within the spleen. No lesions are seen in the liver.

Differential Diagnosis: Metastases, abscesses, multiple hemangiomas or lymphangiomas.

Diagnosis: Lymphoma.

Discussion: Splenic lymphoma can either be primary to the spleen or part of a systemic involvement of all nodal groups. Primary lymphoma without nodal disease is rare and occurs more commonly in an older population (older than 50 years of age). Patients typically have nonspecific symptoms of fever, night sweats, and left upper quadrant pain. These symptoms can mimic an abscess. The CT findings of primary lymphoma can be nonspecific because nodal disease is not present to suggest the diagnosis of lymphoma. Metastases without coexistent liver involvement is unusual, but can be seen in hematogenous metastases especially melanoma. Infectious causes such as Candidiasis can also have this appearance but liver involvement is frequently present. These patients are usually immunocompromised as well.

CASE 25

Clinical History: 16-year-old asymptomatic male being evaluated for a left lower quadrant mass.

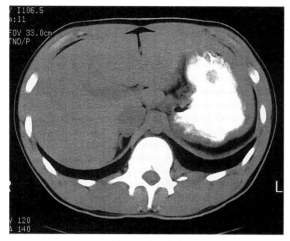

Figure 4.25 A

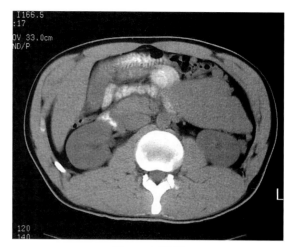

Figure 4.25 B

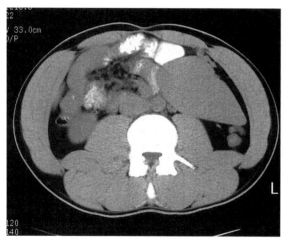

Figure 4.25 C

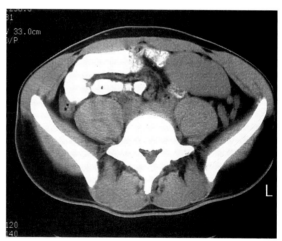

Figure 4.25 D

Findings: NECT demonstrates absence of a spleen in the left upper quadrant. A large well-defined soft issue mass is noted anterior to the left kidney and extends into the left pelvis.

Differential Diagnosis: None.

Diagnosis: Wandering spleen.

Discussion: Wandering or ectopic spleen occurs where there is laxity of the ligaments that fix the spleen in the left upper quadrant, leading to a mobile spleen. One theory on the etiology of a wandering spleen is that it is due to a congenital fusion abnormality of the ligaments, which leads to hypermobility. Another theory suggests that it may be acquired from the effects of hormones. Although most patients are asymptomatic, a complication of a wandering spleen includes torsion that results in chronic intermittent abdominal pain. This can lead to venous congestion and splenic infarcts. Chronic torsion can produce omental and peritoneal adhesions that can form a thick capsule around the spleen. Diagnosis can be made by the absence of the spleen in the normal location and the presence of a mass similar in appearance to a normal spleen in an abnormal location. Diagnosis can be confirmed with a nuclear medicine sulfur colloid scan. Treatment is splenectomy in patients with symptoms of intermittent torsion.

CASE 26

Clinical History: 64-year-old woman from Spain with abdominal pain.*

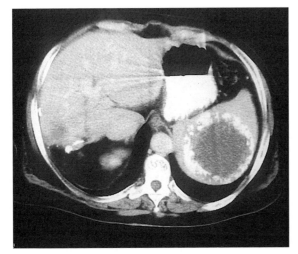

Figure 4.26 A

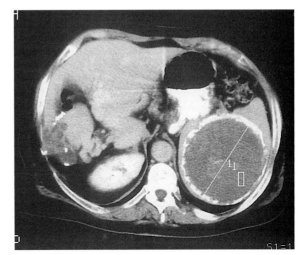

Figure 4.26 B

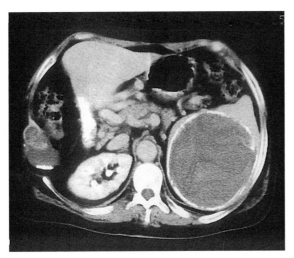

Figure 4.26 C

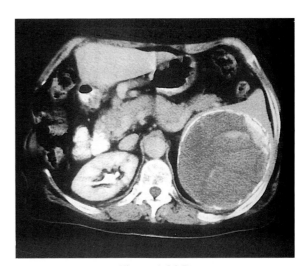

Figure 4.26 D

Findings: CECT demonstrates a 10-cm round cystic lesion within the spleen with peripheral calcifications. Curvilinear calcifications are present centrally within the cyst. Note a second calcified cystic lesion extending off the right lobe of the liver.

Differential Diagnosis: Epidermoid (congenital) cyst, posttraumatic (false) cyst, postinfectious cyst, pancreatic pseudocyst, splenic artery aneurysm, infarct.

Diagnosis: Hydatid cyst.

Discussion: Endemic areas for *Echinococcus granulosus* include Argentina, Greece, Spain, Middle East countries, and Australia. Often, the clinical findings are nonspecific including splenomegaly, fever, and abdominal pain. Available immunologic studies are specific for hydatid disease and can be used to confirm the diagnosis. CT findings of hydatid cysts include a well-defined wall of splenic parenchyma called the pericyst or ectocyst. This can calcify as in this case. Other cystic splenic lesions with peripheral eggshell calcifications include posttraumatic cyst, postinfectious cyst, epidermoid cyst, and pancreatic pseudocyst. The finding of a second lesion in the liver is suggestive of hydatid disease. Another finding in this case suggestive of echinococcal cyst includes daughter cyst formation in the center of the lesion. Low attenuation internal septa are seen representing the daughter cysts, which are budding from the inner germinal layer (endocyst). These can calcify as in this case. The high-attenuation contents of the cyst represent the hydatid sand, which is composed of scolices and debris.

*Case courtesy of Luis Ros, MD, Zaragoza, Spain

CASE 27

Clinical History: 69-year-old man with abdominal pain and elevated serum amylase.

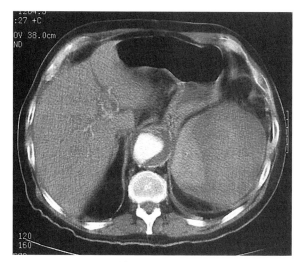

Figure 4.27 A

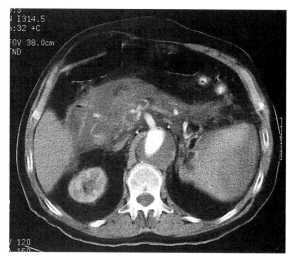

Figure 4.27 B

Findings: CECT demonstrates a large, subcapsular high attenuation splenic fluid collection, which displaces the spleen medially. Extensive pancreatitis is present with thrombosis of the splenic and portal veins. Incidentally noted is an abdominal aortic aneurysm.

Differential Diagnosis: None.

Diagnosis: Subcapsular hematoma secondary to pancreatitis.

Discussion: There are many complications associated with pancreatitis including pancreatic necrosis, abscess formation, pseudoaneurysms, and splenic vein thrombosis. With splenic vein thrombosis, there is formation of collateral circulation and varices in an attempt to reach the superior mesenteric vein. These include gastric varices and omental collaterals. Even with these collateral pathways, venous congestion is present in the spleen, which can lead to infarcts and subsequent hemorrhage. In addition, pancreatic enzymes from pancreatitis can also cause damage to the spleen making it more susceptible to minor injuries.

SUGGESTED READINGS

Trauma

Do HM, Cronan JJ. CT appearance of splenic injuries managed nonoperatively. AJR 1991;157:757–760.

Jeffrey RB, Laing FC, Federle MP, et al. Computed tomography of splenic trauma. Radiology 1981;141:729–732.

Malangoni MA, Cue JI, Fallat ME, et al. Evaluation of splenic injury by computed tomography and its impact on treatment. Ann Surg 1990;211:592–599.

Mirvis SE, Whitley NO, Gens DR. Blunt splenic trauma in adults: CT-based classification and correlation with prognosis and treatment. Radiology 1981;171:33–39.

Naylor R, Coln D, Shires GT. Morbidity and mortality from injuries to the spleen. J Trauma 1974;14:773–778.

Resciniti A, Fink MP, Raptopoulos, et al. Nonoperative treatment of adult splenic trauma: development of a computed tomographic scoring system that detects appropriate candidates for expectant management. J Trauma 1988;128:828–831.

Umlas SL, Cronan JJ. Splenic trauma: Can CT grading systems enable prediction of successful nonsurgical treatment? Radiology 1991;178:481–487.

Wolfman NT, Bechtold RE, Scharling ES, et al. Blunt upper abdominal trauma: evaluation by CT. AJR 1992;158:492–501.

Miscellaneous

Allen KB, Gay BB, Skandalakis JE. Wandering spleen: anatomic and radiologic considerations. South Med J 1992;85:976–984.

Balcar I, Seltzer SE, Davis S, et al. CT patterns of splenic infarction: a clinical and experimental study. Radiology 1984;151:723–729.

Dachman AH, Ros PR, Olmsted WW, et al. Nonparasitic splenic cysts: a report of 52 cases with radiologic-pathologic correlation. AJR 1986;147:537–542.

Darling JD, Flickinger FW. Splenosis mimicking neoplasm in the perirenal space: CT characteristics. J Comput Assist Tomogr 1990;14:839–841.

Gentry LR, Brown JM, Lindgren RD. Splenosis: CT demonstration of heterotopic autotransplantation of splenic tissue. J Comput Assist Tomogr 1982,6.1184–1187.

Gorden DH, Burell MI, Levin DC, et al. Wandering spleen—the radiological and clinical spectrum. Radiology 1977;125:39–46.

Jaroch MT, Broughan TA, Hermann RE. The natural history of splenic infarction. Surgery 1986;100:743–749.

Magid D, Fishman EK, Charache S, et al. Abdominal pain in sickle cell disease: the role of CT. Radiology 1987;163:325–328.

Magid D, Fishman EK, Seigelman SS. Computed tomogrpahy of the spleen and liver in sickle cell disease. AJR 1984;143:245–249.

Shiels WE, Johnson JF, Stephenson SR, et al. Chronic torsion of the wandering spleen. Pediatr Radiol 1989;19:465–467.

Neoplasms

Dawes LG, Malangoni MA. Cystic masses of the spleen. Am Surg 1986;52:333–336.

Duddy MJH, Calder CJ. Cystic haemangioma of the spleen: findings on ultrasound and computed tomography. Br J Radiol 1989;62:180–182.

Ferrozzi F, Bova D, Draghi F, et al. CT findings in primary vascular tumors of the spleen. AJR 1996;166:1097–1101.

Fishman EK, Kuhlman JE, Jones RJ. CT of lymphoma: spectrum of disease. Radiographics 1991;11:647–669.

Glatstein E, Guernsey JM, Rosenberg SA, et al. The value of laparotomy and splenectomy in the staging of Hodgkins's disease. Cancer 1969;24:709–718.

Hahn PF, Weissledger R, Stark DD, et al. MR imaging of focal splenic tumors. AJR 1988;150:823–827.

Ros PR, Moser RP, Dachman AH, et al. Hemangioma of the spleen: radiologic-pathologic correlation in ten cases. Radiology 1987;162:73–77.

Rabushka LS, Kawashima A, Fishman EK. Imaging of the spleen: CT with supplemental MR examination. Radiographics 1994;14:307–332.

Rao BK, AuBuchon J, Lieberman LM, et al. Cystic lymphangiomatosis of the spleen: a radiologic-pathologic correlation. Radiology 1981;141:781–782.

Strijk SP, Wagener DJT, Bogman MJJT, et al. The spleen in Hodgkin disease: diagnostic value of CT. Radiology 1985;154:753–757.

Urrutia M, Mergo, PJ, Ros PR, et al. Cystic masses of the spleen: radiologic-pathologic correlation. Radiographics 1996;16:107–129.

Infection

Callen PW, Filly RA, Marcus FS. Ultrasonogrpahy and computed tomography in the evaluation of hepatic microabscesses in the immunosuppressed patient. Radiology 1980;136:433–434.

Chew FS, Smith PL, Barboriak D. Candidal splenic abscesses. AJR 1981;156:447.

Franquet T, Montes M, Lecumbern FJ, et al. Hydatid disease of the spleen: imaging findings in nine patients. AJR 1990;154:525–528.

Pierkarski J, Federle MP, Moss AA, et al. Computed tomography of the spleen. Radiology 1980;135:683–689.

Shirkhoda A. CT findings in hepatosplenic and renal candidiasis. J Comput Assist Tomogr 1987;11:795–798.

chapter 5

KIDNEYS, URETER, AND BLADDER

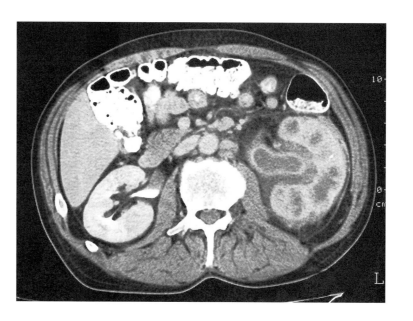

Clinical History: 56-year-old woman with abdominal pain and profound weight loss.

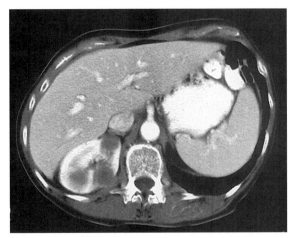

Figure 5.1 A

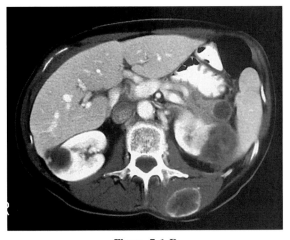

Figure 5.1 B

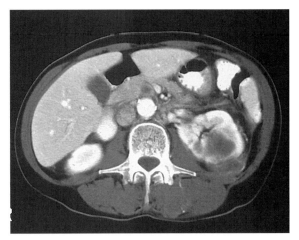

Figure 5.1 C

Findings: CECT demonstrates multiple low attenuation rim-enhancing lesions in both kidneys. A rim-enhancing lesion is seen in the tail of the pancreas and in the left paraspinal muscle.

Differential Diagnosis: Lymphoma, abscess.

Diagnosis: Lung cancer metastases.

Discussion: Metastases to the kidneys are commonly seen at time of autopsy, being nearly four times more common than a primary renal neoplasm. Typically there is widespread metastatic disease when renal metastases are present. The most common primary malignancies include melanoma, lung, breast, and colon cancer. Patients are usually asymptomatic from the renal metastases but can occasionally have hematuria if there is invasion of the collecting system. There is a limited differential diagnosis for multiple renal masses. This includes metastases, lymphoma, multiple renal cell carcinomas, and abscesses. Lymphoma is usually part of a generalized process and widespread lymphadenopathy is usually present. Multiple renal cell carcinomas are rare and is typically seen in patients with von Hippel-Lindau disease. The presence of other lesions in the pancreas and paraspinal muscles makes metastatic disease the best diagnosis.

CASE 2

Clinical History: 23-year-old man with weight loss and night sweats.

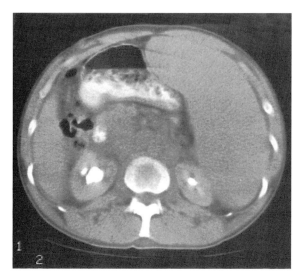

Figure 5.2 A

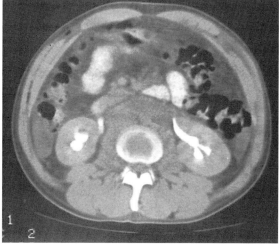

Figure 5.2 B

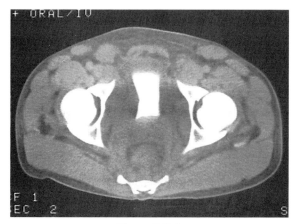

Figure 5.2 C

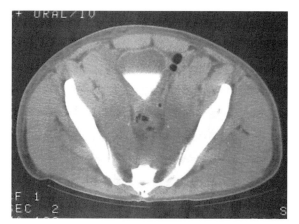

Figure 5.2 D

Findings: (A, B) CECT demonstrates splenomegaly and retroperitoneal adenopathy. (C, D) CECT demonstrates an elongated, triangular-shaped bladder due to surrounding soft tissue masses in the pelvis.

Differential Diagnosis: Pelvic lipomatosis, pelvic hematoma, pelvic fibrosis, pelvic tumor, iliopsoas hypertrophy, normal variant.

Diagnosis: Pelvic lymphoma producing a pear-shaped bladder.

Discussion: A pear- or teardrop-shaped bladder by plain film can be due to multiple etiologies including pelvic lipomatosis, pelvic hematoma or abscess, pelvic neoplasm, and iliopsoas hypertrophy. These can be easily differentiated by CT imaging. The presence of fat surrounding the bladder is diagnostic of pelvic lipomatosis. Pelvic lipomatosis is seen commonly in asymptomatic black men in their fourth decades. Pelvic hematomas are associated with pelvic fractures secondary to trauma with high-density fluid often present. A soft tissue mass in the pelvis compressing the bladder can be due to a pelvic tumor (uterine, prostatic, ovarian) or from adenopathy in patients with lymphoma. In this case, the presence of splenomegaly with retroperitoneal and pelvic adenopathy is diagnostic of lymphoma.

CASE 3

Clinical History: 63-year-old mentally handicapped woman presents with abdominal pain.

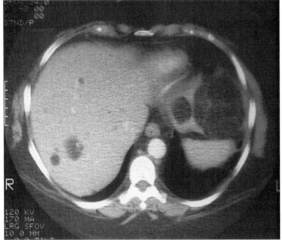

Figure 5.3 A

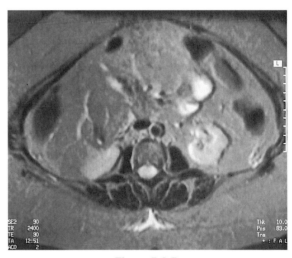

Figure 5.3 B

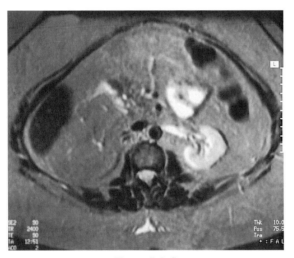

Figure 5.3 C

Figure 5.3 D

Findings: (A, B) CECT demonstrates a 10-cm fatty mass just above the right kidney as well as multiple fatty masses in the liver. (C, D) T2-weighted images demonstrates the fatty signal intensity mass arising from the upper pole of the right kidney.

Differential Diagnosis: None.

Diagnosis: Tuberous sclerosis with hepatic and renal angiomyolipomas.

Discussion: Tuberous sclerosis can involve multiple organ systems in the body including the heart, lungs, and brain. In the abdomen, there can be multiple angiomyolipomas involving most commonly the kidneys but also the liver. Within the angiomyolipomas there will be variable amounts of mature adipose tissue, smooth muscle, and thick-walled blood vessels. Clinically these patients have mental retardation, seizures, and adenoma sebaceum in the face. CT and MR are often diagnostic due to their ability to detect fat. On CT, the lesions will have a negative Houndsfield unit on both NECT and CECT. On MR, the lesions will follow the signal intensity of adjacent fat in the abdomen and subcutaneous tissues. In addition, fat suppression techniques can also be used to aid in the diagnosis. The presence of multiple fat containing lesions within the liver and kidneys is virtually diagnostic of tuberous sclerosis.

CASE 4

Clinical History: 64-year-old woman with left flank pain and fever.

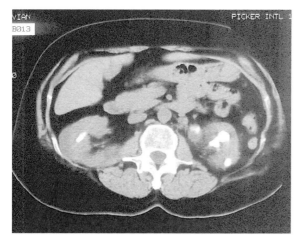

Figure 5.4 A

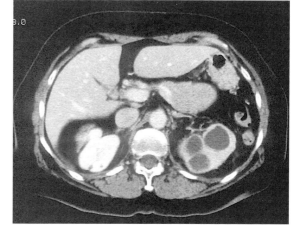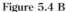

Figure 5.4 B

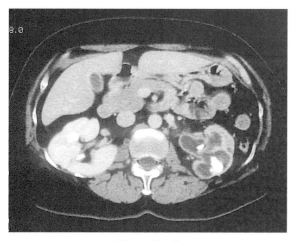

Figure 5.4 C

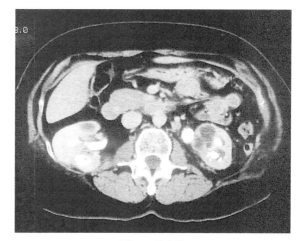

Figure 5.4 D

Findings: (A) NECT demonstrates multiple large calcifications within both kidneys and the left ureter. (B, C, D) CECT demonstrates decreased perfusion to the left kidney. There is severe dilatation of the left calyces, pelvis, and proximal ureter.

Differential Diagnosis: Xanthogranulomatous pyelonephritis.

Diagnosis: Severe left hydronephrosis due to renal calculi.

Discussion: Causes for hydronephrosis are numerous including renal calculi, neoplasms, and trauma. The most common locations for obstruction from a stone are the ureterovesical junction, ureteropelvic junction, and pelvic inlet. Acute hydronephrosis can lead to urinary stasis and infection. CT findings of hydronephrosis include dilatation of the collecting system to the level of obstruction. NECT is useful for detecting stones in the collecting system and finding an obstructing calculi in the ureters. CECT is useful for assessing perfusion to the kidney, which is often diminished in acute obstruction. This case nicely demonstrates on the NECT multiple renal stones in both kidneys including the obstructing stone in the left ureter. The stones could have been missed if only CECT would have been performed. There is no perirenal inflammation present to suggest superimposed infection such as in focal bacterial nephritis or xanthogranulomatous pyelonephritis.

CASE 5

Clinical History: 32-year-old man with a palpable right flank mass.

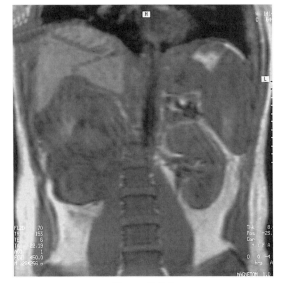

Figure 5.5 A

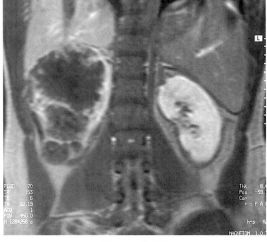

Figure 5.5 B

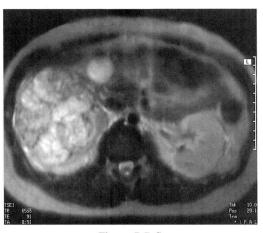

Figure 5.5 C

Findings: (A) Coronal T1WI demonstrates a large 15-cm heterogeneous isointense mass involving the right kidney without any normal kidney seen. (B) Coronal post-gadolinium T1WI demonstrates enhancement of the periphery of the tumor as well as the septations. (C) Axial T2WI demonstrates the lesion to be hyperintense with areas of necrosis.

Differential Diagnosis: Renal abscess, oncocytoma, adenoma.

Diagnosis: Renal cell carcinoma.

Discussion: The use of MRI for renal cell carcinoma has been limited due to the success of CT. CT possesses better spatial resolution than MRI and is better tolerated by most patients. Renal cell carcinoma can be isointense to normal kidney on both T1WI and T2WI. For a small lesion, it can be difficult to separate the neoplasm from the normal renal parenchyma. Because renal cell carcinomas are hypervascular, the use of gadolinium is helpful in detecting these smaller lesions. Often a heterogeneous signal is seen in the tumor due to necrosis and hemorrhage, which is easily detected by MRI. MRI is useful in detecting tumor extension into the perirenal space, involvement of Gerota's fascia, and extension into the renal vein and IVC. Because of its multiplanar capabilities, MRI is helpful in separating renal neoplasms from adrenal or perirenal neoplasms. This case demonstrates the typical findings of a large renal cell carcinoma. It is isointense on T1WI with areas of necrosis and enhancement by gadolinium. A large abscess, oncocytoma, and renal adenoma may have a similar appearance.

CASE 6

Clinical History: 17-year-old woman post automobile accident.

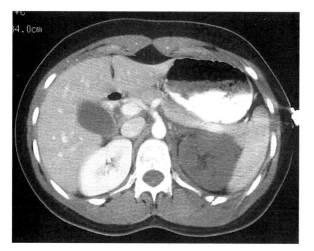

Figure 5.6 A

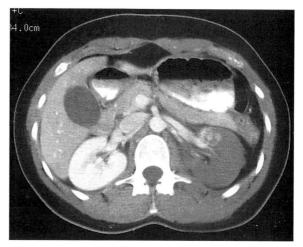

Figure 5.6 B

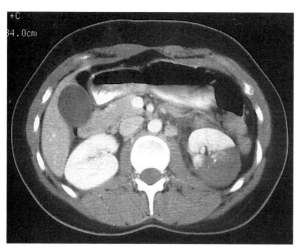

Figure 5.6 C

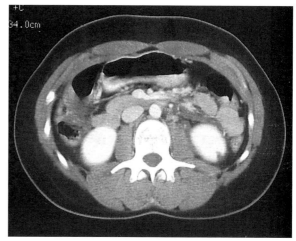

Figure 5.6 D

Findings: Four images from a CECT demonstrate no enhancement of the upper pole of the left kidney with normal enhancement of the lower pole. Note that the renal vein is patent.

Differential Diagnosis: None.

Diagnosis: Posttraumatic left renal artery occlusion in a patient with dual arterial supply.

Discussion: The kidneys are relatively protected from injury by the thoracic cage, vertebral column, perinephric fat, and surrounding fascia. A sign of possible renal injury is fracture of the lower ribs or vertebral bodies. With rapid deceleration from an automobile accident, there is tension placed on the renal pedicle, which can lead to laceration or intimal tear and subsequent occlusion of the renal artery or vein. Blunt trauma can also cause occlusion of the renal vessels. Kidneys can often have dual arterial supply as in this case. The renal artery supplying the upper pole of the left kidney is occluded from the patient's trauma resulting in no blood flow to the upper pole. The second left renal artery supplies the lower pole, which enhances normally. Contrast is seen in the renal vein ruling out a traumatic renal vein thrombosis. Surgery for revascularization is often attempted in these patients to salvage the kidney.

CASE 7

Clinical History: 65-year-old man with hematuria and long history of smoking.

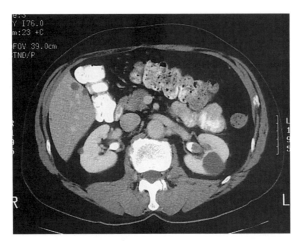

Figure 5.7 A

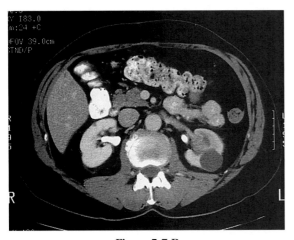

Figure 5.7 B

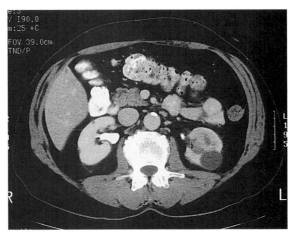

Figure 5.7 C

Findings: CECT demonstrates a 3-cm solid mass in the left renal pelvis with a small filling defect seen in the proximal ureter. Bilateral renal cysts and hepatic cysts are also present.

Differential Diagnosis: Renal cell carcinoma, tuberculosis.

Diagnosis: Transitional cell carcinoma.

Discussion: There are many different etiologies associated with transitional cell carcinoma. These include cigarette smoking, cytoxan therapy, analgesic use (phenacetin), and industrial chemicals (aromatic amines). Transitional cell carcinoma can be single or multiple and is bilateral in approximately 2% of the cases. Treatment is usually radical nephroureterectomy. A filling defect in the proximal ureter can be due to many causes including blood clot, fungus ball, polyp, neoplasm (transitional cell carcinoma), or sloughed papilla in papillary necrosis. The presence of a soft tissue mass in the renal pelvis limits the differential to transitional cell carcinoma, blood clot, and fungus ball. The lesion demonstrates enhancement, which eliminates the latter two choices. A renal cell carcinoma, which can enhance, rarely invades the collecting system. The best diagnosis in this case is transitional cell carcinoma.

CASE 8

Clinical History: 17-year-old male with repeated episodes of hematemesis.

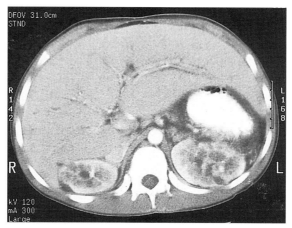

Figure 5.8 A

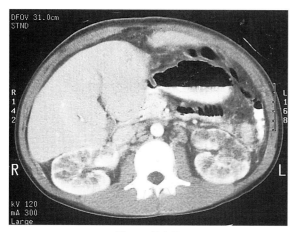

Figure 5.8 B

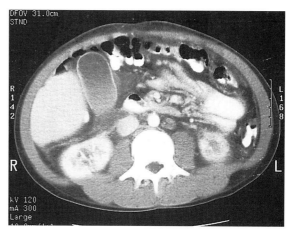

Figure 5.8 C

Findings: CECT demonstrates bilateral enlarged kidneys with poor enhancement of the medullary portion of the kidneys. Note the striated appearance of the kidneys. The liver is also enlarged with attenuated vessels and periportal lucency.

Differential Diagnosis: None.

Diagnosis: Autosomal recessive polycystic kidney disease (ARPCKD).

Discussion: Autosomal recessive polycystic kidney disease constitutes a spectrum of abnormalities that can present either in the newborn period or in childhood. If ARPCKD manifests itself in the newborn, the predominant abnormality is the renal disorder, which leads to death in the first few days of life. The childhood form has a milder renal disease with congenital hepatic fibrosis being the predominant abnormality. These patients die from liver failure and gastrointestinal bleeds secondary to portal hypertension. The kidneys are enlarged but typically function poorly. There are inumerable small cysts (1–2 mm) found primarily in the medullary portion of the kidneys. These small cysts do not enhance with contrast administration. Tubular ectasia is also present, which can lead to contrast stasis giving the kidneys a typically striated appearance. The presence of hepatic fibrosis and enlarged kidneys with a striated appearance is virtually diagnostic of autosomal recessive polycystic kidney disease.

CASE 9

Clinical History: 38-year-old woman with history of pancreatitis.

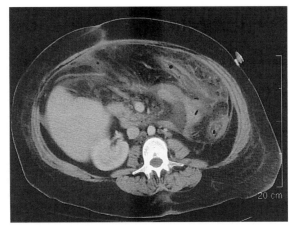

Figure 5.9 A

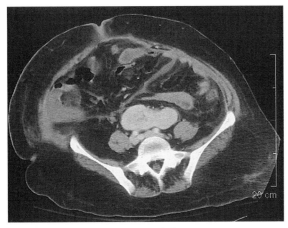

Figure 5.9 B

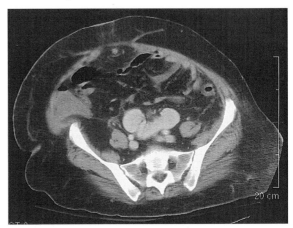

Figure 5.9 C

Findings: (A) CECT of the abdomen demonstrates absence of a kidney in the left renal fossa. Inflammatory changes are noted around the pancreas. (B, C) CECT of the pelvis demonstrates a kidney located in the midline, just anterior to the iliac vessels.

Differential Diagnosis: None.

Diagnosis: Pelvic kidney.

Discussion: The kidney normally migrates cephalad from the pelvis to the upper abdomen. Initially, the kidney receives its blood supply from the iliac artery and then the aorta. If there is an abnormality in the spine or blood supply to the kidney, then cephalad migration will be halted. The most common form of renal ectopy is a pelvic kidney. Pelvic kidney is often associated with hydronephrosis and vesicoureteral reflux, which can lead to repeated infections. Other congenital abnormalities are also associated with a pelvic kidney, including genitourinary malformations (ureteropelvic junction obstruction, cryptorchidism, hypospadia, and vaginal agenesis), gastrointestinal malformations (malrotation, imperforate anus), and cardiac malformations (septal defects). In up to 50% of patients with a pelvic kidney, the contralateral kidney will have an abnormality. Ultrasound and CT is typically diagnostic, obviating further workup.

CASE 10

Clinical History: 36-year-old woman with right flank pain and fever.

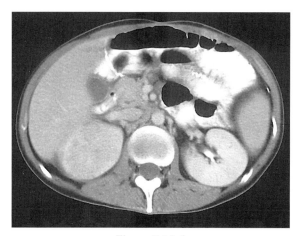

Figure 5.10 A

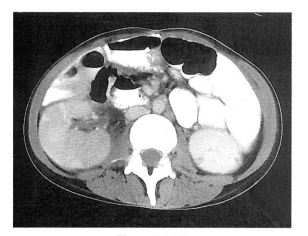

Figure 5.10 B

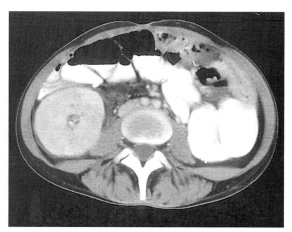

Figure 5.10 C

Findings: CECT demonstrates an enlarged right kidney with slight decreased enhancement.

Differential Diagnosis: Renal vein thrombosis.

Diagnosis: Acute pyelonephritis.

Discussion: Acute pyelonephritis is the most common infection involving the kidney. It is usually the result of an ascending infection from the bladder most commonly by *E. coli*. Colonization of the ureter by *E. coli* results in loss of peristalsis and stasis within the ureter. This allows the infection to reach the kidney in a retrograde manner. By CT, there is typically renal enlargement from edema. There is delayed enhancement after intravenous contrast, and delayed excretion into the collecting system. The degree of contrast enhancement delay is directly proportional to the degree of renal inflammation. Occasionally, striations of decreased attenuation can be seen in the kidney due to renal parenchymal inflammation. This case nicely demonstrates renal enlargement and decreased attenuation of pyelonephritis. Renal vein thrombosis can have a similar CT appearance but in this case the renal vein is patent (as seen on image A) entering the IVC, excluding this as a diagnostic possibility.

Clinical History: 68-year-old man with hematuria.

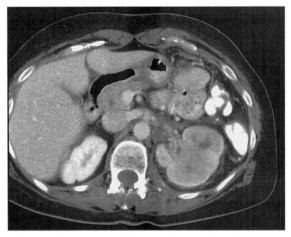

Figure 5.11 A

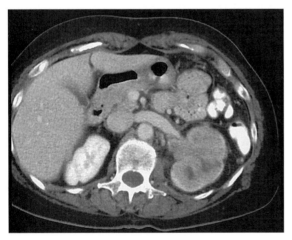

Figure 5.11 B

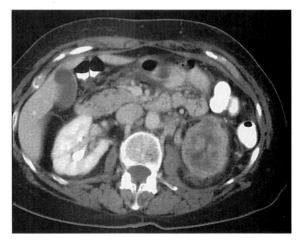

Figure 5.11 C

Findings: CECT demonstrates poor enhancement of the left kidney with a soft tissue mass seen in the renal pelvis. This mass extends into the renal parenchyma and enlarges the left kidney. The renal vein is patent.

Differential Diagnosis: Metastases, renal cell carcinoma, lymphoma, pyelonephritis, renal vein thrombosis.

Diagnosis: Transitional cell carcinoma.

Discussion: Transitional cell carcinoma of the renal pelvis accounts for approximately 4–7% of all renal tumors; 20–40% of these patients have a synchronous-bladder transitional cell carcinoma as well. Transitional cell carcinoma arises in the renal pelvis and can invade the renal parenchyma. This typically leads to diffuse enlargement of the kidney rather than multiple separate masses. The parenchymal involvement by the transitional cell carcinoma accounts for the poor enhancement of the kidney as well. Other tumors can also diffusely involve the kidney. This includes metastases, lymphoma, and less commonly, renal cell carcinoma. Lymphoma is frequently bilateral, which is not seen in this case. A primary neoplasm is commonly known when renal metastases are present. Both pyelonephritis and renal vein thrombosis can cause unilateral renal enlargement with poor enhancement. The renal vein is patent in this case, excluding renal vein thrombosis. Clinical symptoms are helpful in excluding pyelonephritis.

Clinical History: 65-year-old man with history of prostatic hypertrophy presents with microhematuria.

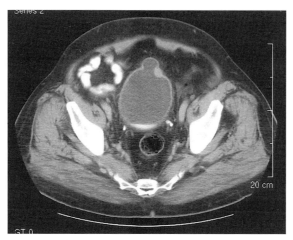

Figure 5.12 A

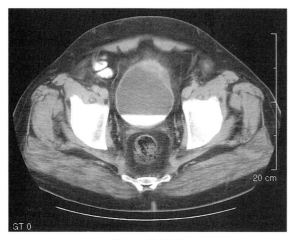

Figure 5.12 B

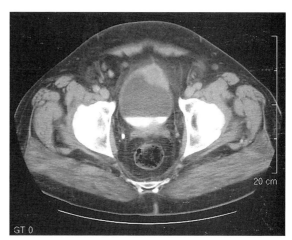

Figure 5.12 C

Findings: CECT demonstrates a small outpouching off the anterior portion of the bladder. There is a soft tissue mass adjacent to the outpouching.

Differential Diagnosis: Urachal diverticulum.

Diagnosis: Bladder diverticulum with transitional cell carcinoma.

Discussion: Bladder diverticula are most commonly due to bladder outlet obstruction rather than a congenital anomaly. The congenital diverticulum or "Hutch" diverticulum results from a musculature defect near the ureterovesical junction. Bladder outlet obstruction can be due to a prostatic disorder (prostatitis, prostate cancer, prostatic hypertrophy), a urethral stricture or cancer, or neurologic dysfunction. Bladder diverticula can be single or multiple and typically arise from the lateral bladder wall. Bladder diverticula can give rise to complications. If the neck of the diverticulum is narrow, urinary stasis can develop leading to stone formation and infection. Neoplasms can also occur and can be either transitional cell carcinoma (since the diverticulum is lined with urothelium) or squamous cell carcinoma (from chronic infection). A urachal diverticulum, although much less common, is another possibility. They occur at the superior and anterior portion of the bladder and may develop adenocarcinomas.

CASE 13

Clinical History: 18-year-old woman with hematuria and left flank mass.

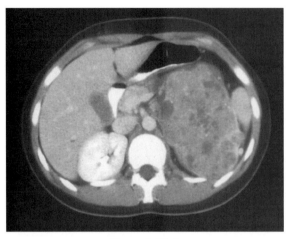

Figure 5.13 A

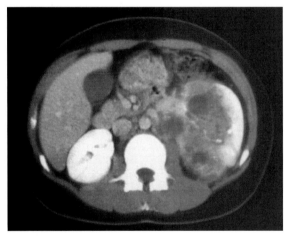

Figure 5.13 B

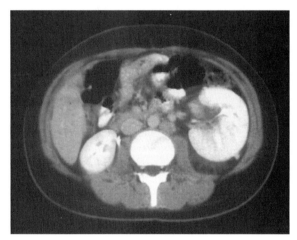

Figure 5.13 C

Findings: CECT demonstrates a 10-cm heterogeneous mass in the upper pole of the left kidney.

Differential Diagnosis: Oncocytoma, renal adenoma, focal bacterial nephritis, metastasis.

Diagnosis: Renal cell carcinoma.

Discussion: Renal cell carcinoma is the most common primary malignancy of the kidney. It arises from the proximal convoluted tubules and approximately 50% of the patients present with hematuria. Other signs inculde a palpable flank mass and flank pain from stretching of the renal capsule. Renal cell carcinoma typically appears as a heterogeneous-enhancing solid tumor of the kidney; 10–20% will have calcifications that tend to be amorphous and centrally located. Areas of necrosis can be seen as in this case. A solid mass in the kidney can also be due to oncocytoma, adenoma, or metastasis. An oncocytoma is considered benign but differentiation from a well-differentiated renal cell carcinoma requires histologic evaluation of the entire tumor. An adenoma is considered premalignant. Therefore, resection is recommended for most solid tumors of the kidney.

CASE 14

Clinical History: 65-year-old man with weight loss and long history of smoking.

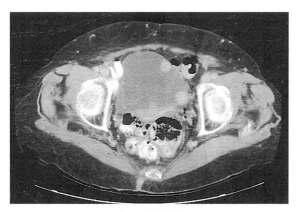

Figure 5.14 A

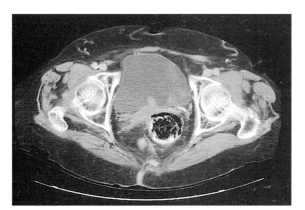

Figure 5.14 B

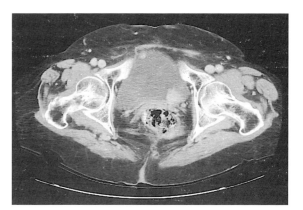

Figure 5.14 C

Findings: CECT demonstrates multiple, round, soft tissue intraluminal masses in the wall of the bladder.

Differential Diagnosis: Transitional cell carcinoma, cystitis cystica, cystitis glandularis, amyloidosis, tuberculosis, schistosomiasis.

Diagnosis: Metastatic lung cancer to the bladder.

Discussion: Metastases to the bladder are unusual unless they are from direct extension from an adjacent organ such as the prostate, uterus, ovary, or colon. Intraperitoneal drop metastases can occur but are usually on the serosal side of the bladder rather than intraluminal as in this case. Hematogenous metastases can occur but are usually widespread throughout the body before bladder metastases are present and therefore do not cause a diagnostic dilemma. The most common primary neoplasms are from breast, lung cancer, and melanoma. Both cystitis cystica and cystitis glandularis are fluid-filled cystic lesions in the wall of the bladder. Cystitis cystica has serous fluid while cystitis glandularis has mucin-filled cysts. They are both a result of chronic inflammation. On a CT scan, cystitis cystica and cystitis glandularis present as fluid density bladder-wall thickening rather than soft tissue density masses as seen in this case. Amyloidosis of the bladder is rare and is associated with amyloidosis in other parts of the body. Multiple transitional cell carcinomas are a good possibility for this case and cannot be excluded without biopsy.

CASE 15

Clinical History: 52-year-old man presents with flank pain and hypotension.

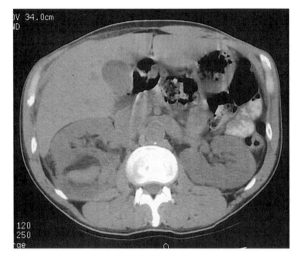

Figure 5.15 A

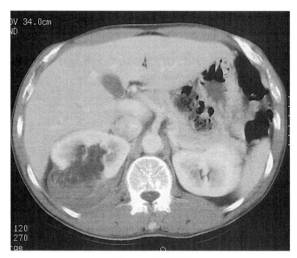

Figure 5.15 B

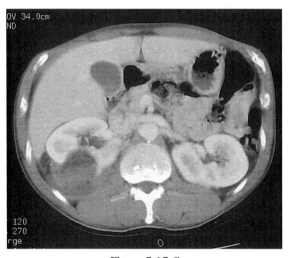

Figure 5.15 C

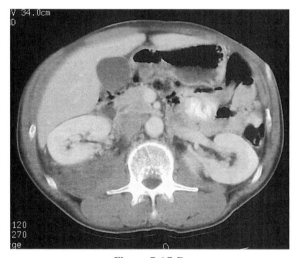

Figure 5.15 D

Findings: (A) NECT demonstrates a fat-containing lesion within the right kidney with hyperdense fluid collections seen within the lesion and in the perirenal space. (B, C, D) CECT demonstrates the lesion to extend outside the kidney. Hemorrhage is seen in the perirenal space.

Differential Diagnosis: None.

Diagnosis: Hemorrhage from an angiomyolipoma.

Discussion: Angiomyolipoma is a benign mesenchymal hamartoma of the kidney containing variable amounts of fat, muscle, and blood vessels. Most of these lesions are found sporadically (80%), but there is a high association of angiomyolipomas with tuberous sclerosis. When the lesion is sporadic, it is typically found in middle-age women. The lesion is usually solitary and found incidentally except when hemorrhage from the lesion occurs as in this case producing flank pain. CT imaging is usually diagnostic due to the presence of fat within the lesion. The absence of fat, however, does not exclude an angiomyolipoma because variable amounts of each mesenchymal component can be present. If the angiomyolipoma arises from the cortical surface, it can be difficult to distinguish from other retroperitoneal fat-containing tumors such as liposarcoma. Therefore, it is crucial to find the organ of origin of the fatty mass. In this example, the lesion is shown to arise from the renal parenchyma confirming the diagnosis of angiomyolipoma.

CASE 16

Clinical History: 40-year-old woman with left flank pain and fever.

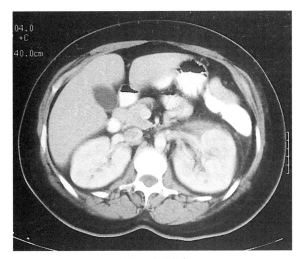

Figure 5.16 A

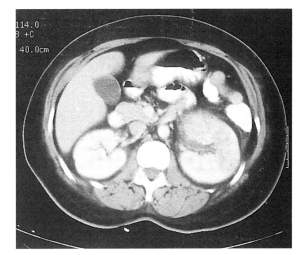

Figure 5.16 B

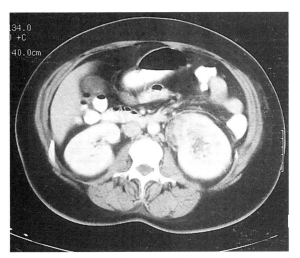

Figure 5.16 C

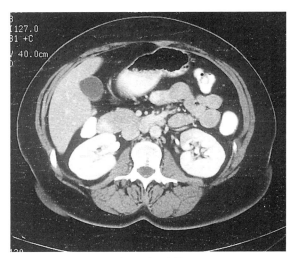

Figure 5.16 D

Findings: (A, B, C) Three images from a CECT demonstrate an enlarged left kidney with a focal area of low attenuation in the anterior portion of the kidney. There is stranding in the perinephric fat and thickening of Gerota's fascia. There is slight decreased enhancement of the entire kidney. (D) An image from a CECT 3 months later after antibiotic therapy demonstrates a normal size left kidney with a small focal low attenuation area anteriorly.

Differential Diagnosis: Renal vein thrombosis, renal infarction.

Diagnosis: Acute focal bacterial nephritis (AFBN).

Discussion: Acute focal bacterial nephritis is a more severe form of acute pyelonephritis. The inflammatory process in acute focal bacterial nephritis has mass effect and can lead to renal necrosis and abscess formation. Diabetic patients are more prone to contracting AFBN, and like pyelonephritis, the most common infecting organisms are Proteus, Klebsiella, and *E. coli*. CT findings of acute focal bacterial nephritis include enlargement of the kidney from the swelling and edema, focal mass with decreased enhancement, which is often wedge shaped, and perinephric inflammatory changes. Often this lesion is difficult to distinguish from a frank abscess or renal neoplasm. Renal vein thrombosis, renal infarction, and a renal neoplasm can enlarge the kidney but will not typically have the inflammatory changes noted in AFBN. The clinical history of fevers ensures the diagnosis. The follow-up CT 3 months later after antibiotic therapy demonstrates resolution of the acute changes in the kidney with a small low attenuation residual scar.

Clinical History: 47-year-old woman with right flank pain.

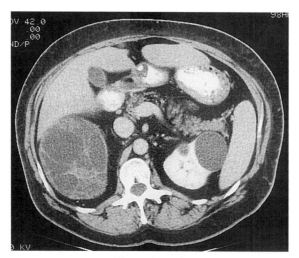

Figure 5.17 A

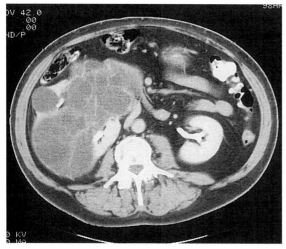

Figure 5.17 B

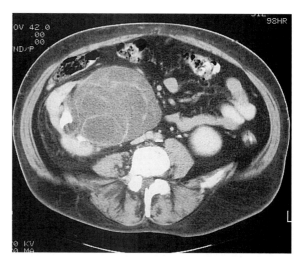

Figure 5.17 C

Findings: CECT demonstrates a large 13-cm multiloculated cystic mass arising from the right kidney. Simple cysts are also seen in the left kidney.

Differential Diagnosis: Renal cell carcinoma with cystic growth.

Diagnosis: Multilocular cystic nephroma (MLCN).

Discussion: Multilocular cystic nephroma is a rare nonhereditary congenital lesion. It typically occurs in children younger than 4 years of age, with approximately 70% being in males. A second peak occurs in women older than 40 years of age. Patients are usually asymptomatic but they can occasionally present with hematuria.

Multilocular cystic nephroma is a large cystic lesion with multiple noncommunicating cysts separated by septations. The lesions are well circumscribed due to a thick fibrous capsule. The cysts contain clear serous fluid and do not usually hemorrhage. Multilocular cystic nephroma is commonly found in the lower pole of the kidney without left or right side predilection. The CT findings of a multiloculated large cystic lesion is characteristic but cannot be differentiated from a renal cell carcinoma with cystic growth. Biopsy or aspiration is inconclusive, frequently requiring local excision or nephrectomy for definitive diagnosis.

CASE 18

Clinical History: 56-year-old man with left flank pain.

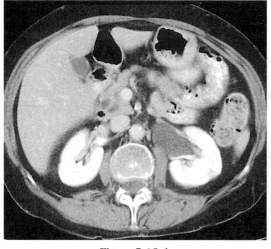

Figure 5.18 A

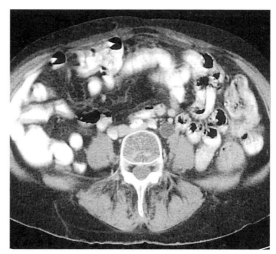

Figure 5.18 B

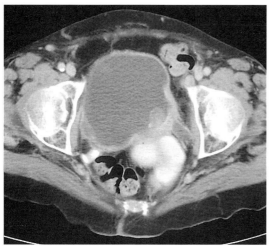

Figure 5.18 C

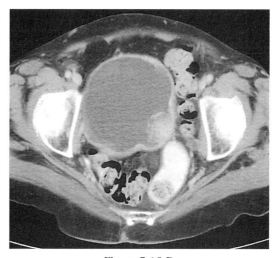

Figure 5.18 D

Findings: (A) CECT demonstrates left hydronephrosis. (B) A dilated left ureter is present anterior to the left psoas muscle. (C, D) There is a large intraluminal bladder mass obstructing the left ureteral orifice. Note the dilated ureter entering into the bladder. The left bladder wall is mildly thickened.

Differential Diagnosis: Primary neoplasm of the bladder (squamous cell carcinoma, adenocarcinoma), schistosomiasis, tuberculosis, hematoma, metastasis.

Diagnosis: Transitional cell carcinoma.

Discussion: Transitional cell carcinoma of the bladder occurs in the sixth decade of life, most commonly in males. They make up 85–90% of bladder tumors followed by squamous cell carcinoma and adenocarcinoma. Transitional cell carcinoma most commonly presents as an intraluminal mass with a broad base. They can be single or multiple and rarely contain calcifications. Hydronephrosis is not frequently seen in transitional cell carcinoma of the bladder unless the ureteral orifice is obstructed as in this case. An intraluminal mass is a nonspecific finding and can be due to any bladder neoplasm or occasionally due to an infection such as tuberculosis or schistosomiasis. CT, however, is excellent in evaluating for lymphadenopathy or extravesicular extension by the tumor and involvement of adjacent organs.

CASE 19

Clinical History: 48-year-old woman with fever, chills, and right flank pain. No history of trauma or surgery.

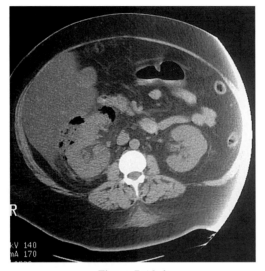

Figure 5.19 A

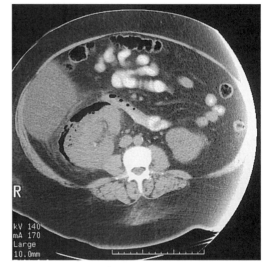

Figure 5.19 B

Findings: NECT demonstrates mottled gas, fluid, and inflammatory changes in the right perirenal space.

Differential Diagnosis: Trauma, instrumentation.

Diagnosis: Perirenal abscess.

Discussion: Air in the perirenal space originates either from a gas-forming organism or is introduced into the perirenal space from either penetrating trauma (stabwound, gunshot) or instrumentation (biopsy, surgery). Air from the latter two causes does not necessarily imply infection. A perirenal abscess, however, requires antibiotics and drainage either percutaneously or surgically. Without a history of trauma or instrumentation, a perirenal abscess is the most likely diagnosis in this case. The most likely cause is pyelonephritis with extension through the renal capsule forming a perirenal abscess. Acute obstruction with a ruptured fornix can also lead to a perirenal abscess but there is no evidence of renal calculi or collecting system obstruction to suggest this diagnosis. The lack of air in the renal parenchyma excludes emphysematous pyelonephritis.

CASE 20

Clinical History: 36-year-old man with severe left flank pain that has improved over the past hour.

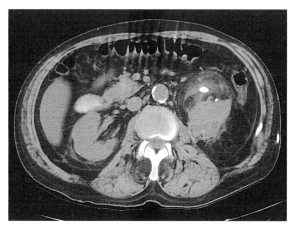

Figure 5.20 A

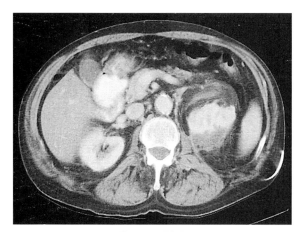

Figure 5.20 B

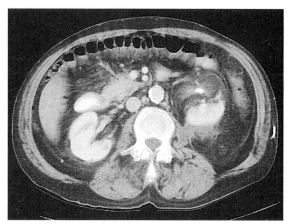

Figure 5.20 C

Findings: (A) NECT demonstrates a large stone in the proximal left ureter. (B, C) CECT demonstrates a posterior sub-capsular fluid collection, perinephric fluid, and inflammation around the left kidney. The enhancement of the left kidney is normal.

Differential Diagnosis: Xanthogranulomatous pyelonephritis, perinephric abscess, trauma.

Diagnosis: Ruptured fornix.

Discussion: Acute obstruction of a collecting system is most commonly due to an obstructing calculus. Plain films are sensitive for detecting most stones because 85–90% are radiopaque. The problem arises in small stones, stones obscured by bowel gas, stones overlying bony structures, and radiolucent stones. Ultrasound is sensitive in detecting stones but is limited in the evaluation of the ureter. A NECT is very sensitive in detecting stones in the kidney and ureter, even those which are radiolucent by plain film. Uric acid, which is the least dense stone, has a houndsfield unit of approximately 125–300 HU. Complications of acute obstruction include loss of renal function and forniceal or renal pelvis rupture, as in this case. The forniceal rupture led to the formation of the subcapsular fluid collection and the fluid in the perirenal space. These patients typically describe relief in the flank pain associated with the obstruction corresponding to decompression of the calyceal system post forniceal or pelvic rupture. This can be misinterpreted clinically as passage of a stone. If the urine is infected, forniceal rupture can lead to a perirenal abscess. The presence of an obstructing stone with subcapsular and perinephric fluid is highly suggestive of the diagnosis of forniceal rupture.

CASE 21

Clinical History: 45-year-old woman with fever and elevated white blood cell count (figures C and D performed months later).

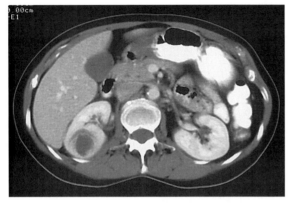

Figure 5.21 A

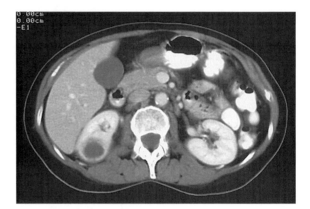

Figure 5.21 B

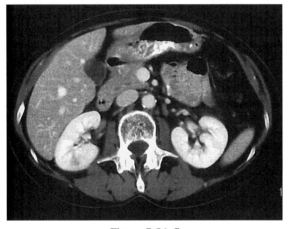

Figure 5.21 C

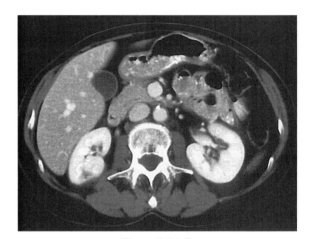

Figure 5.21 D

Findings: (A, B) CECT demonstrates a 2.5-cm cystic lesion with an enhancing rim in the right kidney. (C, D) CECT performed months later demonstrates a small wedge-shaped defect in the location of the prior cystic lesion.

Differential Diagnosis: Renal cell carcinoma, necrotic metastasis.

Diagnosis: Renal abscess.

Discussion: Renal abscesses are commonly the result of obstruction from calculi, tumors, or strictures resulting in an ascending infection. Hematogenous spread can also occur from infection of the skin or endocarditis such as in intravenous drug abusers. These result in microabscesses, which can coalesce and form a large abscess. The most common infecting organisms are *E. coli* and Proteus mirabilis. Renal abscesses can be single or multiple. Multiple abscesses are more common in hematogenous spread. By CT imaging, the lesion is typically of fluid attenuation (10–20 HU) with a thick wall that can demonstrate enhancement. There can be spread of inflammation outside the kidney, with thickening of Gerota's fascia. The presence of air within the fluid is pathognomonic of a renal abscess. A simple cyst would not have a thick wall or fluid of high attenuation. The appearance of this lesion is indistinguishable from a cystic renal cell carcinoma although a neoplasm is excluded with the CT performed 1 month later. Clinical symptoms can usually help differentiate the two entities as in this case.

Clinical History: 56-year-old man with microhematuria on routine physical examination.

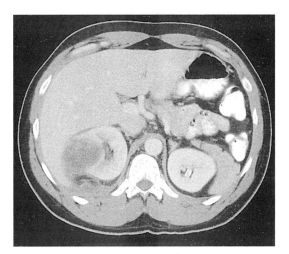

Figure 5.22 A

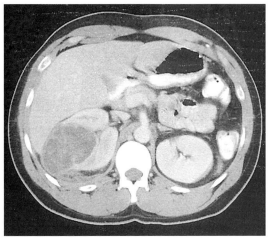

Figure 5.22 B

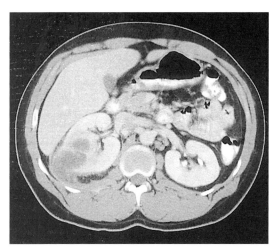

Figure 5.22 C

Findings: CECT demonstrates a cystic lesion in the right kidney, which has thick central-enhancing septa. There is thickening of Gerota's fascia posteriorly.

Differential Diagnosis: Multilocular cystic nephroma, abscess.

Diagnosis: Renal cell carcinoma with cystic growth.

Discussion: Renal cell carcinoma can occur in a wall of a cyst or have central necrosis, resulting in a cystic, complex lesion as in this case. It is critical to closely evaluate a cystic lesion for signs of malignancy. A simple cyst by CT should be round, well defined, with a thin wall. The fluid should be of water density and not enhance with contrast. Thin septations or thin peripheral calcifications can also be seen in benign cysts. Thick and irregular walls or septations, thick calcifications, or a tumor nodule are all suggestive of a malignancy. The lesion in this case demonstrates enhancement of irregular thick septations. In addition, there is extension of the tumor to Gerota's fascia posteriorly. These findings are suggestive of a malignancy, and a renal cell carcinoma was found at surgery. An abscess can have a similar appearance and can also cause thickening of Gerota's fascia. Clinical history is crucial in helping to differentiate the two entities.

CASE 23

Clinical History: 72-year-old woman with hematuria.

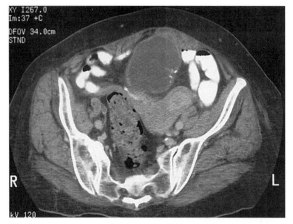

Figure 5.23 A

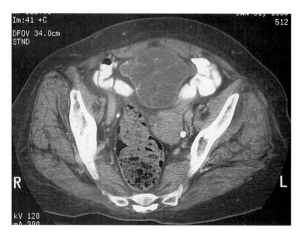

Figure 5.23 B

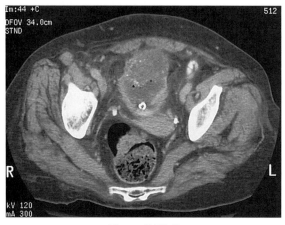

Figure 5.23 C

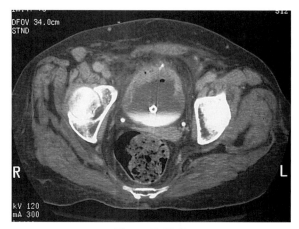

Figure 5.23 D

Findings: CECT demonstrates a large low attenuation mass with septations and calcifications arising from the superior anterior portion of the bladder and extending cranially.

Differential Diagnosis: Transitional cell carcinoma, sarcoma, squamous cell carcinomas.

Diagnosis: Urachal carcinoma.

Discussion: The urachus is a vestigial remnant of the obliterated umbilical arteries and allantoid. It extends from the umbilicus to the anterior superior surface of the bladder. The transitional epithelium of the urachus can undergo metaplasia, dysplasia, and even become malignant and convert to a mucin-producing adenocarcinoma. This accounts for almost 70% of the malignancies in the urachus. Other malignancies of the urachus include sarcomas, transitional cell, and squamous cell carcinomas. Because of the mucin produced, these urachal adenocarcinomas often have stippled or granular calcifications. They are commonly low in attenuation with septations, as in this case. The presence of a calcified mass at the superior anterior surface of the bladder is highly suggestive of a urachal mucinous adenocarcinoma. The other malignancies are less commonly seen but can also arise from the urachus or the bladder. Sarcomas tend to be of higher attenuation than mucin-producing adenocarcinomas and have enhancement with contrast.

CASE 24

Clinical History: 28-year-old man post percutaneous nephrostomy placement.

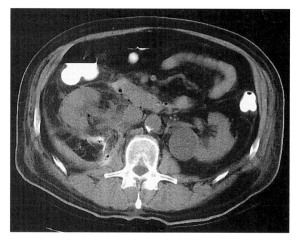

Figure 5.24 A

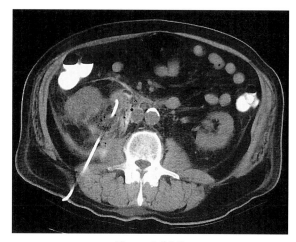

Figure 5.24 B

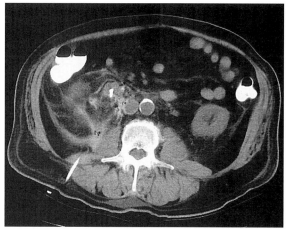

Figure 5.24 C

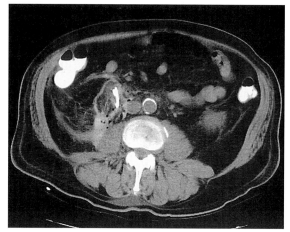

Figure 5.24 D

Findings: NECT demonstrates the nephrostomy tube in th right proximal ureter. Note the high density fluid and air in the perirenal space.

Differential Diagnosis: None.

Diagnosis: Perinephric air secondary to percutaneous nephrostomy.

Discussion: It is often difficult to know the exact location of a nephrostomy tube without cross sectional imaging. In this case, urine returned after the initial pass and contrast was shown within the ureter. The high density fluid in the perirenal space is from the contrast that was administered during the procedure but because only a small amount was extravasated, it was not seen during fluoroscopy. CT is much more sensitive in detecting not only the extravasated contrast but also the perinephric air and urine and the exact location of the nephrostomy tube. A CT was performed in this patient after he complained of persistent pain and fever. There is a limited differential diagnosis for air in the perirenal space. It can be due to a gas forming organism or introduced there by penetrating trauma or instrumentation. Clinical history easily differentiates these possibilities. This case nicely demonstrates perinephric air and fluid without an abscess due to instrumentation.

CASE 25

Clinical History: 38-year-old woman with hypertension and chronic respiratory insufficiency.

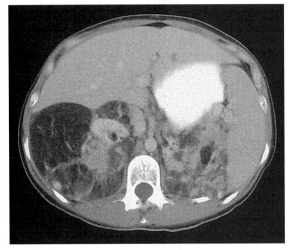

Figure 5.25 A

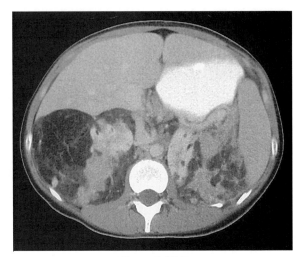

Figure 5.25 B

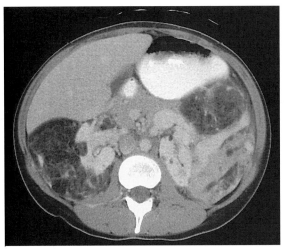

Figure 5.25 C

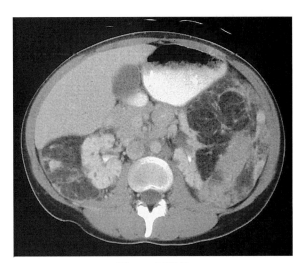

Figure 5.25 D

Findings: CECT demonstrates multiple fatty lesions of varying sizes seen in both kidneys.

Differential Diagnosis: None.

Diagnosis: Tuberous sclerosis with bilateral angiomyolipomas.

Discussion: Angiomyolipomas of the kidneys can be found incidentally in asymptomatic patients as an isolated lesion or as part of tuberous sclerosis. Tuberous sclerosis is a neuroectodermal disorder characterized by multiple renal cysts, bilateral angiomyolipomas, and retinal hamartomas. Approximately 80% of patients with tuberous sclerosis have renal angiomyolipomas that are commonly multiple and bilateral. In tuberous sclerosis, the angiomyolipomas can become very large involving the entire retroperitoneum and deforming the kidney parenchyma, as in this case. Besides the fatty component, a large amount of muscle and/or vascular tissue is also present. Angiomyolipomas are difficult to distinguish from other retroperitoneal sarcomas and specifically from liposarcoma. The key to the diagnosis is to recognize that the fatty lesions arise from the kidney and not the surrounding tissues. The presence of multiple bilateral fat-containing lesions within the kidney as well as in the perirenal space ensures the diagnosis of tuberous sclerosis with angiomyolipomas.

CASE 26

Clinical History: 71-year-old man presents with symptoms of a urinary tract infection.

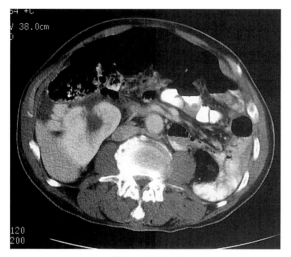
Figure 5.26 A

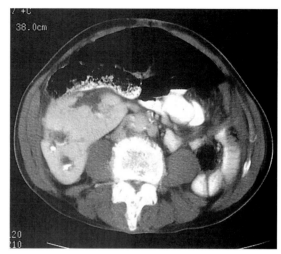
Figure 5.26 B

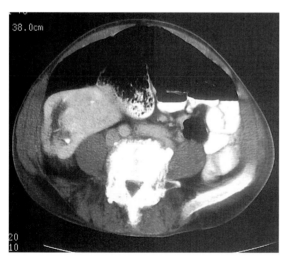
Figure 5.26 C

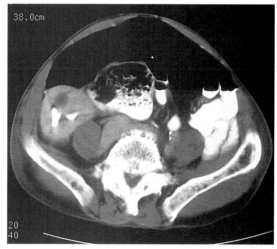
Figure 5.26 D

Findings: CECT demonstrates an abnormally rotated right kidney, which is fused with a second kidney located inferiorly. No left kidney is present.

Differential Diagnosis: None.

Diagnosis: Crossed renal ectopia with fusion.

Discussion: Crossed ectopy occurs when the kidney lies on the side opposite of the ureteral insertion into the bladder. The ureteral insertion is typically normal and the incidence of associated congenital anomalies is rare. The crossed kidney usually lies inferior to the normally positioned kidney and partial fusion is present in 90% of the cases. Males are more commonly affected than females. The left kidney is more commonly ectopic than the right. The etiology is uncertain but may be related to an abnormal umbilical artery, which inhibits the normal cephalad migration of the kidney. These patients are typically asymptomatic with only a slightly higher incidence of stones and urinary tract infections thought to be related to urinary stasis. CT imaging is usually diagnostic and further workup is unnecessary.

CASE 27

Clinical History: 29-year-old man with hypertension.

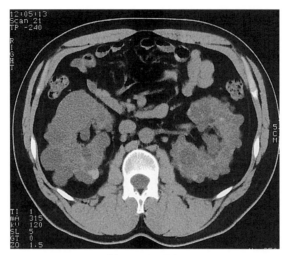

Figure 5.27 A

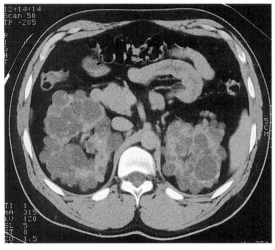

Figure 5.27 B

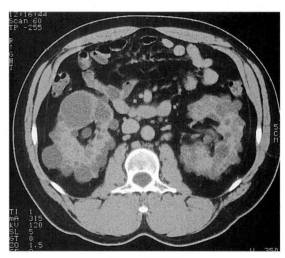

Figure 5.27 C

Findings: (A) NECT demonstrates enlarged kidneys with multiple small cysts some of which are of increased attenuation. (B, C) CECT again demonstrates the multiple renal cysts and the small amount of enhancing parenchyma remaining.

Differential Diagnosis: None.

Diagnosis: Autosomal dominant polycystic kidney disease (ADPCKD).

Discussion: Autosomal dominant polycystic kidney disease commonly presents in the third and fouth decades of life. Patients often complain of hypertension, flank pain, and palpable abdominal masses. All patients will eventually develop renal failure and require either dialysis or renal transplant. Approximately 50% of these patients have berry aneurysms in the circle of Willis, which is one of the leading causes of death in these patients. Diagnosis of ADPCKD is usually not difficult and can be made by family history, CT, or ultrasound. CT is often used to follow these patients to find renal stones and hemorrhagic cysts. A hyperdense cyst on a NECT can be secondary to hemorrhage or infection, which can lead to acute flank pain. Chronic pain is usually due to enlargement of the cysts, causing stretching of the renal capsule. This case nicely demonstrates the bilateral innumerable cysts in enlarged kidneys diagnostic of ADPCKD. Multiple hyperdense cysts are also present from prior hemorrhage.

CASE 28

Clinical History: 56-year-old woman with flank pain, hematuria, and weight loss.

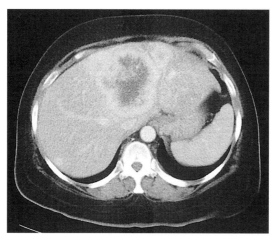

Figure 5.28 A

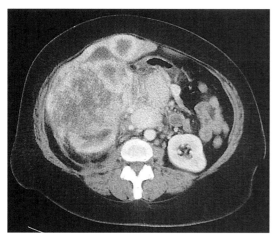

Figure 5.28 B

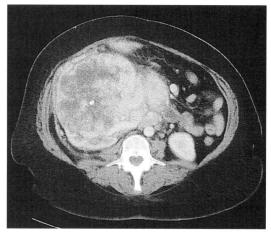

Figure 5.28 C

Findings: CECT demonstrates a large, 10-cm enhancing, necrotic mass arising from the right kidney. There is a small calcification in the center of the lesion. Multple rim enhancing lesions are seen in the liver.

Differential Diagnosis: Metastases.

Diagnosis: Renal cell carcinoma (RCCa) with liver metastases.

Discussion: Renal cell carcinoma is a primary adenocarcinoma arising from the proximal convoluted tubules of the kidney. It is most commonly seen in men in their 6th to 7th decade of life and there is an increased incidence in patients with von Hippel-Lindau disease. Hematuria is the most common sign in patients with renal cell carcinoma occurring in approximately 50% of the patients. Renal cell carcinomas are very vascular tumors and can give rise to hypervascular metastases. They calcify in approximately 15–20 % of the cases. The calcifications are usually central in location while curvilinear calcifications are seen in cystic lesions. A solid-enhancing mass arising from the kidney with hypervascular metastases to the liver is almost certainly renal cell carcinoma. Other lesions that can lead to hypervascular liver metastases include sarcomas and neuroendocrine tumors.

CASE 29

Clinical History: 62-year-old man with gross hematuria.

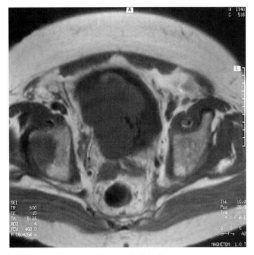

Figure 5.29 A

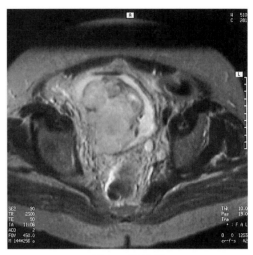

Figure 5.29 B

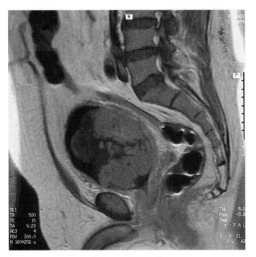

Figure 5.29 C

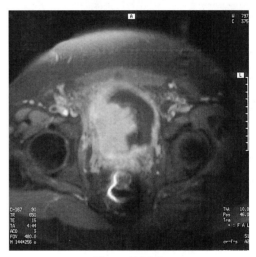

Figure 5.29 D

Findings: (A) Axial T1WI demonstrate a large 10 cm mass in the right side of the bladder that is isointense to muscle. (B) Axial T2WI shows this same lesion to be hyperintense. The lesion extends into the perivesical tissues. (C) Sagittal post gadolinium T1WI demonstrates marked enhancement of this lesion. (D) Axial post gadolinium fat saturated T1WI nicely demonstrates the enhancement of the lesion and the perivesical extension with involvement of the right seminal vesicle.

Differential Diagnosis: Other primary bladder neoplasm (squamous cell carcinoma, adenocarcinoma).

Diagnosis: Transitional cell carcinoma of the bladder.

Discussion: MRI is an excellent modality for evaluating bladder neoplasms. MRI allows visualization of the tumor in multiple planes, which aids in evaluating involvement of adjacent organs, such as the prostate, seminal vesicles, rectum and pelvic sidewall. Lymphadenopathy is also easily detected with MRI. Perivesical extension is critical in the staging of transitional cell carcinoma of the bladder. Perivesical extension changes the tumor staging from a stage B (within the bladder muscle) to a stage C (extension through the bladder muscle and into perivesical tissue). This can be detected with MRI due to the high water content of the tumor (hyperintense on T2WI) and its marked enhancement with gadolinium. The use of fat saturation allows even better contrast resolution between enhancing tumor and perivesical fat. In this case, the hyperintense tumor on T2WI and post gadolinium images is shown to invade through the bladder wall into the perivesical fat and right seminal vesical.

CASE 30

Clinical History: 3-day-old boy with a palpable mass in the right flank.

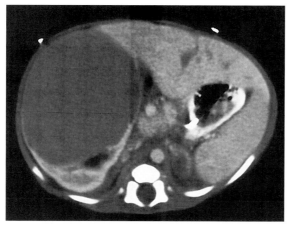

Figure 5.30 A

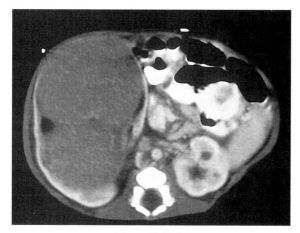

Figure 5.30 B

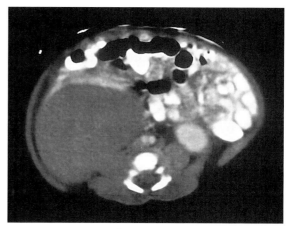

Figure 5.30 C

Findings: CECT demonstrates a large low attenuation homogeneous mass involving the right kidney. Normal parenchyma can be seen surrounding the mass. The mass had an attenuation coefficient of 28 HU.

Differential Diagnosis: Hydronephrosis, Wilm's tumor.

Diagnosis: Mesoblastic nephroma.

Discussion: Mesoblastic nephroma is the most common solid renal neoplasm in a newborn. It is a benign tumor that has also been called a congenital Wilm's tumor and fetal mesenchymal hamartoma. The tumor arises from renal connective tissue and very rarely undergoes sarcomatous transformation (approximately 4%). Patients are typically asymptomatic, and the mass is usually found incidentally by the parents.

By CT imaging, the mass is usually homogeneous and low in attenuation in relation to the normal kidney. This can be mistaken for hydronephrosis so care must be taken to measure houndsfield units. An adrenal mass such as a neuroblastoma can displace the kidney and mimic a renal mass. The presence of renal parenchyma surrounding the mass as in this case ensures the renal origin of the lesion. Treatment is surgical resection and prognosis is typically excellent.

CASE 31

Clinical History: 69-year-old man with left flank pain, fever, and leukocytosis.

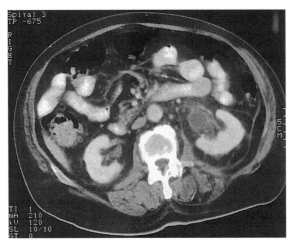

Figure 5.31 A

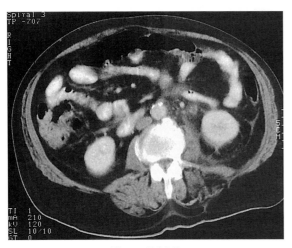

Figure 5.31 B

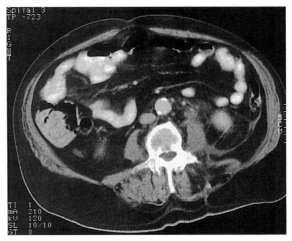

Figure 5.31 C

Findings: CECT demonstrates left hydronephrosis. The dilated ureter can be followed to a small obstructing 12-mm soft tissue mass just anterior to the left psoas muscle. Note inflammatory changes around the ureter and renal pelvis.

Differential Diagnosis: Primary neoplasm (squamous cell carcinoma, adenocarcinoma, papilloma), metastasis, tuberculosis.

Diagnosis: Transitional cell carcinoma of the ureter.

Discussion: Transitional cell carcinoma of the ureter is frequently associated with involvement of other areas of the collecting system. This is thought to be due to the greater amount of uroepithelial surface present in the bladder and renal pelvis in comparison to the ureter. In approximately 25–30% of patients with ureteral transitional cell carcinoma, there is a synchronous lesion in the collecting system.

Transitional cell carcinoma of the ureter can be single or multiple. When multiple, they can be difficult to distinguish from inflammatory conditions such as malakoplakia and leukoplakia. Cystoscopy is often necessary to make the diagnosis. The stranding seen surrounding the renal pelvis and proximal ureter can be due to infection or periureteral extension of tumor. Inflammation and tumor extension are indistinguishable by CT.

CASE 32

Clinical History: 68-year-old man with history of renal calculi presents with fevers and left flank pain.

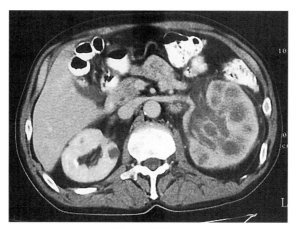

Figure 5.32 A

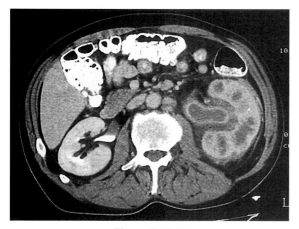

Figure 5.32 B

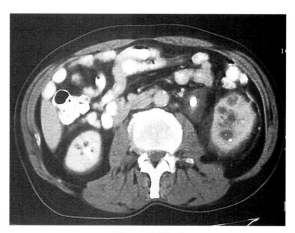

Figure 5.32 C

Findings: CECT demonstrates an enlarged, poorly perfused left kidney. The renal pelvis and calyces are dilated and irregular in appearance. There is stranding in the perinephric space. A more caudal image reveals a dilated ureter with an obstructing calculus. The right kidney is normal.

Differential Diagnosis: Transitional cell carcinoma, lymphoma.

Diagnosis: Xanthogranulomatous pyelonephritis.

Discussion: Xanthogranulomatous pyelonephritis (XGP) is a chronic suppurative granulomatous infection of the kidney secondary to obstruction of the collecting system. As the kidney becomes chronically obstructed, the calyces dilate and fill with purulent material and debris and the kidney itself enlarges. Typically there is an obstructing calculi or a staghorn calculus. On CECT there is a poorly functioning or nonfunctioning kidney, which is diffusely enlarged with dilated calyces filled with higher attenuation pus. An obstructing stone or staghorn calculus is almost always seen as in this example. Simple hydronephrosis would not account for the inflammatory changes around the kidney. An infiltrating malignant process such as TCC or lymphoma can diffusely infiltrate the kidney and globally enlarge it. A dilated collecting system is not commonly seen in these cases unless the tumor involves the ureter. An enlarged kidney with dilated collecting system, perinephric inflammatory changes, and an obstructing stone makes XGP the best diagnosis.

SUGGESTED READINGS

Amendola MA, Glazer GM, Grossman HB, et al. Staging of bladder carcinoma: MRI-CT-surgical correlation. AJR 1986;146:1179–1183.

Banner MP, Pollack HM, Witzleben C. Multilocular renal cysts: radiologic-pathologic correlation. AJR 1981;136:239–247.

Baron RL, McClennan BL, Lee JK, et al. Computed tomography of transitional-cell carcinoma of the renal pelvis and ureter. Radiology 1982;144:125–130.

Bosniak MA. The current radiological approach to renal cysts. Radiology 1986;158:1–10.

Bosniak MA. The small (<3.0 cm) renal parenchymal tumor: detection, diagnosis, and controversies. Radiology 1991;179:307–317.

Bosniak MA, Megibow AJ, Hulnick DH, et al. CT diagnosis of renal angiomyolipoma:the importance of detecting small amounts of fat. AJR 1988;151:497–501.

Brick SH, Friedman AC, Pollack HM, et al. Urachal carcinoma: CT findings. Radiology 1988;169:377–381.

Bree RL, Schultz SR, Hayes R. Large infiltrating renal transitional cell carcinomas: CT and ultrasound features. J Comput Assist Tomogr 1990;14:381–385.

Choyke PL. MR imaging in renal cell carcinoma. Radiology 1988;169:572–573.

Choyke PL, White EM, Zeman RK. Renal metastases: clinicopathologic and radiologic correlation. Radiology 1987;162:359–363.

Curry NS, Schabel SI, Betsill WL. Small renal neoplasms: diagnostic imaging, pathologic features and clinical course. Radiology 1986;158:113–117.

Fein AB, Lee JKT, Balfe DM, et al. Diagnosis and staging of renal cell carcinoma: a comparison of MR imaging and CT. AJR 1987;148:749–753.

Hartman DS, Davis CJ, Goldman SM. Renal lymphoma: radiologic-pathologic correlation of 21 cases. Radiology 1982;144:759–766.

Hartman DS, Lesar MSL, Madewell JE, et al. Mesoblastic nephroma: radiologic-pathologic correlation of 20 cases. AJR 1981;136:69–74.

Hartman DS, Weatherby E, Laskin WB. Cystic renal cell carcinoma: CT findings simulating a benign hyperdense cyst. AJR 1992;159:1235–1237.

Hayden CK, Swischuk LE, Smith TH, et al. Renal cystic disease in childhood. Radiographics 1986;6:97–116.

Johnson CD, Dunnick NR, Cohan RH, et al. Renal adenocarcinoma: CT staging of 100 tumors. AJR 1987;148:59–63.

Kelvin FM, Korobkin M, Heaston DK. The pelvis after surgery for rectal carcinoma: serial CT observations with emphasis on nonneoplastic features. AJR 1983;141:959–964.

Kenney PJ, Stanley, RJ. Computed tomography of ureteral tumors. J Comput Assist Tomogr 1987;11:102–107.

Korobkin M, Cambier L, Drake J. Computed tomography of urachal carcinoma. J Comput Assist Tomogr 1988;12:981–987.

Lupetin AR, Mainwaring BL, Daffner RH. CT diagnosis of renal artery injury caused by blunt abdominal trauma. AJR 1989;153:1065–1068.

Madewell JE, Goldman SM, Davis CJ. Multilocular cystic nephroma: a radiographic-pathologic correlation of 58 patients. Radiology 1983;146:309–321.

Narumi Y, Sato T, Kuriyama K, et al.Vesical dome tumors: significance of extravesical extension on CT. Radiology 1988;169:383–385.

Parienty RA, Pradel J, Imbert MC, et al. Computed tomography of multilocular cystic nephroma. Radiology 1981;140:135–139.

Pollack HM, Wein AJ. Imaging of renal trauma. Radiology 1989;172:297–308.

Silver TM, Kass, EJ, Thornbury JR, et al. The radiological spectrum of acute pyelonephritis in adults and adolescents. Radiology 1976;118:65–71.

Smith SJ, Bosniak MA, Megibow AJ, et al. renal cell carcinoma: earlier discovery and increased detection. Radiology 1989;170:699–703.

Segal AJ, Spataro RF. Computed tomography of adult polycystic disease. J Comput Assist Tomogr 1982;6:777–780.

Senn E, Zaunbauer W, Bandhauer K, et al. Computed tomography in acute pyelonephritis. Br J Urol 1987;59:118–121.

Spataro RF, Davis RS, McLachlan MSF, et al. Urachal abnormalities in the adult. Radiology 1983;149:659–663.

Stillwell TJ, Gomez MR, Kelalis PP. Renal lesions in tuberous sclerosis. J Urol 1987;138:477–481.

Walker FC, Loney LC, Root ER, et al. Diagnostic evaluation of adult polycystic kidney disease in childhood. AJR 1984;142:1273–1277.

Winalski CS, Lipman JC, Tumeh SS. Ureteral neoplasms. Radiographics 1990;10:271–283.

Yousen DM, Gatewood OMB, Goldman SM, et al. Synchronous and metachronous transitional cell carcinoma of the urinary tract: prevalence, incidence, and radiographic detection. Radiology 1988;167:613–618.

chapter 6

PELVIS

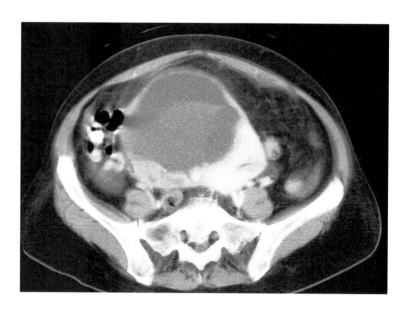

CASE 1

Clinical History: 31-year-old woman with pelvic pain.

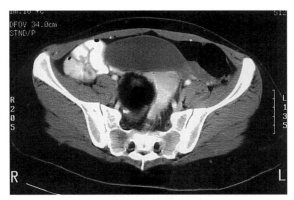

Figure 6.1 A

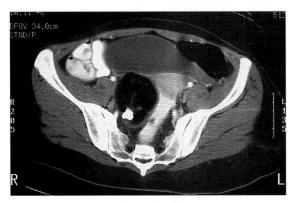

Figure 6.1 B

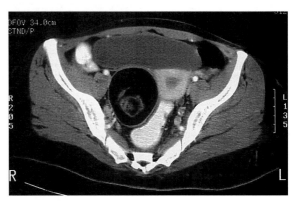

Figure 6.1 C

Findings: CECT demonstrates a 6-cm lesion in the right lower pelvis comprised predominantly of fat with a small soft tissue nodule and calcification.

Differential Diagnosis: None.

Diagnosis: Ovarian teratoma.

Discussion: Ovarian teratoma (dermoid) is the most common ovarian neoplasm in young women. Typically it is easily diagnosed by CT by the presence of fat, fluid, and calcifications. Teratomas can be predominantly cystic in appearance. In these cases, it is crucial to search for a fatty component within the lesion to confirm the diagnosis. In this case, the teratoma is easily diagnosed because it is almost entirely composed of adipose tissue. The presence of the large calcification confirms the diagnosis.

Clinical History: 20-year-old woman post spontaneous vaginal delivery with persistent post-partum fever.

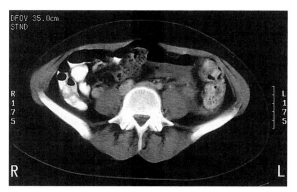

Figure 6.2 A

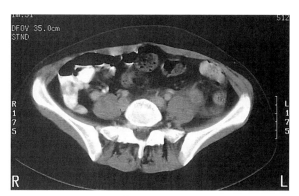

Figure 6.2 B

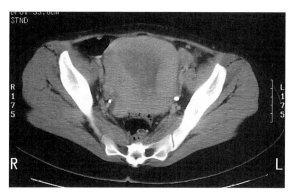

Figure 6.2 C

Findings: CECT demonstrates a large fluid-filled uterus. There is a tubular structure surrounded by inflammatory changes with a low density center anterior and lateral to the left psoas muscle.

Differential Diagnosis: None.

Diagnosis: Ovarian vein thrombophlebitis.

Discussion: The diagnosis of ovarian vein thrombophlebitis is suspected by clinicians due to its classic presentation. This includes lower abdominal and flank pain, fever, and leukocytosis in the first 3 days post-partum, and occasionally a palpable ovarian vein. Many complications can arise from ovarian vein thrombophlebitis including inferior vena cava or renal vein thrombosis, pulmonary embolism, sepsis, and septic emboli. Treatment for ovarian vein thrombosis includes intravenous antibiotics and heparin. If resolution does not occur, then ovarian vein ligation can be performed to halt the spread of the thrombus.

The key to the diagnosis in this case is the extensive inflammatory changes surrounding the left ovarian vein and its low attenuation center. These CT findings in the clinical setting of post-partum fever are highly suggestive of ovarian vein thrombophlebitis.

CASE 3

Clinical History: 37-year-old woman with ESRD on peritoneal dialysis found to have bloody dialysate.

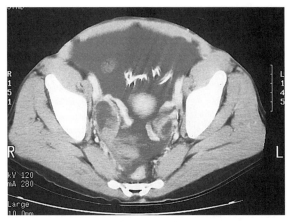

Figure 6.3 A

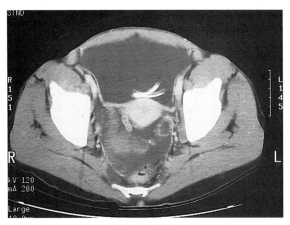

Figure 6.3 B

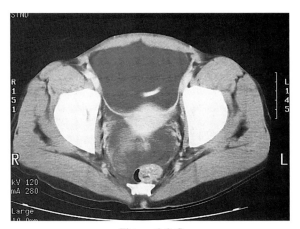

Figure 6.3 C

Findings: CECT demostrates a 4-cm complex right adnexal mass with a soft tissue component seen posteriorly. High attenuation fluid is seen adjacent to the lesion medially. Free intraperitoneal fluid is present secondary to the peritoneal dialysis. A small 2-cm left adnexal cyst is present as well.

Differential Diagnosis: Tubo-ovarian abscess, endometrioma, cystadenoma.

Diagnosis: Hemorrhagic right ovarian cyst.

Discussion: Cystic masses in the adnexa include functional ovarian cyst, tubo-ovarian abscess, endometrioma, and epithelial neoplasms of the ovary. Functional ovarian cysts can be follicular cysts or corpus luteum cyst. Follicular cysts are unruptured follicles that enlarge due to continued stimulation. They are typically greater than 2.5 cm and can be multilocular in appearance. Debris is often seen inside the cyst from prior hemorrhage, which can result in sharp pelvic pain. Follicular cysts will usually regress after one or two menstrual cycles.

In this case, the follicular cyst bled into the peritoneum resulting in hemorrhagic peritoneal fluid. This accounted for the soft tissue component within the cyst and the high attenuation fluid adjacent to the lesion. Follow-up ultrasound 6 weeks later demonstrated resolution of the lesion.

CASE 4

Clinical History: 42-year-old woman with spotting.

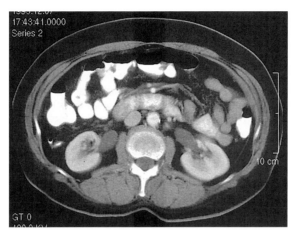

Figure 6.4 A

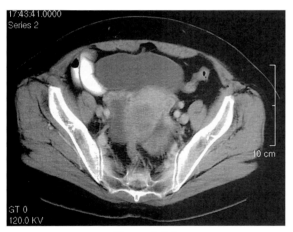

Figure 6.4 B

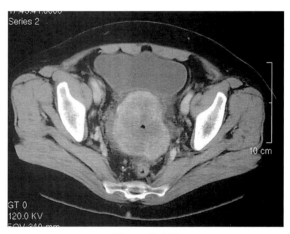

Figure 6.4 C

Findings: CECT demonstrates a large 7-cm heterogeneous mass involving the cervix with stranding in the parametrium with bilateral mild hydronephrosis. A small pocket of air is seen in the mass.

Differential Diagnosis: Endometrial cancer, uterine fibroid.

Diagnosis: Cervical cancer.

Discussion: Cervical cancer is the sixth most common malignancy in women with a peak age of presentation between 45–55 years old; 95% of cervical cancers are squamous cell carcinomas, with the remaining 5% adenocarcinomas. Risk factors include multiparity, multiple sexual partners, and early onset of sexual activity. CT imaging is usually not helpful in stages up to IIa (extension beyond the cervix but not the lower ⅓ of the vagina) because of inaccuracy in evaluating lower vaginal involvement by cervical cancer. Pelvic examination is more accurate than CT. CT, however, is useful for detecting parametrial involvement, enlarged lymph nodes, and hydronephrosis. This case demonstrates a large mass involving the cervix with peritumoral stranding representing extension of the tumor into the parametrium. Hydronephrosis is also present. This is a crucial finding because the presence of hydronephrosis even without pelvic sidewall involvement places the patient in a stage IIIb category.

CASE 5

Clinical History: 44-year-old woman with bladder outlet obstruction.

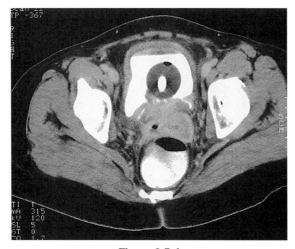

Figure 6.5 A

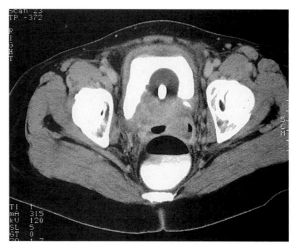

Figure 6.5 B

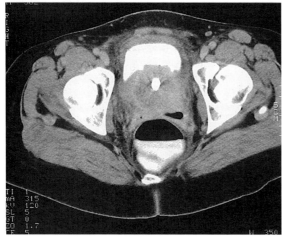

Figure 6.5 C

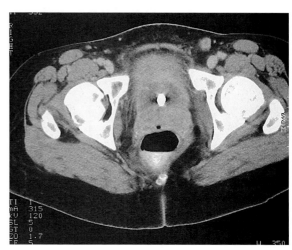

Figure 6.5 D

Findings: CECT demonstrates a large mass that involves the base of the bladder and extends distally surrounding a foley catheter balloon. There is extension of the mass to the vagina.

Differential Diagnosis: Transitional cell carcinoma, sarcoma, metastasis.

Diagnosis: Urethral cancer (squamous cell carcinoma).

Discussion: Carcinoma of the urethra is much more common in females than in males. The most common histology is squamous cell carcinoma followed by adenocarcinoma and transitional cell carcinoma. The peak age is in the sixth decade of life. The etiology is thought to be secondary to prior infections or trauma. Urethral cancers can be divided based on their location. Cancers arising from the distal urethra are typically low grade and have a good prognosis. The proximal urethral tumors, however, present later in life and are usually more advanced with a poor prognosis. This case demonstrates an aggressive proximal urethral squamous cell carcinoma. This lesion involves the periurethral tissues and extends into the base of the bladder and the vagina. This lesion is similar in appearance to a transitional cell carcinoma of the bladder or an aggressive sarcoma. The key to the diagnosis is following the extent of the lesion distally into the perineum suggestive of a urethral carcinoma.

CASE 6

Clinical History: 38-year-old woman with cervical cancer and fever.

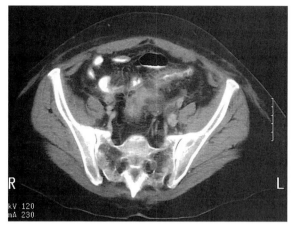

Figure 6.6 A

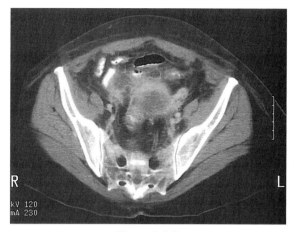

Figure 6.6 B

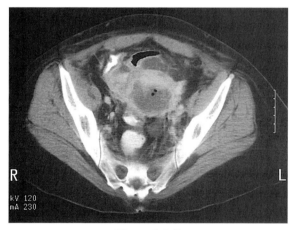

Figure 6.6 C

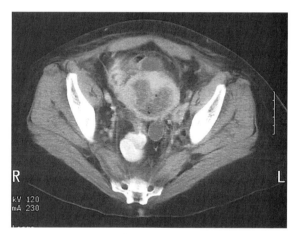

Figure 6.6 D

Findings: CECT demonstrates an enlarged uterus filled with high attenuation fluid and air. There is extension into the right fallopian tube and a small extrauterine fluid collection is present as well. Note the thickening of the adjacent bowel and the inflammatory changes around the uterus.

Differential Diagnosis: Hematometra, hydrometra.

Diagnosis: Pyometra (obstructed uterus from cervical cancer).

Discussion: Fluid within the uterus can be due to several causes including pus (pyometra), sterile fluid (hydrometra), and blood (hematometra). Intrauterine fluid can be seen normally in menstruating and pregnant women. Abnormal causes for intrauterine fluid include submucosal leiomyomas, endometritis, endometrial cancer, and cervical cancer. Larger fluid collections (pyometra and hematometra) commonly occur in an obstructed uterus. In women of reproductive age, this can be due to cervical cancer, uterine leiomyoma, endometrial cancer, radiation therapy, and postsurgical scarring and stenosis. In this case, the uterus was obstructed from a cervical cancer resulting in pyometra with high attenuation pus and air in the endometrial cavity. The infected fluid can escape from the uterus via the fallopian tubes as in this case leading to the formation of a pelvic abscess and subsequent thickening of the adjacent small bowel.

CASE 7

Clinical History: 19-year-old woman with a palpable pelvic mass.

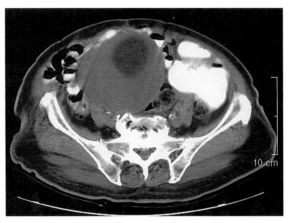

Figure 6.7 A

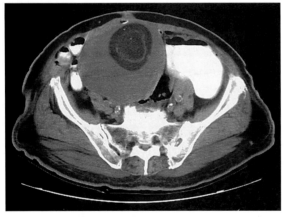

Figure 6.7 B

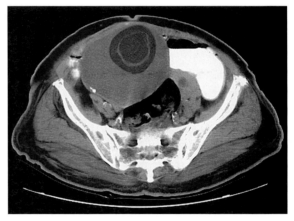

Figure 6.7 C

Findings: CECT demonstrates a large (12 cm) cystic lesion in the right pelvis with a small peripheral calcification. Within the cystic component, there is a 5-cm area of fat attenuation.

Differential Diagnosis: None.

Diagnosis: Ovarian teratoma (Dermoid cyst).

Discussion: Ovarian teratomas commonly occur in young women and are benign. Less than 1% of these lesions have malignant degeneration, which typically occurs within the soft tissue component of the lesion (dermoid plug). Dermoid cysts are usually asymptomatic except when they grow to be large and exert pressure causing pelvic pain or hydronephrosis. Teratomas are also at risk for torsion and therefore are usually surgically removed. Cystic dermoids typically are homogeneously cystic in appearance except for a possible fat-fluid level within them. In this case, the round fatty component is floating within the cystic lesion. The presence of fat and peripheral calcifications is virtually diagnostic of a cystic teratoma.

CASE 8

Clinical History: 35-year-old woman with a palpable mass by pelvic examination.

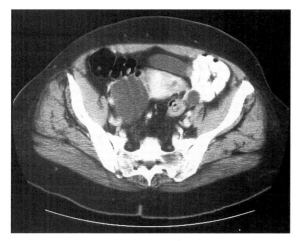

Figure 6.8 A

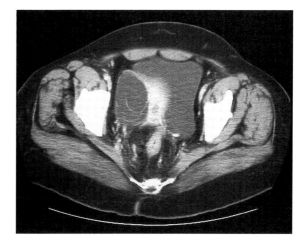

Figure 6.8 B

Findings: CECT demonstrates a 4-cm cystic lesion in the right adnexa with a thin wall and thin septations. A small 1-cm cyst is seen in the left adnexa.

Differential Diagnosis: Mucinous cystadenoma, cystadenocarcinoma, functional ovarian cyst, endometrioma, tubo-ovarian abscess.

Diagnosis: Serous cystadenoma.

Discussion: The majority of ovarian tumors are of epithelial origin. Benign epithelial tumors of the ovary can be classified as serous or mucinous cystadenomas. Serous cystadenomas occur between the ages of 20–50 years old with malignant transformation occurring in 30–45% of the cases, typically in older patients. By CT imaging, typically there is a unilocular or multilocular cystic lesion with thin walls and septations. Serous cystadenomas can range in size from 4 to 15 cm. Bilateral cystadenomas can occur in up to 30–50% of the cases. The presence of a soft tissue component (mural nodule) or of a thick wall suggests that the lesion may be a cystadenocarcinoma. The CT appearance of this lesion with thin walls and septations is nonaggressive and suggests a cystadenoma. No lymphadenopathy, peritumoral stranding, or ascites is present to suggest a malignancy. A mucinous cystadenoma can have a similar appearance but the fluid is frequently of attenuation higher than water. Tubo-ovarian abscess and cystadenocarcinoma typically have a thicker wall and more aggressive appearance. An endometrioma or functional ovarian cyst could be indistinguishable from this lesion by CT imaging.

Clinical History: 48-year-old woman with pelvic pain.

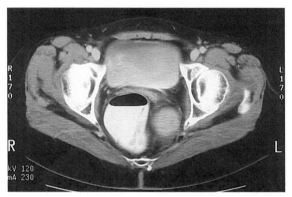

Figure 6.9 A

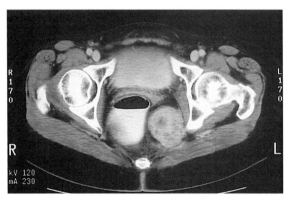

Figure 6.9 B

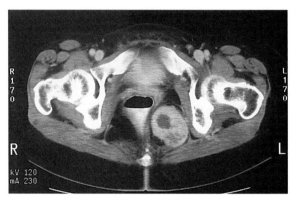

Figure 6.9 C

Findings: CECT demonstrates a 5-cm enhancing solid mass with small internal areas of low density located to the left of the rectum displacing it to the right.

Differential Diagnosis: Metastases, sarcoma, lymphoma.

Diagnosis: Perirectal hemangiopericytoma.

Discussion: Hemangiopericytoma is a rare tumor arising from the capillary pericytes, which can be found in the lower extremities, retroperitoneum, and brain (dura). The lesion tends to be hypervascular with marked enhancement after intravenous contrast administration. As with other retroperitoneal and extraperitoneal masses, hemangiopericytoma can grow to be large (>10 cm) before being detected. Symptoms usually do not occur until the lesion compresses an adjacent organ causing pain or decrease in function. A mass in the perirectal tissue is typically a neoplasm arising from the rectum. This lesion, however, appears to be separate from the rectum and uterus making a rectal malignancy (adenocarcinoma, lymphoma) or pedunculated uterine leiomyoma unlikely. The tumor can also arise from the perirectal tissue. A mesenchymal tumor such as a sarcoma would be a good possibility in the differential diagnosis as well as a lymphoma. Metastases, especially from an aggressive neoplasm such as melanoma, could also have this appearance.

Clinical History: 54-year-old woman with a palpable pelvic mass.

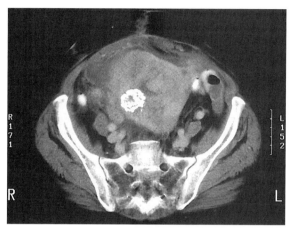

Figure 6.10 A

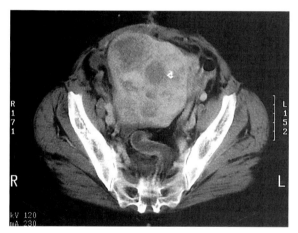

Figure 6.10 B

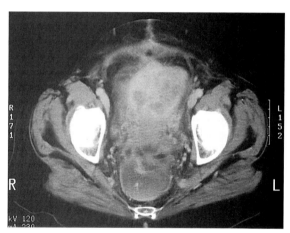

Figure 6.10 C

Findings: CECT demonstrates a large 10-cm heterogeneous mass with multiple coarse calcifications in the region of the uterus.

Differential Diagnosis: Uterine cancer.

Diagnosis: Uterine leiomyomas (fibroids).

Discussion: Uterine leiomyoma is the most common solid neoplasm of the uterus and occurs in 20–40% of women of reproductive age. Uterine leiomyomas are commonly multiple and are usually found incidentally on CT or ultrasound. They can also present as a palpable mass or with bleeding and pelvic pain. Leiomyomas can be classified by their location as submucosal, intramural, or subserosal. Intramural leiomyomas are the most common type, the submucosal type the most likely to present with bleeding. On CT, the leiomyomas can be hypodense, isodense, or hyperdense relative to the normal uterus depending on the degree of internal hemorrhage and necrosis. They will commonly distort the uterine contour and displace the endometrial cavity. A characteristic feature of uterine leiomyomas is calcification that can be rimlike, amorphous, popcornlike, or coarse as in this case. Uterine fibroids are often difficult to distinguish from a uterine or cervical cancer (if located in the lower uterine segment) and biopsy or curettage may be necessary to confirm the diagnosis.

CASE 11

Clinical History: 73-year-old woman with weight loss.

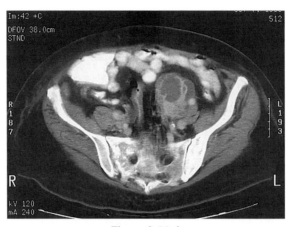

Figure 6.11 A

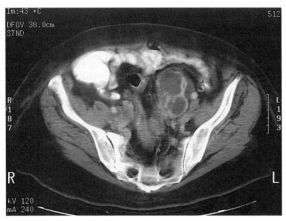

Figure 6.11 B

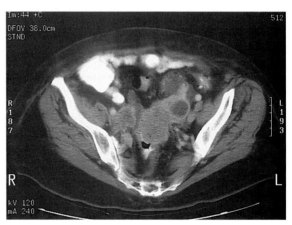

Figure 6.11 C

Findings: CECT demonstrates a 5-cm multilocular cystic lesion in the left adnexa with thick walls and septations. A 4-cm low attenuation mass is present medial to the lesion as well as a 2.5-cm necrotic right iliac lymph node.

Differential Diagnosis: Metastasis.

Diagnosis: Serous cystadenocarcinoma.

Discussion: Approximately 90–95% of ovarian cancers are from epithelial origin and can be divided histologically into serous, mucinous, endometrioid, clear cell, and Brenner cell tumors. The most common types are serous and mucinous cystadenocarcinomas. Serous tumors are more likely to be malignant and bilateral than mucinous tumors. Epithelial neoplasms can spread locally to involve the fallopian tubes, uterus, bowel, and contralateral ovary. Lymphangitic spread to pelvic and retroperitoneal lymph nodes as well as peritoneal metastases and ascites can also occur. This case demonstrates a complex cystic adnexal mass with thick walls and septations suggestive of an epithelial neoplasm. The presence of an adjacent soft tissue mass and pelvic adenopathy confirms the diagnosis of a malignancy. A tubo-ovarian abscess, endometrioma, and hemorrhagic ovarian cyst would not produce adenopathy or an adjacent soft tissue mass as in this case. A metastasis, possibly from the gastriontestinal tract, could have a similar appearance.

CASE 12

Clinical History: 28-year-old woman post cesarean section with fever and leukocytosis.

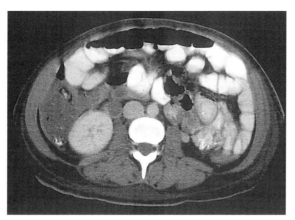

Figure 6.12 A

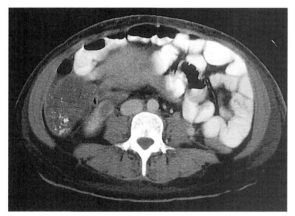

Figure 6.12 B

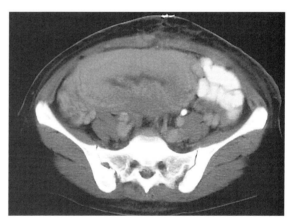

Figure 6.12 C

Findings: CECT demonstrates an enlarged uterus with fluid in the endometrial cavity. A 1.5-cm round lesion with a low attenuation center is seen on multiple images anterior to the right psoas muscle.

Differential Diagnosis: None.

Diagnosis: Ovarian vein thrombophlebitis.

Discussion: Ovarian vein thrombophlebitis occurs when there is bacterial seeding from endometritis. Endometritis can occur after a cesarean section or vaginal delivery. Since during pregnancy and puerperium, patients are in a hypercoaguable state, thrombosis may occur in the ovarian veins secondarily infected from the endometritis. Although this can occur any time in the puerperium, most commonly it occurs in the first 3 days post partum. The right ovarian vein is affected more frequently than the left. This case demonstrates the classic findings of ovarian vein thrombophlebitis. There is a post-partum uterus with a tubular structure in the location of the right ovarian vein with a low attenuation center representing the thrombus. Inflammatory changes are present around the vessel and that vessel appears enlarged due to the thrombosis. A normal caliber ovarian vein is present on the left side for comparison.

CASE 13

Clinical History: 22-year-old woman with a pelvic mass detected by ultrasound.

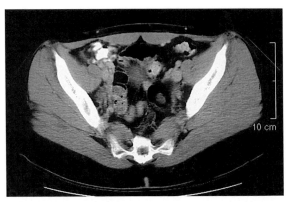

Figure 6.13 A

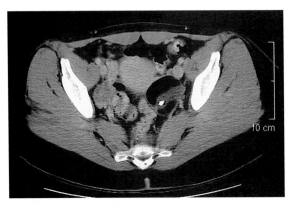

Figure 6.13 B

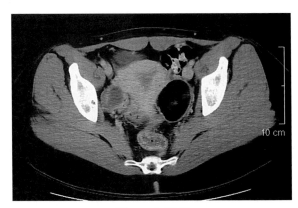

Figure 6.13 C

Findings: CECT demonstrates a 4.5-cm left adnexal mass composed primarily of fat with a central soft tissue component. A small calcification is seen in the soft tissue component. A small right ovarian cyst is present.

Differential Diagnosis: None.

Diagnosis: Ovarian dermoid.

Discussion: Germ cell tumors of the ovary account for 15–25% of all ovarian tumors. The most common germ cell neoplasm is the mature teratoma or dermoid. An ovarian teratoma will contain tissue from the ectoderm, mesoderm, and endoderm. The majority of these lesions will be comprised of adipose tissue and squamous epithelial tissue. Occasionally, a tooth or part of a bone will be present within a teratoma. Diagnosis can be made on plain film if a mature tooth is present in the pelvis. The presence of a calcification in the pelvis is not diagnostic on a plain film because it can correspond to a uterine leiomyoma or represent a phlebolith. CT, however, is often diagnostic. The presence of fat, soft tissue density, and a calcification in an adnexal mass is diagnostic of an ovarian dermoid as is seen in this case.

CASE 14

Clinical History: 60-year-old woman with postmenopausal bleeding.

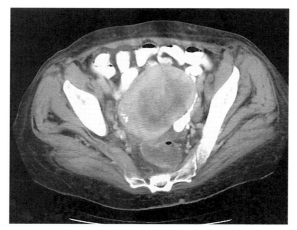

Figure 6.14 A

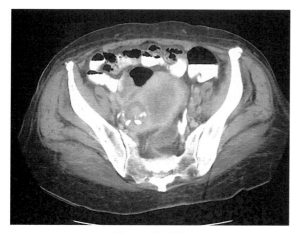

Figure 6.14 B

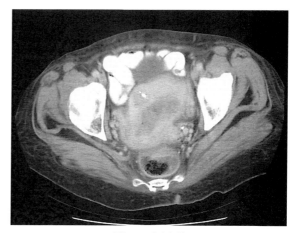

Figure 6.14 C

Findings: CECT demonstrates an enlarged uterus with a central hypodense region (measuring 25 HU) of approximately 5 cm. Two calcified low attenuation lesions are present in the uterine wall.

Differential Diagnosis: Uterine fibroid, cervical cancer, pyometra, hematometra.

Diagnosis: Endometrial cancer.

Discussion: Adenocarcinomas account for 95% of all endometrial cancers with the remaining 5% corresponding to sarcomas. The majority of uterine adenocarcinomas occur in the sixth and seventh decades of life and present with intermenstrual or postmenopausal bleeding. Risk factors for endometrial carcinoma include nulliparity, hormonal replacement, late menopause, and obesity.

CT findings of endometrial carcinoma include a hypodense mass in the uterine wall or endometrial cavity. Less commonly the neoplasm can appear as an enhancing mass in the wall of the uterus. Fluid can be seen in the uterine cavity due to obstruction of the uterus especially if the tumor involves the lower uterine segment. Invasion of the myometrium can be seen as infiltration of the hypodense mass into the normally enhancing uterine wall. This case demonstrates a large low attenuation mass in the uterus that represents a combination of blood and tumor involving the endometrial cavity. Because calcified leiomyomas are present in the uterus, the differential diagnosis should include a degenerating fibroid. Diagnosis was made by dilatation and curettage.

CASE 15

Clinical History: 56-year-old woman with weight loss and pelvic pain.

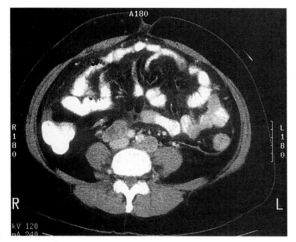

Figure 6.15 A

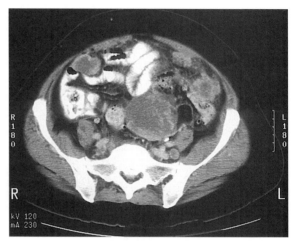

Figure 6.15 B

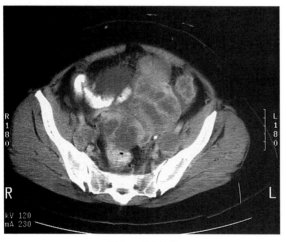

Figure 6.15 C

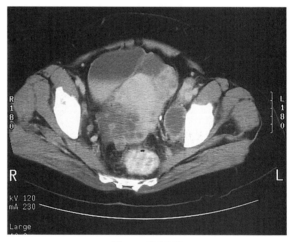

Figure 6.15 D

Findings: (A) CECT demonstrates paraaortic and juxtacaval lymphadenopathy. (B) Low-density soft tissue masses are seen in the omentum. The superior extent of a large pelvic mass is seen. (C, D) Images of the pelvis demonstrate a large heterogeneous bilobed mass extending cephalad from the cervix. Bilateral (2 cm) iliac adenopathy is present.

Differential Diagnosis: Endometrial cancer.

Diagnosis: Cervical cancer.

Discussion: CT is excellent in detecting large lymphadenopathy and intraperitoneal metastases. In this case, the iliac lymphadenopathy (>1.5 cm) stages this patient in a IIIb category. However, the presence of omental metastases and paraaortic lymphadenopathy upgrades the patient to a stage IVb. This information is crucial in determining treatment and prognosis. The 5-year survival in patients with stage IV disease is approximately 14% as opposed to 36% in IIIb disease. Treatment consists of radiation therapy and/or surgery. Radiation therapy is typically used in patients with stages above IIa.

CASE 16

Clinical History: 49-year-old woman with pelvic pain and weight loss. Patient is status post hysterectomy.

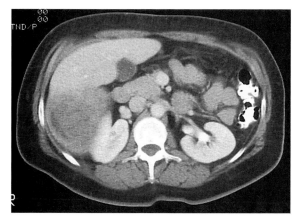

Figure 6.16 A

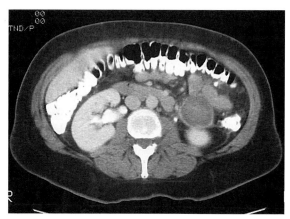

Figure 6.16 B

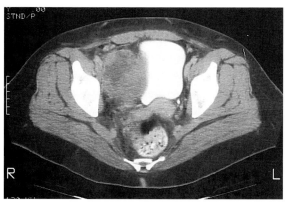

Figure 6.16 C

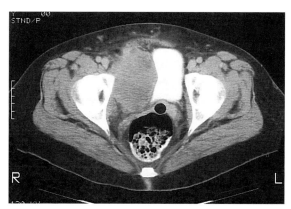

Figure 6.16 D

Findings: (A, B) CECT demonstrates a large heterogeneous complex mass in Morrison's pouch as well as a second mass in Gerota's fascia on the left side. (C, D) A 7-cm complex mass is seen in the right adnexa with displacement of the bladder to the left.

Differential Diagnosis: Cystadenocarcinoma, metastases.

Diagnosis: Granulosa cell tumor.

Discussion: Granulosa cell tumor and Sertoli-Leydig tumor are stromal cell (sex cord) tumors and account for 3% of all ovarian neoplasms. They are hormonally active and patients can present with precocious puberty. Granulosa cell tumors are considered to be malignant but have a good prognosis because most cases are diagnosed as a stage I lesion. The prognosis is worse, however, in perimenopausal women in whom the lesion tends to be larger with metastatic disease frequently present. Granulosa cell tumors tend to be multilocular cystic lesions with a variable amount of solid component. They can grow to be large and are often confused with uterine leiomyomas or ovarian cystadenoma/cystadenocarcinoma. The presence of peritoneal implants in this case excludes uterine fibroids from the differential diagnosis. An ovarian malignancy (cystadenocarcinoma, granulosa cell tumor) and metastases are the best diagnoses for this case.

CASE 17

Clinical History: 48-year-old woman with an abnormal bimanual examination.

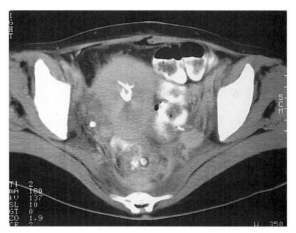

Figure 6.17 A

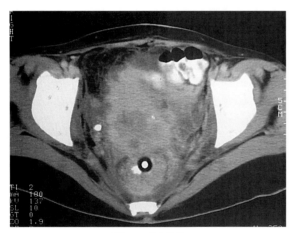

Figure 6.17 B

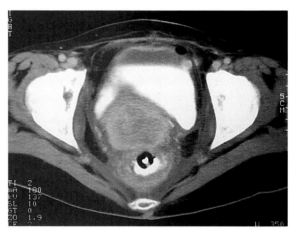

Figure 6.17 C

Findings: CECT demonstrates a large (5 cm) heterogeneous mass involving the cervix with extension to both pelvic sidewalls. Incidentally, there is an IUD in the endometrial cavity.

Differential Diagnosis: Endometrial cancer.

Diagnosis: Cervical cancer.

Discussion: CT imaging is useful in staging of cervical cancer. The FIGO staging classification is as follows:

0	carcinoma in situ
I	confined to cervix
II	extension beyond the cervix without involvement of the pelvic sidewall or lower ⅓ of the vagina
IIa	invasion of upper ⅔ of the vagina only
IIb	parametrial invasion without extension to the sidewall
III	involvement of pelvic sidewall and lower ⅓ of vagina
IIIa	invasion of lower ⅓ of the vagina
IIIb	involvement of pelvic sidewall or hydronephrosis
IVa	involvement of bladder and rectum
IVb	distant disease (paraaortic and inguinal adenopathy, peritoneal metastases)

CT is not accurate in stages up to IIa but is useful in evaluating for parametrial spread and adenopathy. A normal cervix measures 3 cm and has fairly uniform enhancement. The borders of the cervix should be well defined without soft tissue stranding, masses, or adenopathy. A secondary sign of cervical cancer is an obstructed uterus. This case demonstrates a large heterogeneous mass with extension to the pelvic sidewall indicating a stage IIIb lesion.

CASE 18

Clinical History: 71-year-old man with a large mass at the base of the penis.

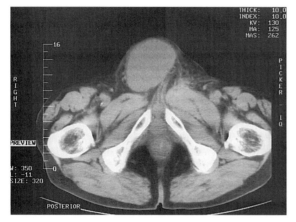

Figure 6.18 A

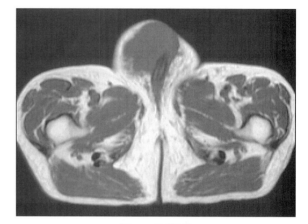

Figure 6.18 B

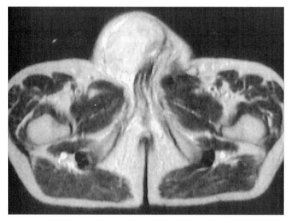

Figure 6.18 C

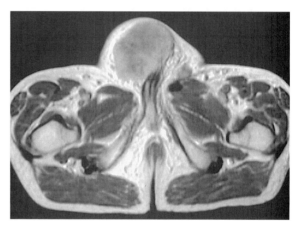

Figure 6.18 D

Findings: (A) NECT demonstrates an 8-cm well defined solid mass to the right of the base of the penis. It appears to be displacing the penile muscles to the left. (B) T1WI shows the mass to be isointense to muscle. The penile muscles are intact. (C) T2WI shows the mass to be hyperintense relative to muscle. (D) Post gadolinium T1WI shows the mass to have heterogeneous enhancement.

Differential Diagnosis: Penile cancer, metastases.

Diagnosis: Leiomyosarcoma of the spermatic cord.

Discussion: The key to the diagnosis in this case is to recognize that the large mass is displacing the penis rather than arising from it. A primary penile neoplasm such as a squamous cell carcinoma would tend to infiltrate the muscles and the skin of the penis. Inguinal adenopathy would probably be present with a neoplasm of this size. Instead, this mass arises from the spermatic cord. The most common neoplasm of the spermatic cord is a sarcoma, either malignant fibrous histiocytoma or leiomyosarcoma. This lesion appears to be separate from the testicle and is too medial to represent inguinal lymphadenopathy. Metastasis would be a good diagnostic consideration.

CASE 19

Clinical History: 47-year-old woman with pelvic pain and hypotension.

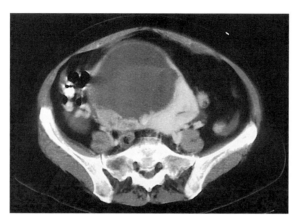

Figure 6.19 A

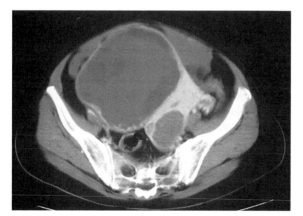

Figure 6.19 B

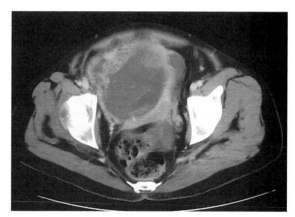

Figure 6.19 C

Findings: CECT demonstrates a large (12 cm) cystic lesion in the pelvis, which displaces the uterus to the left. There is fluid of higher attenuation within the lesion. A smaller 3.5 cm cystic lesion is present posterior to the uterus.

Differential Diagnosis: Ovarian neoplasm (cystadenoma, cystadenocarcinoma), hemorrhagic ovarian cyst, endometrioma, tubo-ovarian abscess.

Diagnosis: Hemorrhagic uterine leiomyoma.

Discussion: A uterine leiomyoma (fibroid) is a benign tumor of smooth muscle in the uterus. It typically occurs in women of reproductive age and is stimulated by estrogens. Uterine leiomyomata, therefore, regress after menopause. By CT imaging, uterine fibroids typically appear similar in density to the normal uterus. Diagnosis is made by contour deformity of the uterus or the presence of calcifications. Occasionally, as in this case, there is hemorrhagic necrosis, which accounts for the high attenuation fluid seen within the lesion. When a leiomyoma becomes large, it becomes difficult to differentiate it from an adnexal mass. The differential diagnosis would therefore include cystic adnexal lesions such as ovarian neoplasms (cystadenoma and cystadenocarcinoma), endometriomas, hemorrhagic ovarian cysts, and tubo-ovarian abscesses. If the patient has a positive HCG level, ectopic pregnancy must be included in the differential diagnosis as well.

CASE 20

Clinical History: 54-year-old woman with incontinence and dysuria.

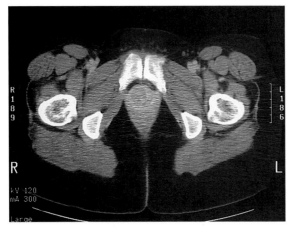

Figure 6.20 A

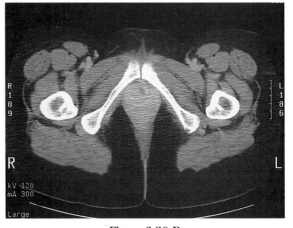

Figure 6.20 B

Findings: CECT of the perineum demonstrates a small (less than 1 cm) cystic lesion in the region of the urethra. An enhancing soft tissue component is in the periphery of the cystic lesion.

Differential Diagnosis: Obstructed urethra, squamous cell carcinoma of the urethra.

Diagnosis: Urethral diverticulum with an adenocarcinoma.

Discussion: Urethral diverticulum is considered an acquired anomaly of the urethra thought to originate from the periurethral glands. Urethral diverticula are typically located adjacent to the urethra and are best visualized by voiding cystourethrogram where they appear as small outpouchings from the urethra. The urothelium inside a urethral diverticulum may undergo dysplasia due to chronic infections and/or calculi. Eventually, malignancies may develop. This case is unusual because the most common malignant neoplasm of the urethra is a squamous cell carcinoma rather than an adenocarcinoma. Other tumors of the urethra include transitional cell carcinomas and metastases. The small fluid-filled structure represents the diverticulum from which an adenocarcinoma developed. Other fluid-filled structures in the lower pelvis include an obstructed urethra and an obstructed periurethral gland. The soft tissue component (or mural nodule) is suggestive of a malignancy.

SUGGESTED READINGS

Affre J, de Peyronnet MR, Deltour F, et al. Secondary foci of primary tumors of the bladder in the upper urinary tract. Urol Radiol 1981;3:7–12.

Amendola MA, Walsh JW, Amendola BE, et al. Computed tomography in the evaluation of carcinoma of the ovary. J Comput Assist Tomogr 1981;5:179–186.

Balfe DM, Van Dyke J, Lee JKT, et al. Computed tomography in malignant endometrial neoplasms. J Comput Tomogr 1983;7:677–681.

Bolduan JP and Farah RN. Primary urethral neoplasms: review of 30 cases. J Urol 1981;125:198–200.

Buy JN, Ghossain MA, Moss AA, et al. Cystic teratoma of the ovary: CT detection. Radiology 1989;171:69–701.

Buy JN, Ghossain MA, Sciot C, et al. Epithelial tumors of the ovary: CT findings and correlation with US. Radiology 1991;178:811–818.

Casillas J, Joseph RC, Guerra JJ. CT appearance of uterine leiomyomas. Radiographics 1990;10:999–1007.

Fukuda T, Ikeuchi M, Hashimoto H, et al. Computed tomography of ovarian masses. J Comput Assist Tomogr 1986;10:990–996.

Ghossain MA, Buy JN, Ligneres C. Epithelial tumors of the ovary: comparison of MR and CT findings. Radiology 1991;181:863–870.

Ginaldi S, Wallace S, Jing BS, et al. Carcinoma of the cervix: lymphangiography and computed tomography. AJR 1981;136:1087–1091.

Goldman SM, Davidson AJ, Neal J. Retroperitoneal and pelvic hemangiopericytomas: clinical, radiologic, and pathologic correlation. Radiology 1988;168:13–17.

Hadar H, Gadoth N, Gillon G. Computed tomography of renal agenesis and ectopy. J Comput Assist Tomogr 1984;137–143.

Katsuhiko H, Matsuzawa M, Chen HF, et al. Computed tomography in the evaluation and treatment of endometrial carcinoma. Cancer 1982;50:904–907.

Karasick S, Lev-Toaff SA, Toaff ME. Imaging of uterine leiomyomas. AJR 1992;158:799–805.

Kilcheski, TS, Arger PH, Mulhern CB, et al. Role of computed tomography in the presurgical evaluation of carcinoma of the cervix. J Comput Assist Tomogr 1981;5:378–383.

Kim SH, Choi BI, Lee HP, et al. Uterine cervical carcinoma: comparison of CT and MR findings. Radiology 1990;175:45–52.

Levine RL, Urethral cancer. Cancer 1980;45:1965–1972.

Megibow AJ, Hulnick DH, Bosniak MA, et al. Ovarian mestatases: computed tomographic appearance. Radiology 1985;165:161–164.

Savader SJ, Otero RR, Savader BL. Puerperal ovarian vein thrombosis: evaluation with CT, US and MR imaging. Radiology 1988;167:637–639.

Sawyer RW, Vick CW, Walsh JW, et al. Computed tomography of benign ovarian masses. J Comput Assist Tomogr 1985;9:784–789.

Stern AJ, Patel SK. Diverticulum of the female urethra. Radiology 1976;121:222.

Tada S, Tsukioka M, Ishii C, et al. Computed tomographic features of uterine myoma. J Comp Assist Tomogr 1981;5:866–869.

Vick CW, Walsh JW, Wheelock JB, et al. CT of the normal and abnormal parametria in cervical cancer. AJR 1984;143:597–603.

Walsh JW, Goplerud DR. Computed tomography of primary, persistent and recurrent endometrial malignancy. AJR 1982;139:1149–1154.

Walsh JW, Goplerud DR. Prospective comparison between clinical and CT staging in pirmary cervical carcinoma. AJR 1981;137:997–1003.

chapter 7

RETROPERITONEUM
AND ADRENAL

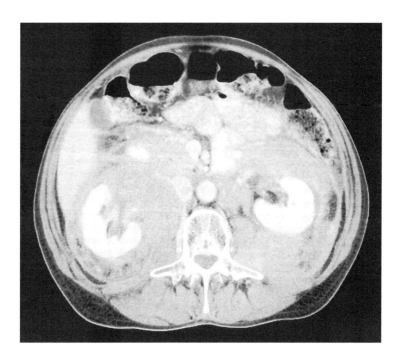

CASE 1

Clinical History: 66-year-old woman with hypotension.

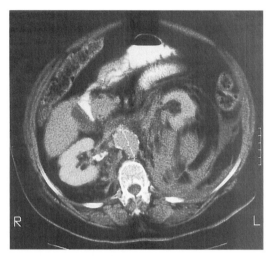

Figure 7.1 A

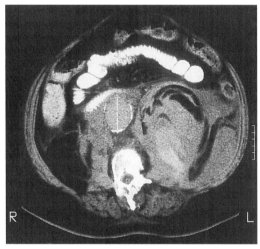

Figure 7.1 B

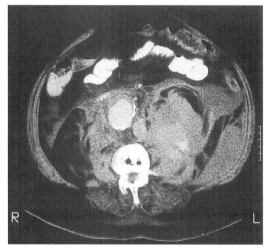

Figure 7.1 C

Findings: CECT demonstrates acute hemorrhage in the para-aortic region, left perirenal space, and left anterior and posterior pararenal space. A 5-cm abdominal aortic aneurysm is present.

Differential Diagnosis: None.

Diagnosis: Aortic aneurysm rupture.

Discussion: Untreated aortic aneurysm ruptures have a mortality rate between 50–90%. Most patients die before reaching the hospital due to the rapid blood loss. Those patients who reach surgery still have a poor prognosis, with less than half surviving 30 days. CT is not necessary in patients with a pulsatile mass or known aneurysm who present with hypotension or back pain. These patients typically go directly to surgery. Patients who are hemodynamically stable without a history of an aneurysm often undergo a CECT; CECT is sensitive in detecting aneurysm rupture. In most cases, high attenuation fluid is present around the aorta and spreads along fascial planes into the perinephric space. Fluid/fluid levels are often present as well as hyperdense fluid representing acute hemorrhage or extravasated contrast. In this case, the hyperdense fluid represents acute hemorrhage, which forms a "hematocrit" or fluid/fluid level in the perinephric space.

CASE 2

Clinical History: 56-year-old woman taking coumadin for a replaced heart valve.

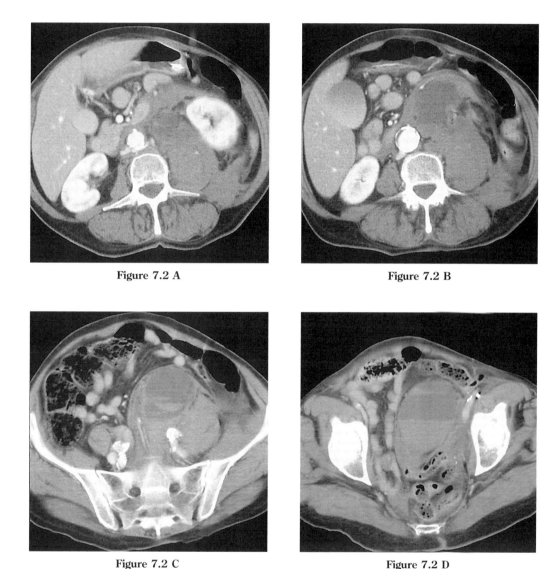

Figure 7.2 A

Figure 7.2 B

Figure 7.2 C

Figure 7.2 D

Findings: CECT demonstrates a large retroperitoneal soft tissue density mass anterior to and involving the left psoas muscle, displacing the kidney anteriorly. A fluid/fluid level is present.

Differential Diagnosis: None.

Diagnosis: Retroperitoneal hemorrhage.

Discussion: Retroperitoneal hemorrhage can be due to multiple etiologies including anticoagulants, trauma, penetrating injury, leaking aortic aneurysms, and bleeding disorders. The hemorrhage tends to spread along the retroperitoneal fascial planes and will therefore spare the perirenal space if the posterior renal fascia has not been interrupted (penetrating injury, prior surgery). Also, hemorrhage will not cause bone destruction as can be found with neoplasms. In the acute and early subacute phases of a hemorrhage, a fluid/fluid level can be present. The denser blood products will settle to the bottom of the fluid collection forming a "CT-hematocrit level." This is nearly diagnostic of hemorrhage. With time, the fluid collection will become less dense and cystic in appearance. It is important to exclude an underlying hemorrhagic neoplasm; therefore, close follow-up scans are necessary as well as correlation with clinical history.

CASE 3

Clinical History: 35-year-old man with severe hypertension refractory to medications.

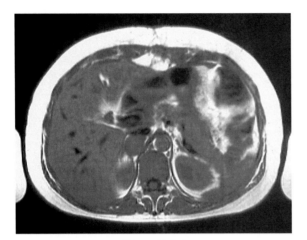

Figure 7.3 A

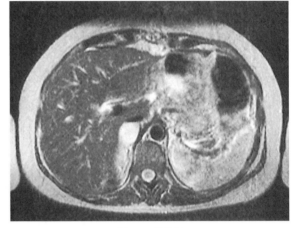

Figure 7.3 B

Findings: (A) T1WI demonstrates a 3-cm round lesion in the right adrenal gland that is isointense to liver. Note the displacement of the IVC anteriorly. (B) T2WI demonstrates the same lesion to be hyperintense relative to liver.

Differential Diagnosis: Adenoma, metastasis, hemorrhage, granulomatous infection (tuberculosis, histoplasmosis).

Diagnosis: Pheochromocytoma.

Discussion: Pheochromocytoma is a rare tumor arising from the chromaffin cells in the adrenal medulla. The rule of "10's" for pheochromocytomas states that 10% are extra-adrenal (para-aortic, organ of Zuckerkandl, perivesical), 10% are multicentric, and 10% are malignant. The most common finding in patients with pheochromocytomas is hypertension due to excess catecholamine release. Other symptoms include tachycardia, sweating, nausea, and chest pain. Imaging of pheochromocytoma includes CT and MRI. CT is very sensitive in detecting small adrenal lesions. Contrast, however, may be contraindicated in patients with suspected pheochromocytomas because it can cause a hypertensive crisis. MRI is very sensitive as well and adds multiplanar capabilities. Pheochromocytomas are typically slightly hypointense on the T1WI and markedly hyperintense on the T2WI as in this case. This appearance is nonspecific because there is overlap with other adrenal lesions such as adenocarcinoma and metastases. With an appropriate clinical picture (hypertension and elevated urinary VMA) and an adrenal mass, the diagnosis of pheochromocytoma is almost certain.

CASE 4

Clinical History: 50-year-old man with severe intractable hypertension.

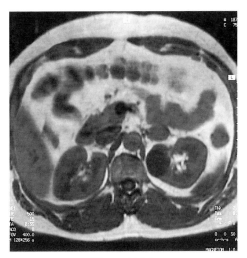

Figure 7.4 A

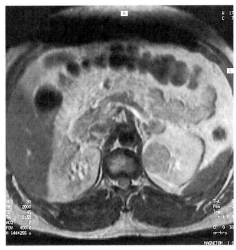

Figure 7.4 B

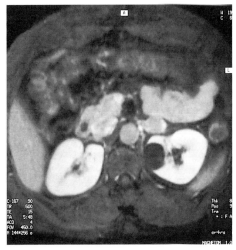

Figure 7.4 C

Findings: (A) T1WI demonstrates a hypointense (relative to liver) 2.5-cm left adrenal lesion. (B) Proton-weighted image demonstrates the lesion to be slightly hyperintense to liver. (C) Post gadolinium fat-saturation T1WI shows the lesion to be isointense to liver (mild enhancement). Incidentally, there is a cyst in the left kidney.

Differential Diagnosis: Metastasis, pheochromocytoma.

Diagnosis: Functioning adenoma (Aldosteronoma).

Discussion: The most common benign functioning adenoma of the adrenal produces ACTH and therefore is associated with Cushing's syndrome. The second most common kind is aldosteronoma, producing primary aldosteronism (Conn's syndrome). These patients present with hypertension, hypokalemia, and low plasma renin levels. In the majority of cases, primary aldosteronism is due to an adenoma, with the remainder of cases due to adrenal hyperplasia. MRI of aldosteronoma is similar to that of nonfunctioning adenoma. Aldosteronomas are typically small (less than 4 cm), round or oval, and well defined. The lesion tends to be iso- or hypointense on the T1WI relative to liver. On post gadolinium fat-saturated images, the lesion is usually isointense to liver with mild enhancement relative to liver and kidneys. On T2WI, aldosteronomas are iso- to hypointense as opposed to metastases and pheochromocytomas, which are hyperintense relative to liver. In a patient with symptoms and laboratory data suggestive of hyperaldosteronism, a small adrenal mass is likely to be an aldosteronoma.

CASE 5

Clinical History: 48-year-old woman with history of multiple pulmonary emboli.

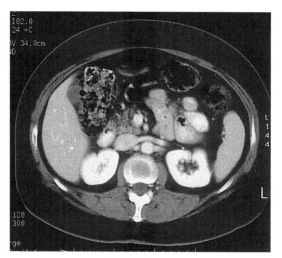

Figure 7.5 A

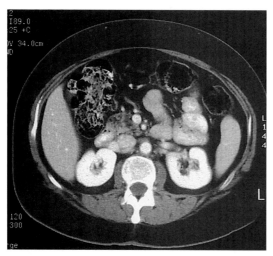

Figure 7.5 B

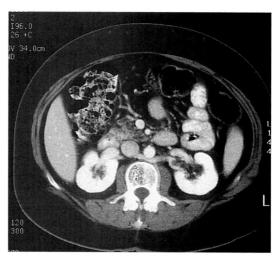

Figure 7.5 C

Findings: CECT demonstrates a left renal vein anterior and posterior to the aorta.

Differential Diagnosis: None.

Diagnosis: Circumaortic left renal vein.

Discussion: Circumaortic left renal vein is a common developmental anomaly of the IVC occurring in approximately 4% of patients. The ventral renal vein is usually in the normal location and the dorsal renal vein is typically several centimeters caudal to it. The ventral renal vein drains the inferior and anterior portions of the left kidney and the dorsal renal vein drains the superior and posterior aspects of the left kidney. Circumaortic left renal vein is usually asymptomatic and of little clinical significance except in placement of an IVC filter or surgery. Placement of the filter should not occlude the orifice of the renal vein or renal vein thrombosis can occur. Placement should be caudal to the most inferior renal vein, which is usually the dorsal renal vein. Alternatively, the filter can be placed cephalad to both renal veins. This will prevent emboli from reaching the lung from the lower extremities.

CASE 6

Clinical History: 57-year-old woman with left flank pain.

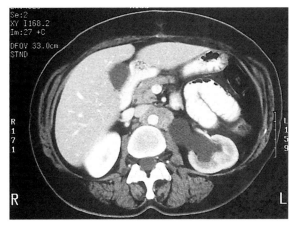

Figure 7.6 A

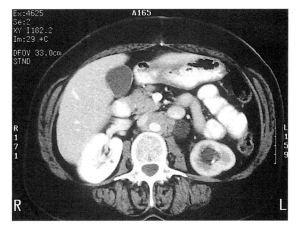

Figure 7.6 B

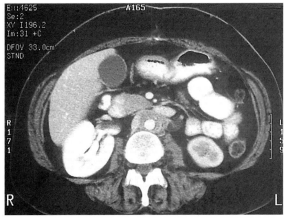

Figure 7.6 C

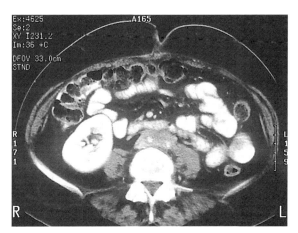

Figure 7.6 D

Findings: CECT demonstrates a soft tissue density mass surrounding the aorta. Left hydronephrosis is present.

Differential Diagnosis: Lymphoma, infectious lymphadenopathy, metastatic lymphadenopathy.

Diagnosis: Retroperitoneal fibrosis (RPF).

Discussion: Retroperitoneal fibrosis is an uncommon process composed histologically by fibroblasts, inflammatory cells, and collagen. It typically encases the aorta and the IVC and can involve the ureters, leading to hydronephrosis. The majority of cases of retroperitoneal fibrosis are idiopathic possibly due to an autoimmune process. Benign causes of retroperitoneal fibrosis include medications (methysergide, beta blockers), infections (tuberculosis, syphilis), and aortic aneurysm. Malignancies can also elicit a desmoplastic reaction leading to retroperitoneal fibrosis as well. The CT findings of RPF are nonspecific, ranging from stranding in the retroperitoneum (without a mass) to a large soft tissue density mass. RPF enhances after contrast administration and usually begins in the lower part of the abdomen. Infectious and metastatic lymphadenopathy as well as lymphoma can have a similar appearance. Although the CT findings are not diagnostic, CT is helpful in following these patients after surgery or steroid treatment.

CASE 7

Clinical History: 56-year-old man with a lung mass.

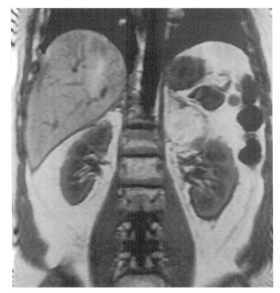

Figure 7.7 A

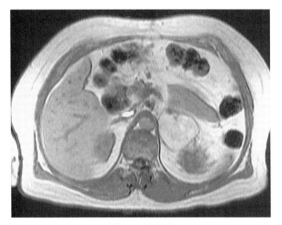

Figure 7.7 B

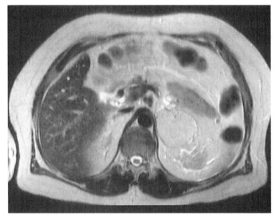

Figure 7.7 C

Findings: (A) Coronal T1WI demonstrates a 4.5-cm mass above the left kidney that is isointense to fat. (B) Axial proton-weighted image demonstrates the lesion to be isointense to fat. (C) T2WI shows the same lesion to again be isointense to fat.

Differential Diagnosis: None.

Diagnosis: Adrenal myelolipoma.

Discussion: Myelolipoma is a benign tumor arising from the adrenal cortex. It is composed of mature fat and cells similar to those found in the bone marrow such as myelocytes, megakaryocytes, erythrocytes, and lymphocytes. These lesions are typically asymptomatic and found incidentally on imaging. Adrenal myelolipomas can have a variable amount of fat present within the lesion. The presence of fat in an adrenal lesion is diagnostic of a myelolipoma. Myelolipomas can also hemorrhage and calcify, which can give the lesion a heterogeneous appearance. This can mimic other adrenal masses such as adrenal carcinomas and metastases. MRI is useful in detecting myelolipomas due to the characteristic signal fat has on various pulse sequences. In addition, fat suppression sequences can be used to identify fat within an adrenal lesion.

CASE 8

Clinical History: 35-year-old man with night sweats and weight loss.

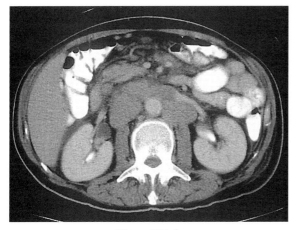

Figure 7.8 A

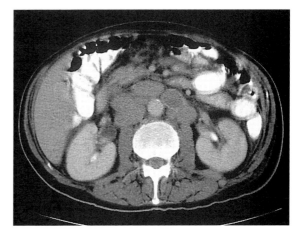

Figure 7.8 B

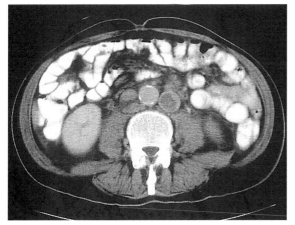

Figure 7.8 C

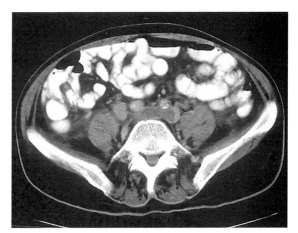

Figure 7.8 D

Findings: CECT demonstrates extensive retroperitoneal adenopathy. There is a vascular structure to the left of the aorta with a low attenuation thrombus.

Differential Diagnosis: Necrotic lymph node.

Diagnosis: Thrombosis of a left-sided IVC in a patient with lymphoma.

Discussion: Left-sided IVC or transposition of the IVC is a relatively uncommon developmental anomaly of the IVC. The infrarenal IVC lies to the left of the aorta and drains into the left renal vein. The suprarenal IVC is in its normal position and location. The infrarenal IVC can be mistaken for adenopathy if its extent is not followed superiorly and inferiorly. The key to the diagnosis is following the vessel as it drains into the left renal vein or bifurcates into the iliac veins. In this case, the low attenuation center could be mistaken for a necrotic lymph node rather than thrombosis of the IVC, which can lead to lethal complications such as pulmonary emboli. This case was further complicated by the enlarged retroperitoneal lymph nodes from the patient's lymphoma.

CASE 9

Clinical History: 26-year-old man post surgery from a prior gunshot wound to the back.

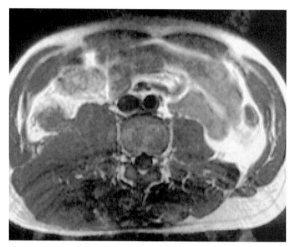

Figure 7.9 A

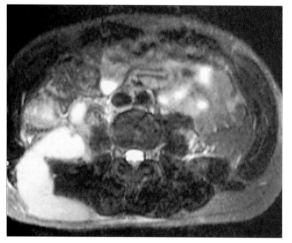

Figure 7.9 B

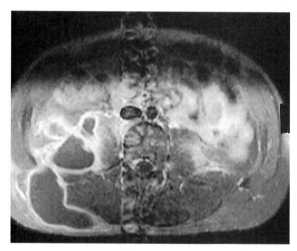

Figure 7.9 C

Findings: (A) T1WI demonstrates a soft tissue mass that is isointense to muscle arising from the right psoas muscle with extension posteriorly. (B) T2WI shows this lesion to be hyperintense similar to water intensity. (C) This same lesion is rim-enhancing on the T1WI post gadolinium.

Differential Diagnosis: Necrotic metastasis.

Diagnosis: Retroperitoneal abscess.

Discussion: Nearly 50% of the masses arising from the iliopsoas muscle are inflammatory in nature. These inflammatory processes typically arise from adjacent organs such as the kidneys, spine (tuberculosis), colon, or pancreas. Penetrating injuries or postsurgical complications can also lead to iliopsoas infections as well. The majority of these inflammatory masses are pyogenic in nature, with abscesses resulting from tuberculous spondylitis less commonly seen.

As with abscesses in other parts of the body, these masses are of water intensity on T1WI and T2WI. Abscesses are often difficult to detect on the T1WI because they are isointense to muscle. Often asymmetry is the only clue to their presence, as in this case. They are easily seen on the T2WI and on the post gadolinium images. On the T1WI post gadolinium, abscesses usually have an enhancing rim, with the central portion being isointense to muscle. The lack of enhancement centrally and the hyperintense signal on T2WI is suggestive of an abscess. A necrotic metastasis could have a similar appearance but it typically has a thick irregular enhancing rim.

CASE 10

Clinical History: 35-year-old man with weight loss and low-grade fever.

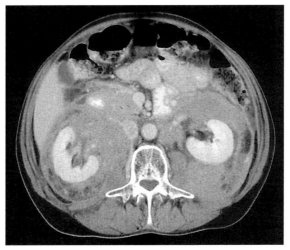

Figure 7.10 A

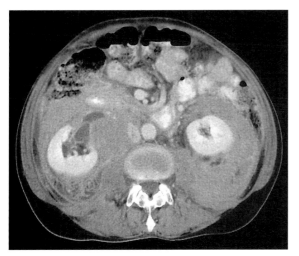

Figure 7.10 B

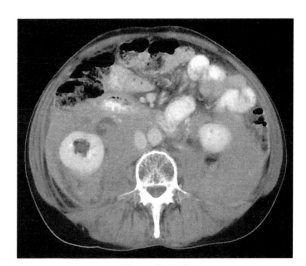

Figure 7.10 C

Findings: CECT demonstrates massive bilateral perinephric soft tissue masses. The soft tissue mass surrounds the kidneys with minimal involvement of the para-aortic and juxtacaval regions as well. Right hydronephrosis is present.

Differential Diagnosis: Hemorrhage, sarcoma.

Diagnosis: Perinephric lymphoma.

Discussion: Perinephric lymphoma can occur by extension of retroperitoneal lymphoma into the perinephric space. In approximately 10% of cases, however, perinephric disease without significant parenchymal disease or retroperitoneal lymphadenopathy is predominant. Perinephric lymphoma typically surrounds the kidney and conforms to the perirenal space. As the lymphoma progresses, it can enlarge the perirenal space and occasionally cause hydronephrosis, as in this case.

Hemorrhage can also involve the perinephric space but fluid attenuation material is usually present as well. A sarcoma will typically be a large well-defined mass that displaces the kidney rather than surrounds the kidney and conforms to fascial boundaries.

CASE 11

Clinical History: 17-year-old girl with back pain.

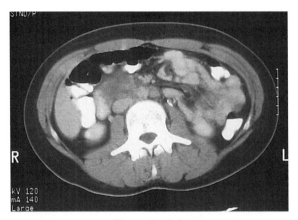

Figure 7.11 A

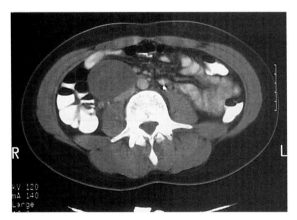

Figure 7.11 B

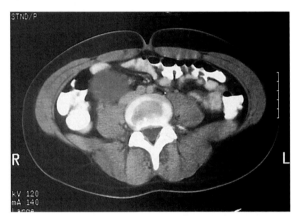

Figure 7.11 C

Findings: CECT demonstrates a cigar-shaped low attenuation enhancing mass located in the right paraspinal region just anterior to the IVC.

Differential Diagnosis: Schwannoma, neurilemomas, sarcoma.

Diagnosis: Ganglioneuroma.

Discussion: The majority of benign primary neoplasms of the retroperitoneum are from neural crest remnants or neural tissue. Neurogenic tumors of the retroperitoneum include schwannoma, neurilemoma, and ganglioneuroma. Ganglioneuromas histologically are mature ganglion cells without metastatic potential. They may represent a mature neuroblastoma. They occur most commonly in children and can be found in the posterior mediastinum as well as in the paraspinal retroperitoneum. On imaging, ganglioneuromas can calcify, which differentiates them from a neurofibroma, which rarely calcifies. They are typically round or elongated and well defined. If no calcifications are present, then it is difficult to distinguish a ganglioneuroma from other retroperitoneal tumors.

CASE 12

Clinical History: 29-year-old woman with a family history of hypertension and thyroid cancer.

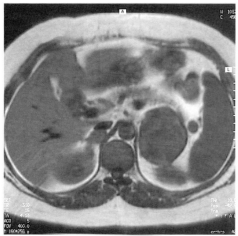

Figure 7.12 A

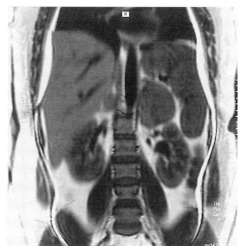

Figure 7.12 B

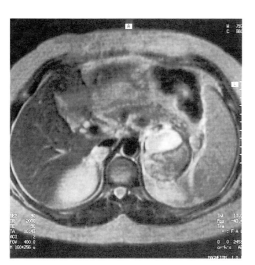

Figure 7.12 C

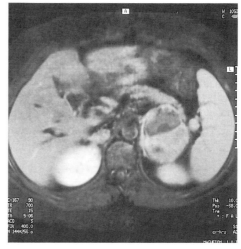

Figure 7.12 D

Findings: (A, B) Axial and coronal T1WI demonstrates a 2-cm right adrenal mass hypointense to the liver. A 6-cm left adrenal mass is present with similar signal characteristics. (C) T2WI demonstrates the lesions to be hyperintense with an area of necrosis in the left adrenal gland. (D) Post gadolinium fat-saturated T1WI demonstrates enhancement of both lesions. A nonenhancing central area corresponds to central necrosis in the left adrenal.

Differential Diagnosis: Metastases, hemorrhage, infection (tuberculosis, histoplasmosis).

Diagnosis: MEN II and bilateral pheochromocytomas.

Discussion: Multiple endocrine neoplasia type II consists of pheochromocytomas (often multiple), medullary carcinoma of the thyroid, and parathyroid adenoma. Because MEN II is autosomal dominant, other family members may also have similar findings and symptoms. Diagnosis is usually made by the presence of elevated urinary vanillylmandelic acid (VMA) levels. MRI has been useful in the evaluation of pheochromocytomas. Because pheochromocytomas are usually symptomatic, they often present early when the lesion is small. The multiplanar capability of MRI is useful in evaluating for small adrenal lesions. Pheochromocytomas are usually iso- or slightly hypointense relative to the liver on T1WI, whereas the lesion is very hyperintense on T2WI. This overlaps with MR findings in other adrenal neoplasms (metastases, adenocarcinoma). Because pheochromocytomas are very vascular, they enhance with gadolinium, as in this case. Hemorrhage tends to have a hyperintense signal on T1WI due to blood products. Both infection and metastases could have this appearance too.

CASE 13

Clinical History: 51-year-old man with dull back pain.

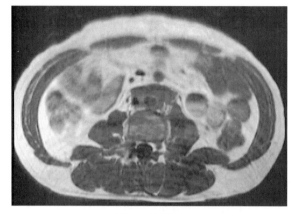

Figure 7.13 A

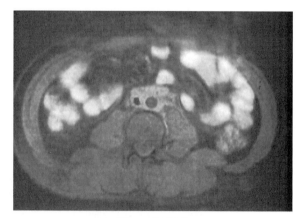

Figure 7.13 B

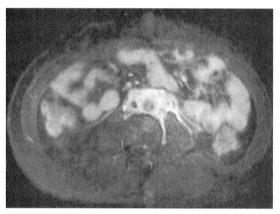

Figure 7.13 C

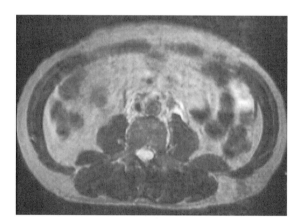

Figure 7.13 D

Findings: (A) T1WI demonstrates a muscle intensity mass surrounding the aorta and IVC. (B) T1WI with fat suppression shows the same lesion to be slightly hyperintense compared with muscle. (C) Fat-suppressed T1WI post gadolinium shows marked enhancement of the retroperitoneal mass. (D) T2WI shows the lesion to be heterogeneously hyperintense relative to muscle.

Differential Diagnosis: Lymphoma, metastatic lymphadenopathy, infectious lymphadenopathy.

Diagnosis: Retroperitoneal fibrosis (RPF).

Discussion: Nearly 70% of cases of retroperitoneal fibrosis are idiopathic, occurring in men between the ages of 40–60 years. Most patients are asymptomatic unless there is involvement of the ureters, leading to hydronephrosis. Rarely, the IVC can be encased causing lower extremity swelling and deep venous thrombosis. Treatment is with steroids and/or surgery. Surgery is performed to free up the ureters and relieve the hydronephrosis. MR imaging is slightly more specific than CT in making this diagnosis. Occasionally, mature RPF will be hypointense on both the T1WI and the T2WI due to the collagen formation. When this occurs, the findings are rather specific for retroperitoneal fibrosis. However, a hyperintense signal on a T2WI or T1WI post gadolinium image, however, is nonspecific. It can be due to acute or active RPF, desmoplastic reaction from a malignant cause, or lymphadenopathy either secondary to a malignancy (testicular cancer, lymphoma) or infectious etiology (tuberculosis, MAI).

CASE 14

Clinical History: 78-year-old woman with abdominal bloating.

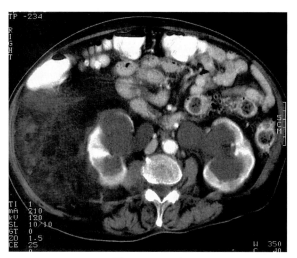

Figure 7.14 A

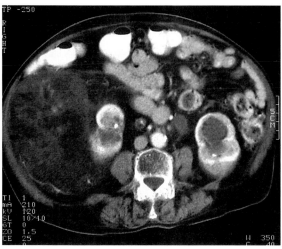

Figure 7.14 B

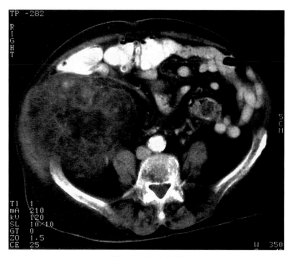

Figure 7.14 C

Findings: CECT demonstrates a massive 12-cm predominantly fatty mass in the right perirenal space, displacing the kidney medially. Note the radiating strands of soft tissue throughout the mass. Bilateral hydronephrosis is present as well.

Differential Diagnosis: None.

Diagnosis: Liposarcoma.

Discussion: Primary retroperitoneal neoplasms arise almost entirely from mesenchymal tissue. The most common retroperitoneal neoplasm is liposarcoma followed by leiomyosarcomas. On CT imaging, liposarcomas can present in several manners. Histologically, liposarcomas can be well differentiated, intermediate or poorly differentiated, with poorer prognosis for the most undifferentiated forms. By CT, well-differentiated liposarcomas are predominantly of fatty density, whereas the undifferentiated ones are of soft tissue density without detectable fat. Microscopically, however, fat is present. The presence of fat and soft tissue in a retroperitoneal tumor is nearly diagnostic of a liposarcoma.

CASE 15

Clinical History: 45-year-old man with abdominal pain.

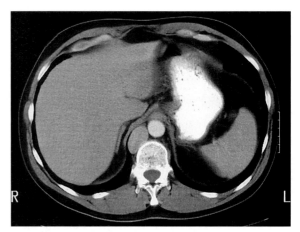

Figure 7.15 A

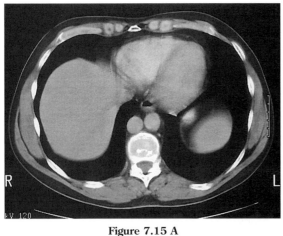

Figure 7.15 B

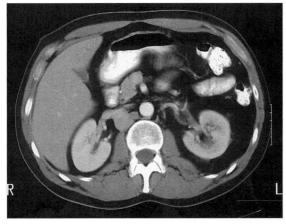

Figure 7.15 C

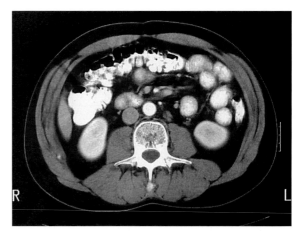

Figure 7.15 D

Findings: CECT demonstrates an enlarged azygous vein with no identifiable IVC.

Differential Diagnosis: None.

Diagnosis: Interrupted IVC with azygous continuation.

Discussion: Interrupted IVC with azygous continuation is a relatively uncommon developmental anomaly of the IVC. It is due to failure in forming the suprarenal portion of the IVC. Below the renal veins, there is a normal IVC to the right of the aorta formed from the confluence of the iliac veins. Above the renal veins, the normal IVC (including the intrahepatic IVC) is not present. Instead there is an enlarged azygous vein seen in its normal location in the retrocrural space, draining into the SVC. The hepatic veins, which normally drain into the IVC, drain directly into the right atrium via the suprahepatic segment of the IVC. It is important to recognize azygous continuation because the azygous vein could be mistaken for an enlarged retrocrural lymph node. It is also important to diagnose this anomaly in patients undergoing shunting procedures for portal hypertension or IVC filter placement.

CT AND MRI OF THE ABDOMEN AND PELVIS

CASE 16

Clinical History: 56-year-old man with a lung mass.

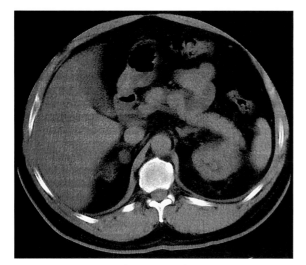

Figure 7.16 A

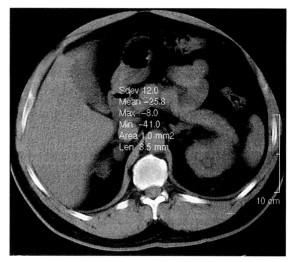

Figure 7.16 B

Findings: NECT demonstrates a 1.5-cm right adrenal mass with an attenuation value of – 25.8 HU.

Differential Diagnosis: Metastasis, pheochromocytoma.

Diagnosis: Adrenal adenoma.

Discussion: The evaluation of adrenal masses is critical in the workup of a patient with a known primary malignancy. Adrenal adenomas are common with an incidence of approximately 8% in autopsy series. The decision to proceed with curative therapy often rests on the characterization of an adrenal mass to exclude distant metastasis. Therefore, a method to noninvasively diagnose adenomas with confidence is needed. Adenomas have a preponderance of lipid-laden cells that give them a lower attenuation value than nonadenomas (metastasis, pheochromocytoma, adenocarcinoma). Using an attenuation value of 10 HU as the cutoff for an adenoma on a NELT, the specificity of diagnosing an adrenal adenoma ranged from 92–100%. Using less than 0 HU, the specificity was 100%. Therefore, an adrenal mass with a negative attenuation value is diagnostic for an adrenal adenoma.

Clinical History: 21-year-old man post surgery for a gunshot wound in the pelvis.

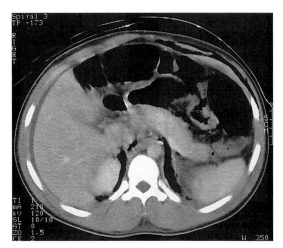

Figure 7.17 A

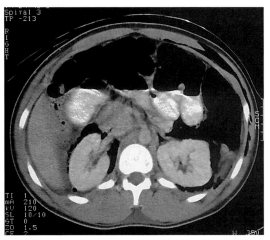

Figure 7.17 B

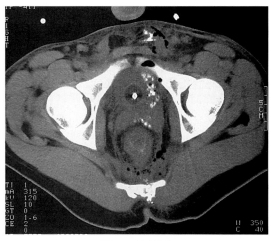

Figure 7.17 C

Findings: CECT demonstrates extensive retroperitoneal air surrounding both kidneys. Mottled air and soft tissue is seen posterior to the rectum. A path of bone fragments and air is seen from the sacrum to the left groin, marking the path of the bullet.

Differential Diagnosis: None.

Diagnosis: Pneumoretroperitoneum.

Discussion: Pneumoretroperitoneum can be due to several causes including perforated bowel, recent surgery, penetrating wound, or gas-forming organism. Portions of the GI tract that are retroperitoneal/extraperitoneal include the duodenal sweep, ascending and descending colon, and rectum. Perforation of any of these loops of bowel can lead to pneumoretroperitoneum. Pneumoretroperitoneum is often difficult to detect by plain film because the air will not collect under the diaphragm or around the liver as in pneumoperitoneum. CT, however, is excellent for evaluating even small amounts of retroperitoneal air. Retroperitoneal air tends to collect on the underside of Gerota's fascia and posterior peritoneum or along the psoas muscle. This is easily detected by CT. The retroperitoneal spaces (anterior and posterior pararenal and perirenal space) become one space in the lower abdomen and are contiguous with the extraperitoneal space in the pelvis. In this case, the retroperitoneal air tracked superiorly from the perforated rectum due to a gunshot wound.

CASE 18

Clinical History: 2-year-old girl with hypertension and an abdominal mass.

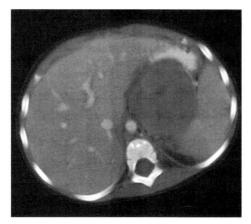

Figure 7.18 A

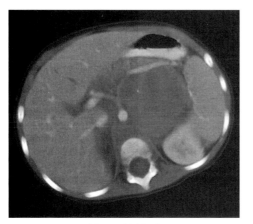

Figure 7.18 B

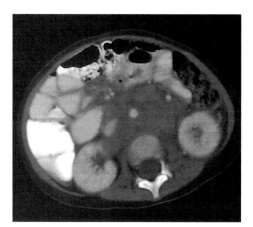

Figure 7.18 C

Findings: CECT demonstrates a large 6-cm heterogeneous mass arising from the left suprarenal region. This mass displaces the splenic vein anteriorly and appears separate from the kidney. Note extensive retroperitoneal adenopathy.

Differential Diagnosis: Wilms tumor.

Diagnosis: Neuroblastoma.

Discussion: Neuroblastoma is the most common solid abdominal mass of infancy arising from the neural crest. The majority occur in children less than 4 years of age but can occur up to 9 years of age. Most neuroblastomas occur in the adrenal gland but they can be found in the chest, abdomen, and pelvis. Patients can present with a palpable mass, hypertension, nystagmus, and abdominal pain.

In a child younger than 5 years of age, the most common solid retroperitoneal masses are a Wilms tumor and neuroblastoma. It is critical to try to determine the organ of origin of these masses. In this case, the mass is separated from the kidney by a cleft of fat and displaces the kidney posteriorly and laterally, suggesting an adrenal origin. Retroperitoneal adenopathy is also present, which is commonly seen in neuroblastoma. Diagnosis can be confirmed by the presence of elevated urinary VMA levels.

CASE 19

Clinical History: 36-year-old man with right testicular pain and swelling.

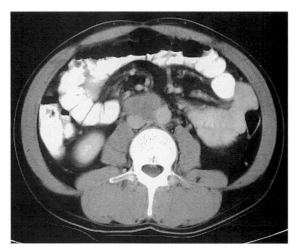

Figure 7.19 A

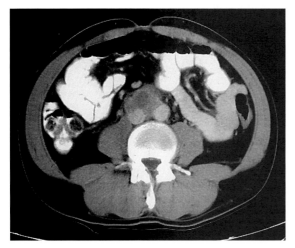

Figure 7.19 B

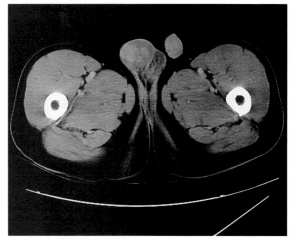

Figure 7.19 C

Findings: CECT demonstrates a low attenuation soft tissue mass surrounding the aorta and IVC. An enlarged right scrotal sac with fluid is present.

Differential Diagnosis: Lymphoma, retroperitoneal fibrosis, infectious lymphadenopathy (tuberculosis, MAI).

Diagnosis: Metastatic seminoma.

Discussion: Testicular cancer is the most common cancer in men between 15 and 35 years of age. Testicular cancer can be divided into germ cell and nongerm cell types. Germ-cell neoplasms constitute nearly 95% of all cases. Of the germ-cell types, the most common is a seminoma. Because seminomas are extremely radiosensitive, they have an excellent prognosis. Workup for testicular cancer typically includes an abdominal CT scan to evaluate for retroperitoneal adenopathy. Testicular cancers spread via lymphatics, following the course of the gonadal veins. Therefore, a left-sided testicular cancer would spread to lymph nodes in the left renal hilum, whereas right-sided testicular cancers spread to the right paraaortic and juxtacaval regions, as in this case. A soft tissue mass surrounding the aorta and IVC can be due to both lymphoma and retroperitoneal fibrosis. In this age group, AIDS-related diseases, such as MAI adenopathy, must also be considered. The history of a swollen right testicle, the age of the patient, and the retroperitoneal adenopathy are highly suggestive of the diagnosis of metastatic testicular cancer.

CASE 20

Clinical History: 57-year-old woman with an enlarging abdomen.

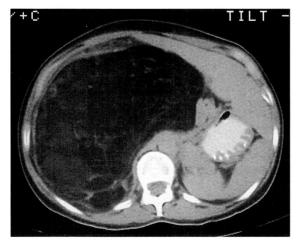
Figure 7.20 A

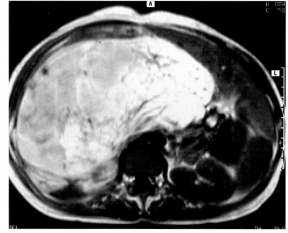
Figure 7.20 B

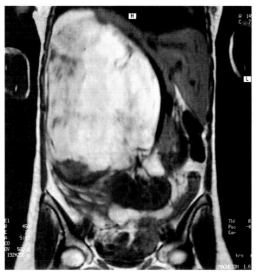
Figure 7.20 C

Findings: (A) CECT demonstrates a 20-cm fatty tumor arising from the retroperitoneum. Strands of soft tissue course through the lesion. (B, C) Axial and coronal T1WI demonstrates this large lesion to be hyperintense to liver and isointense to fat. The soft tissue strands seen on CT are of low signal intensity on the MRI. Note the displacement of the right kidney, liver, and IVC.

Differential Diagnosis: None.

Diagnosis: Liposarcoma.

Discussion: Liposarcoma is the most common primary malignancy of the retroperitoneum in patients younger than 60 years of age. CT cannot differentiate between the various types of sarcomas except for a liposarcoma, which contains fat. MRI is extremely useful in evaluating a liposarcoma because it can show the extent of tumor and its relationship to adjacent organs and vessels in various planes. Because liposarcomas contain fat, portions of the lesion will be hyperintense on T1WI. In this example, almost the entire lesion is composed of fat and appears hyperintense on the axial and coronal T1WI. Low intensity strands are seen radiating through the lesion, which represent the soft tissue component. This appearance is nearly diagnostic of a liposarcoma.

CASE 21

Clinical History: 25-year-old man with multiple skin lesions.

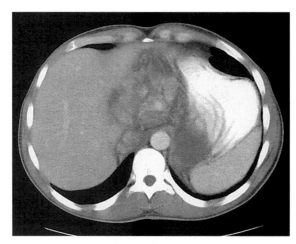

Figure 7.21 A

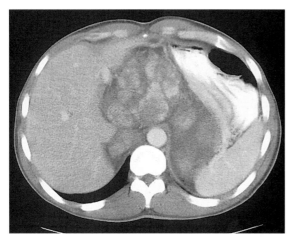

Figure 7.21 B

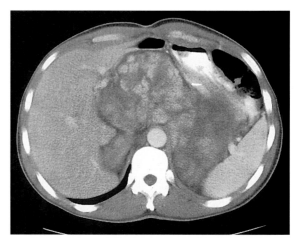

Figure 7.21 C

Findings: CECT demonstrates a large serpiginous-enhancing mass encompassing the entire retroperitoneum and displacing the stomach and bowel anteriorly.

Differential Diagnosis: Lymphoma, sarcoma.

Diagnosis: Neurofibromatosis (type I).

Discussion: Neurofibromatosis type I or von Recklinghausen disease is often referred to as peripheral neurofibromatosis because many of the findings are outside the central nervous system. This includes involvement of the skin (cafe-au-lait spots), bone (sphenoid wing dysplasia, ribbon ribs), and GI tract (multiple neurofibromas). Neurofibromatosis is characterized by dysplasia of neuroectodermal and mesodermal tissues, which can result in multiple neurofibromas. Neurofibromas are tumors of the nerve sheath, with nerves and nerve fibers coursing through it. Therefore, it is difficult to surgically remove a neurofibroma without injuring the underlying nerve. Plexiform neurofibroma is composed of tortuous fusiform enlargement of small peripheral nerves intermixed with connective tissue. These can grow to be very large, surrounding adjacent structures without causing obstruction or constriction. They are typically low in attenuation but can demonstrate mild enhancement, as seen in this case. The location and appearance can occasionally make neurofibromatosis difficult to distinguish from lymphoma.

CASE 22

Clinical History: 36-year-old man with hypertension.

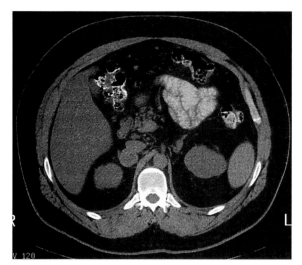

Figure 7.22 A

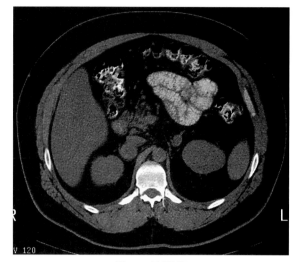

Figure 7.22 B

Findings: NECT demonstrates bilateral adrenal masses measuring 3 cm on the right and 1.5 cm on the left.

Differential Diagnosis: Metastases, infection (tuberculosis, histoplasmosis), bilateral adenomas, hemorrhage.

Diagnosis: Bilateral pheochromocytoma in a patient with multiple endocrine neoplasia type II (MEN II).

Discussion: Multiple endocrine neoplasia is an autosomal-dominant disorder involving organs that stem from the neural crest. These cells produce a polypeptide hormone and are known as APUD cells (amine precursors uptake and decarboxylation). MEN II or Sipple disease consists of medullary carcinoma of the thyroid, parathyroid adenoma, and pheochromocytoma. The pheochromocytomas in MEN II are often bilateral. Bilateral adrenal masses can be due to several etiologies. Metastases are fairly common especially in lung cancer but also in other hematogenous metastases, such as melanoma and breast cancer. The primary malignancy is typically known when adrenal metastases are found. Granulomatous infections (tuberculosis, histoplasmosis) can involve the adrenal glands, usually presenting with bilateral adrenal calcifications. Adrenal hemorrhage is uncommon in adults and usually occurs during severe stress (surgery, trauma), hypotension, or sepsis. This is more commonly seen in neonates. The history of hypertension and family history of MEN II makes bilateral pheochromocytomas the best diagnosis.

CASE 23

Clinical History: 39-year-old man with chronic renal insufficiency post a motor vehicle accident.

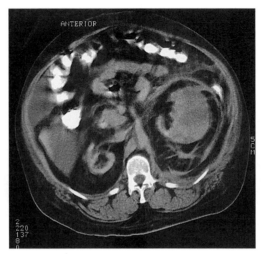

Figure 7.23 A

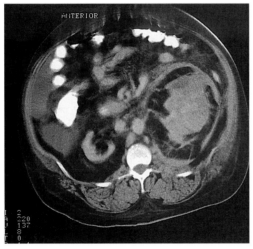

Figure 7.23 B

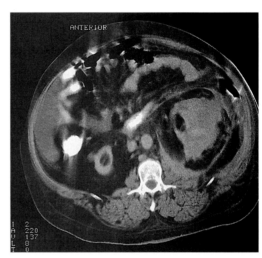

Figure 7.23 C

Findings: CECT demonstrates a high attenuation subcapsular fluid collection involving the left kidney. Fluid and stranding is seen in the left perirenal space. Both kidneys appear small.

Differential Diagnosis: Lymphoma, abscess.

Diagnosis: Perirenal hemorrhage.

Discussion: Hemorrhage in the perirenal space can be due to blunt or penetrating trauma, anticoagulant therapy, or a hypervascular neoplasm (angiomyolipoma, renal cell carcinoma). The high attenuation fluid is suggestive of an acute or subacute hemorrhage. If Gerota's fascia has not been disrupted, the hemorrhage will often be contained within the perirenal space, as in this case. Purulent material from an abscess can also be high in attenuation. Clinical history and the patient's symptoms are usually able to distinguish between the two diagnoses. Lymphoma can often involve the perirenal space but tends to be of soft tissue density. An underlying neoplasm should be excluded in this case with a follow-up CT scan after the hemorrhage has resolved.

CASE 24

Clinical History: 65-year-old man with a lung mass.

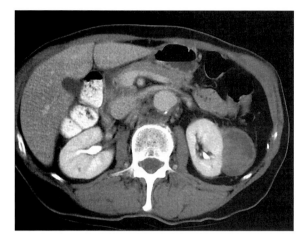

Figure 7.24 A

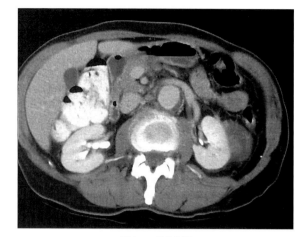

Figure 7.24 B

Findings: CECT demonstrates a 4-cm heterogeneous enhancing mass in the left perirenal space that displaces the kidney medially.

Differential Diagnosis: Sarcoma, renal cell carcinoma, lymphoma.

Diagnosis: Lung cancer metastasis.

Discussion: Metastases to the retroperitoneum are commonly seen in pelvic malignancies (cervix, prostate, and bladder) and testicular tumors. These usually spread to retroperitoneal lymph nodes in the para-aortic, juxtacaval, and aortocaval chains. Metastases to the perirenal space, as in this case, is much less common. These are typically hematogenous metastases from lung, breast, and melanoma.

The appearance of a metastasis on a CECT is similar to most solid retroperitoneal tumors. The heterogeneous appearance makes lymphoma less likely because they tend to have homogeneous enhancement. The mass does not appear to arise from the kidney so a renal cell carcinoma is unlikely as well. A solid heterogeneous mass in the perirenal space is most likely to be a metastasis or primary retroperitoneal neoplasm such as a sarcoma or neurogenic tumor.

CASE 25

Clinical History: 65-year-old woman with a history of lung cancer.

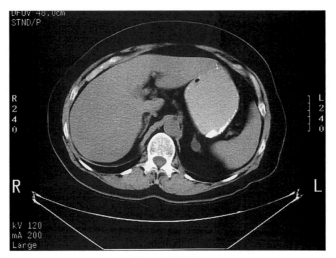

Figure 7.25 A

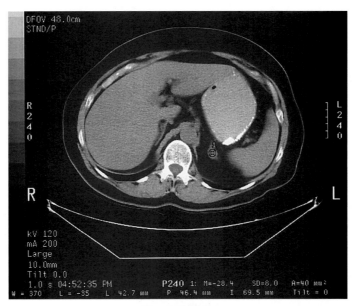

Figure 7.25 B

Findings: NECT demonstrates a 1.5-cm left adrenal mass with an attenuation coefficient of −28.4 HU.

Differential Diagnosis: Metastasis, pheochromocytoma.

Diagnosis: Adrenal adenoma.

Discussion: Adrenal adenomas can be nonfunctioning and functioning (associated with Cushing's disease or primary hyperaldosteronism). Nonfunctioning adrenal adenomas are the most common neoplasm of the adrenal gland. Adenomas are typically less than 3 cm, solitary, and unilateral. Typical characteristics of an adrenal adenoma include a round or oval shape, good delineation, and lack of growth on serial CT scans. Adrenal masses that are smaller than 3 cm are almost always benign. The attenuation value for an adenoma can be less than zero due to lipid-laden adrenocortical cells. A metastasis, adenocarcinoma, and pheochromocytoma have a positive attenuation value, usually greater than 18 HU. The small size of the lesion and negative attenuation value, in this case, are diagnostic of an adrenal adenoma.

CASE 26

Clinical History: 65-year-old man with back pain and hypotension.

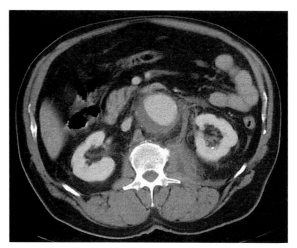

Figure 7.26 A

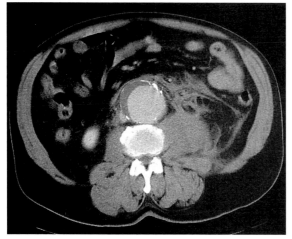

Figure 7.26 B

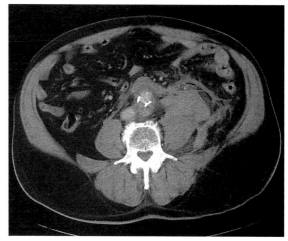

Figure 7.26 C

Findings: CECT demonstrates a large 6-cm infrarenal abdominal aortic aneurysm. A soft-tissue attenuation mass is seen in the left perinephric space, involving the left psoas muscle as well.

Differential Diagnosis: None.

Diagnosis: Abdominal aortic aneurysm rupture.

Discussion: Abdominal aortic aneurysms occur in approximately 4% of the population. Most commonly, the aneurysms are due to atherosclerosis. Other etiologies include infection, trauma, cystic medial necrosis, and syphilis. CECT is excellent in evaluating aneurysms because it gives not only the size of the lumen but also the outer dimension of the aneurysm as well. CECT can also demonstrate the extent of the aneurysm (suprarenal vs. infrarenal) and the involved vessels (SMA, IMA, renal arteries). CECT is rarely performed in patients with ruptured aneurysms due to the high mortality rate and hemodynamic instability of the patient. When imaged, however, high attenuation fluid corresponding to periaortic hemorrhage is present in the paraaortic region, often extending into the perinephric space, as in this case. The presence of retroperitoneal hemorrhage in a patient with an aneurysm is a surgical emergency with a poor prognosis, even with a prompt diagnosis.

Clinical History: 56-year-old man with weight loss.

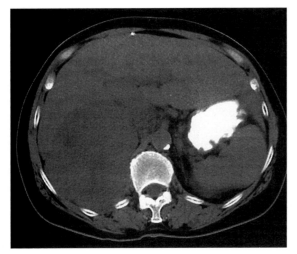

Figure 7.27 A

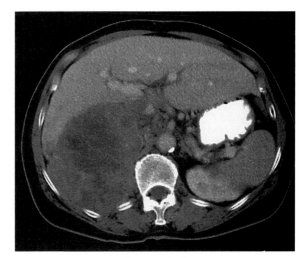

Figure 7.27 B

Findings: (A) NECT demonstrates a large 10-cm mass in the right adrenal gland. (B) CECT shows this lesion to have heterogeneous enhancement.

Differential Diagnosis: Metastasis, hemorrhage, pheochromocytoma, infection (tuberculosis, histoplasmosis), sarcoma.

Diagnosis: Adrenal carcinoma.

Discussion: Adrenal carcinomas arise from the adrenal cortex where hormones are produced such as cortisol, aldosterone, androgen, and estrogen. Most adrenal carcinomas produce hormones (most commonly cortisol) but the hormone produced is often incomplete and not fully functional. This accounts for the large size of these lesions before they are clinically symptomatic. The lesion is typically larger than 5 cm and can be up to 25 cm. Adrenal carcinomas are easily seen on CT. They demonstrate enhancement with contrast but the enhancement is often heterogeneous due to areas of necrosis. Adrenal carcinomas can invade adjacent organs such as the kidney, liver, and spleen. Vascular invasion can also occur into the adrenal vein, which drains into the IVC. Differential diagnosis includes metastases, which are typically smaller, and hemorrhage, which does not enhance centrally. Pheochromocytomas are clinically symptomatic and present when the lesion is much smaller. Biopsy of the adrenal gland can easily be performed in most situations to confirm the diagnosis.

CASE 28

Clinical History: 56-year-old man with back pain.

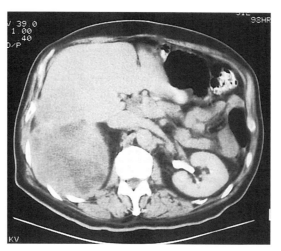

Figure 7.28 A

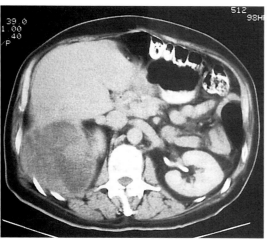

Figure 7.28 B

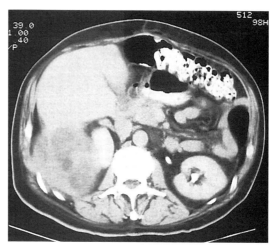

Figure 7.28 C

Findings: CECT demonstrates a large 9-cm enhancing heterogeneous mass arising from the right perirenal space.

Differential Diagnosis: Metastasis, lymphoma, neurogenic tumor.

Diagnosis: Leiomyosarcoma.

Discussion: The majority of primary retroperitoneal tumors are malignant and of mesenchymal origin. The most common are liposarcomas, leiomyosarcomas, and malignant fibrous histiocytomas (MFH). Leiomyosarcomas are typically large heterogeneous tumors, often with central areas of necrosis. They can occur anywhere in the retroperitoneum and will often grow to be large before being detected. Leiomyosarcomas do not contain fat, which differentiates them from liposarcomas. The heterogeneous appearance on a CECT is typical of a leiomyosarcoma or MFH. This is in contrast to the homogeneous appearance of lymphoma. Large metastases to the retroperitoneum are rare. When they do occur, the primary malignancy is usually melanoma, breast, or lung cancer. Neurogenic tumors are usually homogeneous and low in attenuation. A large heterogeneous mass in the retroperitoneum is most suggestive of a sarcoma (MFH or leiomyosarcoma).

CASE 29

Clinical History: 61-year-old man with palpable axillary lymphadenopathy.

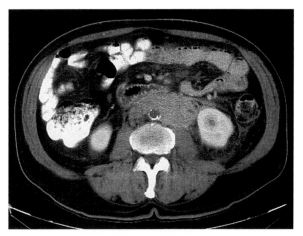

Figure 7.29 A

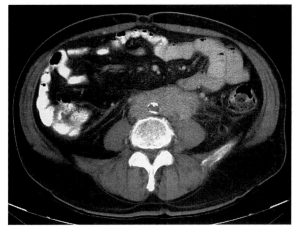

Figure 7.29 B

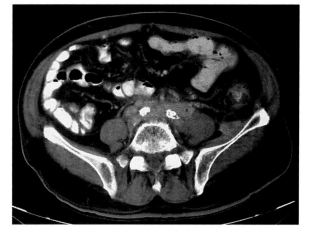

Figure 7.29 C

Findings: CECT demonstrates a soft tissue mass in the retroperitoneum, which surrounds the aorta, IVC, and iliac vessels.

Differential Diagnosis: Retroperitoneal fibrosis, metastatic lymphadenopathy, infectious lymphadenopathy (tuberculosis).

Diagnosis: Non-Hodgkin lymphoma (NHL).

Discussion: The majority of patients with non-Hodgkin lymphoma will have abdominal involvement at the time of diagnosis. CT is the imaging modality of choice for evaluating adenopathy. These enlarged lymph nodes can present as discrete masses or a large confluent mass surrounding and obliterating the retroperitoneal fat planes around the aorta and inferior vena cava, as in this case. Lymph nodes are measured in the short axis to prevent confusion between two adjacent lymph nodes mistaken for a single enlarged lymph node. Lymph nodes are considered enlarged if they measure greater than 6 mm in the retrocrural region, 11 mm in the paraaortic region, or 15 mm in the pelvis. Retroperitoneal adenopathy can be secondary to a variety of causes. Lymphoma is a common etiology especially if disease is elsewhere. Metastatic lymphadenopathy from testis, ovary, uterus, bladder, and GI tract primary malignancies can have a similar appearance. Infectious lymphadenopathy from tuberculosis and MAI are becoming more prevalent due to AIDS and HIV-related diseases.

SUGGESTED READINGS

Amis ES. Retroperitoneal fibrosis. AJR 1991;157:321–329.

Bousvaros A, Kirks DR, Grossman H. Imaging of neuroblastoma: an overview. Pediatric Radiol 1986;16:89–106.

Bullock N. Idiopathic retroperitoneal fibrosis. Br Med J 1988;297:240–241.

Cohan RH, Baker ME, Moore JO, et al. Computed tomography of primary retroperitoneal malignancies. J Comput Assist Tomogr 1988;12:804–810.

Cohan RH, Dunnick NR, Leder RA, et al. Computed tomography of renal lymphoma. J Comput Assist Tomogr 1990;14:933–938.

Degesys GE, Dunnick NR, Silverman PM, et al. Retroperitoneal fibrosis: use of CT in distinguishing among possible causes. AJR 1986;146:57–60.

Dorfman RE, Alpern MB, Gross BH, et al. Upper abdominal lymph nodes: criteria for normal size determined with CT. Radiology 1991;180:319–322.

Dunnick NR, Heston D, Halvorsen R, et al. CT appearance of adrenal cortical carcinoma. J Comput Assist tomogr 1982;6:978–982.

Einstein DM, Singer, AA, Chilcote, WA, et al. Abdominal lymphadenopathy: spectrum of CT findings. Radiographics 1991;11:457–472.

Ellis JH, Bies JR, Kenyon K, et al. Comparison of NMR and CT imaging in the evaluation of metastatic retroperitoneal lymphadenopathy from testicular carcinoma. J Comput Assist Tomogr 1984;8:709–719.

Feldberg MAM, Koehler PR, van Waes PFGM. Psoas compartment disease studied by computed tomography. Radiology 1983;148:505–512.

Hopper KD. Rupture into retroperitoneum. AJR 1985;145:435–437.

Johnson K, Kohler TR, Nicholls SC, et al. Ruptured abdominal aortic aneurysm: the harborview experience. J Vasc Surg 1991;13:240–247.

Jones JH, Ross EJ, Matz LR, et al. Retroperitoneal fibrosis. Am J Med 1970;48:203–208.

Kellman GM, Alpern MB, Sandler MA. Computed tomography of vena caval anomalies with embryologic correlation. Radiographics 1988;8:533–556.

Korobkin M, Brodeur FJ, Yutzy, et al. Differentiation of adrenal adenomas from nonadenomas using CT attenuation values. AJR 1996;166:531–536.

Kvilekval KH, Best IM, Mason RA, et al. The value of computed tomography in the management of symptomatic abdominal aortic aneurysms. J Vasc Surg 1990;12:28–33.

Lane RH, Stephens DH, Reiman HM. Primary retroperitoneal neoplasms: CT findings in 90 cases with clinical and pathologic correlation. AJR 1989;152:83–89.

Lee MJ, Hahn PF, Papanicolaou N, et al. Benign and malignant adrenal masses: CT distinction with attenuation coefficients, size, and observer analysis. Radiology 1991;179:415–418.

Mayo J, Gray R, St Louis E, et al. Anomalies of the inferior vena cava. AJR 1983;140:339–345.

Musante F, Derchi LE, Bazzocchi M, et al. MR imaging of adrenal myelolipomas. J Comput Assist Tomogr 1991;15:111–114.

Quint LE, Glazer GM, Francis IR, et al. Pheochromocytoma and paraganglioma: comparison of MR imaging with CT and I-131 MIBG scintigraphy. Radiology 1987;165:89–93.

Reed MD, Friedman AC, Nealey P. Anomalies of the left renal vein: analysis of 433 CT scans. J Comput Assist Tomogr 1982;6:1124–1126.

Reinig JW, Doppman JL, Dwyer AJ, et al. Adrenal masses differentiated by MR. Radiology 1986;158:81–84.

Rosen A, Korobkin M, Silverman PM, et al. CT diagnosis of ruptured abdominal aortic aneurysm. AJR 1984;143:265–268.

Scatarige JC, Fishman EK, Kuhajda FP, et al. Low attenuation nodal metastases in testicular carcinoma. J Comput Assist Tomogr 1982;7:682–687.

van Erkel AR, van Gils PG, Lequin M, et al. CT and MR distinction of adenomas and nonadenomas of the adrenal gland. J Comput Assist Tomogr 1994;18:432–438.

Vick CW, Zeman RK, Mannes R, et al. Adrenal myelolipoma: CT and ultrasound findings. Urol Radiol 1984;7–13.

Wilms, GE, Baert AL, Kint EJ, et al. Computed tomographic findings in bilateral adrenal tuberculosis. Radiology 1983;146:729–730.

Wolverson MK, Kanneglesser H. CT of bilateral adrenal hemorrhage with acute adrenal insufficiency in the adult. AJR 1984;142:311–314.

chapter 8

MESENTERY, OMENTUM, AND PERITONEUM

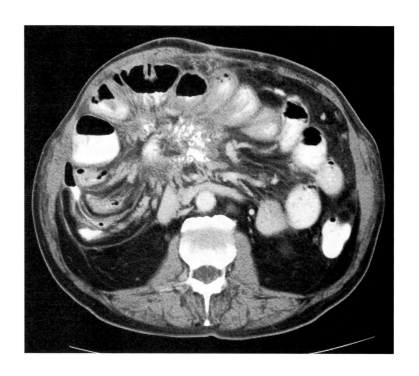

CASE 1

Clinical History: 56-year-old man with vague abdominal pain.

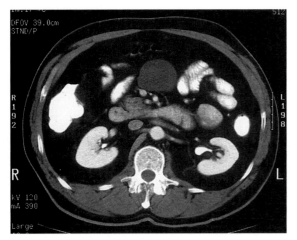

Figure 8.1 A

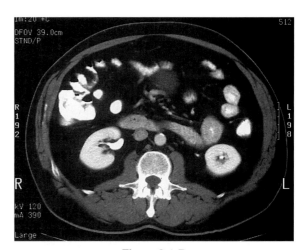

Figure 8.1 B

Findings: CECT demonstrates a small 5-cm cystic lesion in the mesentery.

Differential Diagnosis: Duplication cyst, pancreatic pseudocyst, lymphangioma.

Diagnosis: Mesenteric cyst.

Discussion: Mesenteric cyst can be lined by either epithelial (duplication cyst and enteric cyst subtypes), endothelial (lymphangioma), or mesothelial (mesothelial cyst subtype) cells. If there is absence of a lining in a cyst of the mesentery, it is classified as a pseudocyst (nonpancreatic). Mesenteric cyst, regardless of the histologic subtype, is typically filled with fluid either serous (duplication, enteric, or mesothelial cyst), fatty or chylous (lymphangioma), hemorrhagic (pseudocyst), or purulent (pseudocyst). Mesenteric cysts are usually unilocular (except lymphangioma, which is usually multilocular) and thin walled (except duplication cyst and pseudocyst that usually have a thick wall, visible by US and CT). Lymphangioma is intimately attached to the bowel wall because it originates from it and therefore is the only mesenteric cyst subtype that will require bowel resection to remove it. Because of the same reason, lymphangiomas may produce bowel dilatation and obstruction.

CASE 2

Clinical History: 69-year-old woman with weight loss and bloody stools.

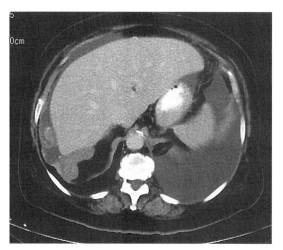

Figure 8.2 A

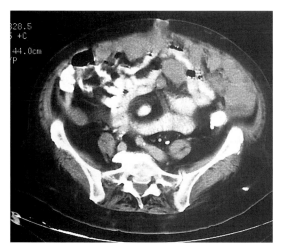

Figure 8.2 B

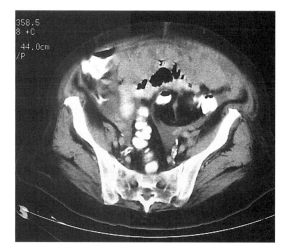

Figure 8.2 C

Findings: CECT demonstrates a soft tissue mass along the peritoneal surface in the perihepatic space. Ascites is also present. Thick soft tissue masses are seen in the omentum as well.

Differential Diagnosis: Mesothelioma, tuberculosis, lymphoma.

Diagnosis: Peritoneal carcinomatosis from colon adenocarcinoma.

Discussion: Metastatic disease involving the peritoneum is commonly seen in patients with primary neoplasms of the ovary, colon, pancreas, and stomach. The metastases can have a variety of appearances. They can present as soft tissue nodules varying in size from a few millimeters to several centimeters, large plaque-like lesions along the peritoneum, and thickening of the mesentery. If the primary tumor is mucinous (ovary and colon adenocarcinoma), then the metastases can be cystic in appearance. These metastases can often be difficult to distinguish from normal unopacified or fluid-filled bowel loops. Good contrast opacification of the bowel is necessary to distinguish between normal bowel loops and metastases. Delayed imaging is often helpful as well as decubitus scanning.

CASE 3

Clinical History: 25-year-old woman with a slow-growing abdominal wall mass.

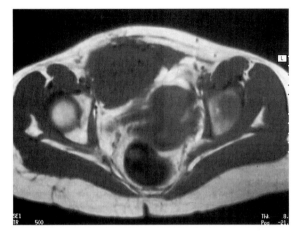

Figure 8.3 A

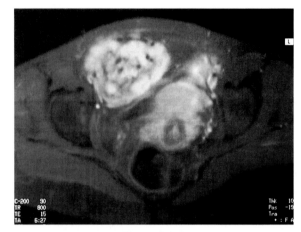

Figure 8.3 B

Findings: (A) T1WI demonstrates a 7-cm mass arising from the right rectus muscle, which is isointense to muscle. (B) Post gadolinium fat saturation T1WI demonstrates marked enhancement of this lesion.

Differential Diagnosis: Metastasis, sarcoma.

Diagnosis: Abdominal wall desmoid tumor (fibromatosis).

Discussion: Desmoid tumor is a benign fibrous tumor that arises from muscle or the muscular aponeurosis. Desmoid tumors do not metastasize but are locally aggressive and will typically recur after resection. They occur most commonly in young women between the ages of 20–40 years and are associated with multiple pregnancies. Less commonly desmoid tumors can also be associated with a history of trauma and Gardner syndrome. By MR imaging, desmoid tumors tend to be iso- or slightly hypointense to muscle on T1WI. They have a variable appearance on T2WI and can enhance with gadolinium, as in this case. Occasionally, low intensity areas are seen on both the T1WI and T2WI corresponding to fibrous tissue. Because they are locally aggressive and can infiltrate adjacent structures, they can be confused with a malignant neoplasm. Treatment is with surgical resection and radiation therapy.

CASE 4

Clinical History: 78-year-old man with abdominal pain.

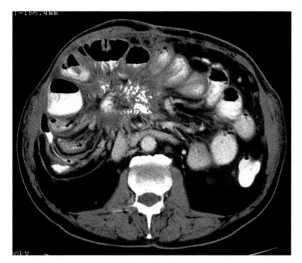

Figure 8.4 A

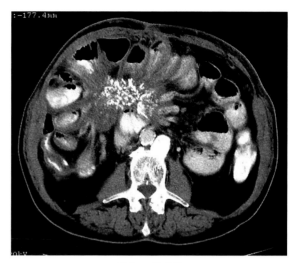

Figure 8.4 B

Findings: CECT demonstrates a soft tissue mass infiltrating the mesentery with extensive coarse calcifications within it.

Differential Diagnosis: Fibromatosis, metastasis, carcinoid, lymphoma, sarcoma.

Diagnosis: Retractile mesenteritis (fibrosing mesenteritis, mesenteric panniculitis).

Discussion: Retractile mesenteritis is a rare disorder of unknown etiology that results in diffuse inflammation, fatty infiltration, and fibrosis of the mesentery. This disorder is usually confined to the mesentery and can calcify as in this case. By CT, there is a soft tissue mass that can contain fat and calcifications that extends from the root of the mesentery toward the bowel. This can lead to retraction and kinking of the bowel clinically, resulting in crampy abdominal pain. Other entities that can involve the mesentery include lymphoma, metastases, and sarcomas. These do not usually cause bowel obstruction or calcify. Carcinoid tumor can cause a desmoplastic reaction and bowel kinking as well, similar to retractile mesenteritis. This would be the best differential diagnosis in this example.

CASE 5

Clinical History: 76-year-old man post motor vehicle accident.

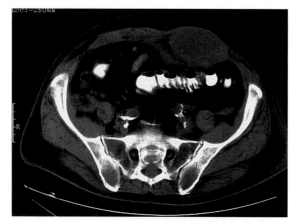

Figure 8.5 A

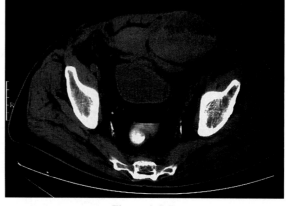

Figure 8.5 B

Findings: NECT demonstrates a 7-cm elliptical cystic lesion in the anterior abdominal wall arising from the rectus muscle. A fluid-fluid level is present.

Differential Diagnosis: Cystic metastasis, sarcoma, desmoid.

Diagnosis: Hematoma.

Discussion: An abdominal wall hematoma can be due to trauma, instrumentation, or anticoagulation and can usually be diagnosed by clinical history. Tumors can also occur in the anterior abdominal wall and must be excluded. Primary tumors (sarcoma) can become necrotic and also present with a fluid-fluid level ("hematocrit level"). Fibromatosis (desmoid tumor) is typically a solid mass with little necrosis. Necrotic/ cystic metastases can have this appearance as seen in metastases from melanoma, renal cell carcinoma, or mucinous adenocarcinoma from the GI tract or ovary.

CASE 6

Clinical History: 71-year-old man with hematuria.

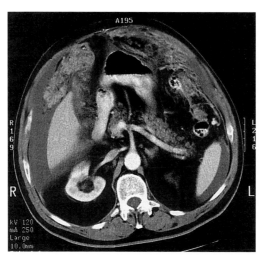

Figure 8.6 A

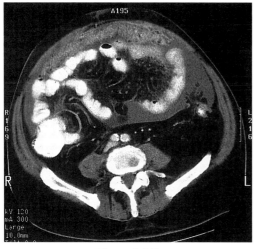

Figure 8.6 B

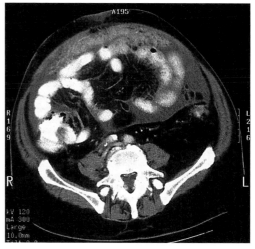

Figure 8.6 C

Findings: CECT demonstrates plaque-like soft tissue masses and thickening of the greater omentum.

Differential Diagnosis: Tuberculosis, mesothelioma, lymphoma.

Diagnosis: "Omental caking" in a patient with transitional cell carcinoma.

Discussion: "Omental caking" is a term used to describe peritoneal metastases or other processes (i.e., tuberculosis) that replace the normal fat of the greater omentum. Normally, the greater omentum constitutes the structure existing between the transverse colon and the anterior abdominal wall. Metastases in this fat plane can thicken or replace the fatty density of the omentum with a soft tissue density, as in this case. The most common neoplasms that present with peritoneal metastases include the GI tract and ovaries. Other entities can simulate peritoneal metastases such as lymphoma, tuberculosis, and mesothelioma. Transitional cell carcinoma is a rare cause of omental caking and other causes of a thickened omentum needs to be excluded. Biopsy can easily be performed through the anterior abdominal wall if necessary.

CASE 7

Clinical History: 67-year-old man with fever and abdominal pain.

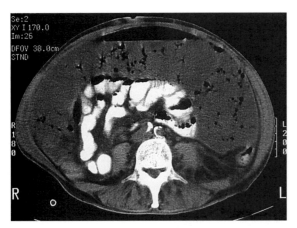

Figure 8.7 A

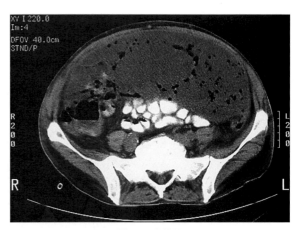

Figure 8.7 B

Findings: NECT demonstrates a large low attenuation mass encompassing most of the anterior peritoneum. Multiple pockets of air are present within the mass as well as pneumoperitoneum.

Differential Diagnosis: None.

Diagnosis: Abdominal abscess.

Discussion: This case is difficult because of the large size of the abscess and its anterior location. The presence of pneumoperitoneum and mottled air within the lesion excludes pseudomyxoma peritonei and ascites. This mass could easily be confused with a dilated stool-filled colon as is seen in institutionalized patients. The colon, however, is displaced posteriorly by this large abscess and no identifiable bowel wall is seen surrounding the abscess. Pneumoperitoneum, which is contiguous with the lumen of the abscess confirms the diagnosis of a large intra-abdominal abscess.

CASE 8

Clinical History: 48-year-old woman with generalized abdominal pain.

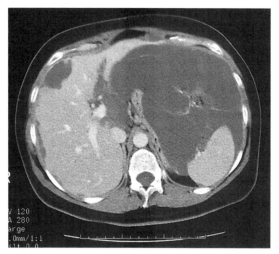

Figure 8.8 A

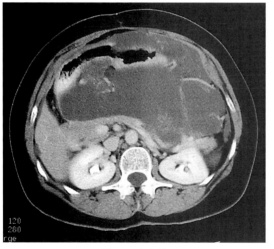

Figure 8.8 B

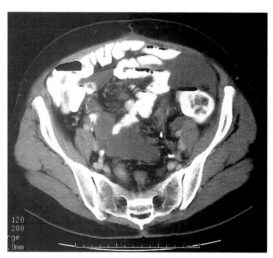

Figure 8.8 C

Findings: CECT demonstrates multiple large loculated fluid collections in the omentum, mesentery and serosal surface of the liver. Multiple septations are present within these cystic lesions.

Differential Diagnosis: Ascites, omental cyst, cystic mesothelioma, cystadenoma of the ovary.

Diagnosis: Pseudomyxoma peritonei.

Discussion: Pseudomyxoma peritonei is the result of diffuse spread of mucinous material throughout the abdomen due to rupture of a low-grade mucinous adenocarcinoma. This is most commonly due to an appendiceal or ovarian neoplasms but less commonly can be due to a urachal or endometrial carcinomas. Patients present with a slow increase in abdominal girth and abdominal pain. By CT imaging, pseudomyxoma peritonei can present as a large fluid-filled exerting mass effect on adjacent organs. Septations and rarely calcifications can occur within pseudomyxoma peritonei, which appears as loculated ascites. Pseudomyxoma peritonei can also present as multiple cystic lesions of variable size found scattered throughout the peritoneum. They can be found in peritoneal recesses where ascites or cells tend to collect, such as on the serosal surface of the liver, omentum, mesentery, subhepatic space, and pouch of Douglas.

CASE 9

Clinical History: 59-year-old woman with abdominal pain.

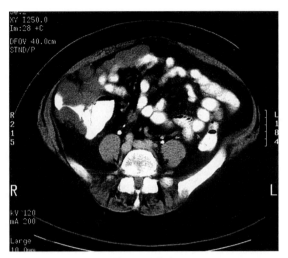

Figure 8.9 A

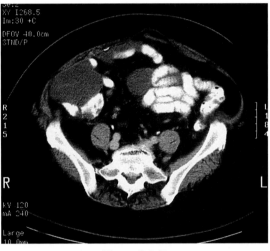

Figure 8.9 B

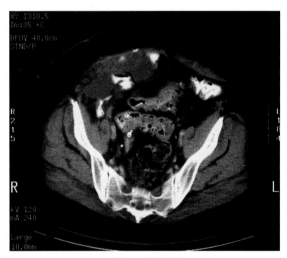

Figure 8.9 C

Findings: CECT demonstrates multiple loculated fluid collections surrounding multiple bowel loops and the anterior peritoneal surface. No bowel obstruction is seen.

Differential Diagnosis: Mesothelial cyst, cystic metastases, duplication cysts, pseudomyxoma peritonei.

Diagnosis: Cystic mesothelioma.

Discussion: Cystic mesothelioma is an uncommon form of peritoneal mesothelioma. It is more commonly seen in females and local recurrence is common after treatment. By CT imaging, there are multiple loculated cystic lesions found on the bowel surface, mesentery, and peritoneal surfaces. Although these lesions surround and demonstrate mass effect on the bowel, obstruction is rare. The cysts in cystic mesothelioma are filled with clear fluid and is of water density by CT. Multiple cystic lesions in the abdomen can be due to cystic metastases, such as from the ovary or appendix. Pseudomyxoma peritonei is a low-grade peritoneal carcinomatosis and can have a similar appearance. Multiple duplication cysts and mesothelial cysts are extremely rare and would be unlikely in this case.

CASE 10

Clinical History: 23-year-old woman with polyarthralgias.

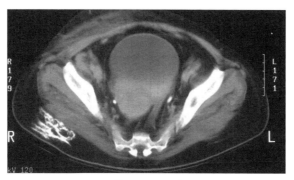

Figure 8.10 A

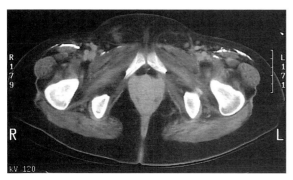

Figure 8.10 B

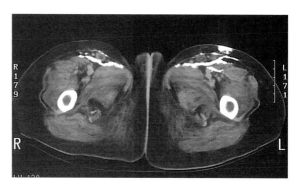

Figure 8.10 C

Findings: CECT demonstrates plaque-like calcifications in the subcutaneous fat in the right buttock and in the right and left groin.

Differential Diagnosis: Hyperparathyroidism, scleroderma, systemic lupus erythematosus, calcinosis universalis.

Diagnosis: Dermatomyositis.

Discussion: Dermatomyositis is an idiopathic inflammatory process of muscles, resulting in muscle atrophy and infiltration by inflammatory cells. It occurs in childhood and late adulthood with female predominance. It results in proximal muscle weakness, interstitial lung disease, inflammatory arthropathy, and an erythematous rash. Plaquelike calcifications can be found in soft tissues of the extremities, abdominal and chest wall, axilla, and inguinal region. Other causes include hyperparathyroidism, calcinosis universalis, and collagen vascular diseases such as scleroderma and SLE. Treatment is with steroids and cytotoxic agents such as methotrexate.

CASE 11

Clinical History: 38-year-old woman receiving coumadin with an enlarging mass in the right abdomen after physical therapy.

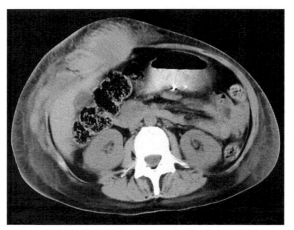

Figure 8.11 A

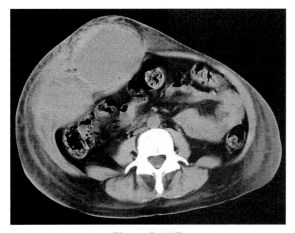

Figure 8.11 B

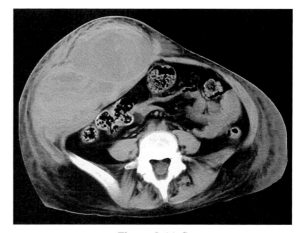

Figure 8.11 C

Findings: NECT demonstrates two large cystic lesions, each measuring approximately 6 cm arising from the right anterior abdominal wall. High attenuation material is present centrally with a fluid-fluid level.

Differential Diagnosis: Cystic metastasis, sarcoma (MFH, leiomyosarcoma), desmoid tumor.

Diagnosis: Hematoma.

Discussion: When a patient is taking anticoagulants such as coumadin or heparin even trivial trauma can result in massive hemorrhage. Occasionally, spontaneous rectus abdominis bleeding can also occur. The presence of high attenuation material centrally with a fluid-fluid level suggests an acute hematoma. Metastasis, desmoid, or sarcoma would be unlikely due to the clinical history but an underlying mass needs to be excluded. This could be performed with a follow-up scan after the hematoma has resolved.

CASE 12

Clinical History: 60-year-old woman with increasing abdominal girth.

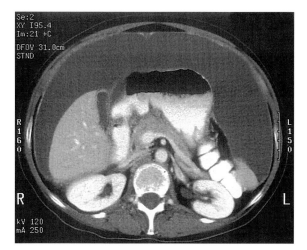

Figure 8.12 A

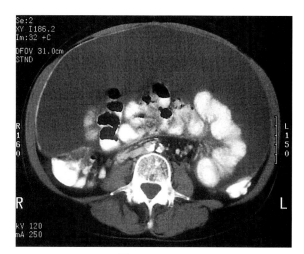

Figure 8.12 B

Findings: CECT demonstrates a large cystic lesion in the anterior abdomen displacing bowel centrally.

Differential Diagnosis: Ascites, omental cyst, cystic mesothelioma, cystadenoma of the ovary.

Diagnosis: Pseudomyxoma peritonei.

Discussion: Pseudomyxoma peritonei is an uncommon disorder resulting from rupture of a low-grade mucinous adenocarcinoma typically from the ovary or appendix. This allows diffuse spread of mucinous material in the peritoneal cavity, resulting in massive ascites-like carcinomatosis. Because the process is indolent with slow accumulation of gelatinous material in the peritoneum, there is often a delay in diagnosis. The key to the diagnosis is the mass effect exerted by this cystic-like lesion on the bowel and solid organs. In contradistinction, ascites will flow around bowel loops without causing displacement of the bowel. An omental cyst and cystic mesothelioma are rare, usually smaller in size, and localized rather than a diffuse process. Cystadenoma of the ovary can grow to be large but it will arise from the pelvis. This lesion appears to arise from the mid abdomen. This appearance is very suggestive of pseudomyxoma peritonei.

CASE 13

Clinical History: 75-year-old man with weight loss and a palpable abdominal mass.

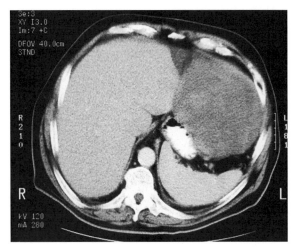

Figure 8.13 A

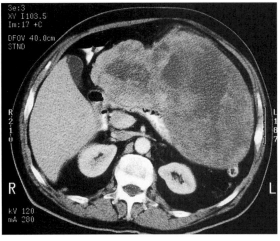

Figure 8.13 B

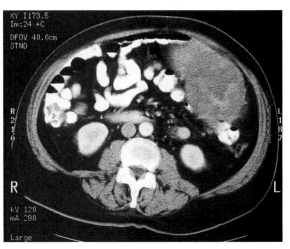

Figure 8.13 C

Findings: CECT demonstrates a massive well-defined 30-cm heterogeneous enhancing mass in the left abdomen beginning near the diaphragm and extending caudally to the pelvis.

Differential Diagnosis: Metastasis, lymphoma, fibromatosis.

Diagnosis: Malignant fibrous histiocytoma (MFH).

Discussion: Malignant fibrous histiocytoma is a soft tissue sarcoma that most commonly arises in the soft tissue of the proximal portions (thigh, arm) of the extremities followed by the ones that originate from the retroperitoneum. Rarely MFH arises from the mesentery, as in this case. As with most sarcomas, MFH tends to be a well defined and a large mass before it presents clinically. MFHs are hypervascular and enhance with contrast administration. Other solid masses in the mesentery can be due to lymphoma, metastases, and fibromatosis. There is no adenopathy to suggest lymphoma, and metastases tend to be smaller multiple masses. Pancreatic pseudocyst and mesenteric cyst are excluded due to the central enhancement. Fibromatosis and one of the various sarcomas (such as MFH) are the best diagnositic possibilities in this case.

CASE 14

Clinical History: 62-year-old woman with chronic lung disease.

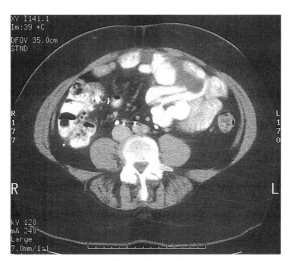

Figure 8.14 A

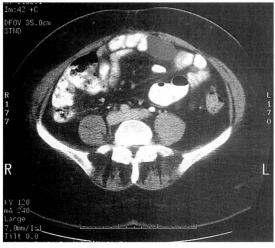

Figure 8.14 B

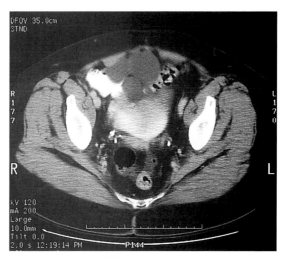

Figure 8.14 C

Findings: CECT demonstrates multiple cystic lesions in the omentum and on the surface of multiple loops of small bowel.

Differential Diagnosis: Mesothelial cyst, cystic metastases, duplication cysts, pseudomyxoma peritonei.

Diagnosis: Cystic mesothelioma.

Discussion: Peritoneal mesothelioma is an uncommon neoplasm arising from the peritoneum of the abdomen. It typically occurs in women between the ages of 30–45 years of age. Cystic mesothelioma is unrelated to malignant peritoneal mesothelioma and asbestos exposure. By CT imaging, the lesions are multilocular and of water density. They are found along the peritoneal surface and the surface of the bowel. The walls of the cyst are typically thin, with occasional thin septations. Cystic mesothelioma will usually compress the bowel without causing obstruction.

SUGGESTED READINGS

Bernardino ME, Jing, BS, Wallace S. Computed tomography diagnosis of mesenteric masses. AJR 1979;132:33–36.

Berquist TH, Ehman RL, King BF, et al. Value of MR imaging in differentiating benign from malignant soft-tissue masses: study of 95 lesions. AJR 1990;155:1251–1255.

Crim JR, Seeger LL, Yao L, et al. Diagnosis of soft-tissue masses with MR imaging: can benign masses be differentiated from malignant ones? Radiology 1992;185:581–586.

Dach J, Patel N, Patel S, et al. Peritoneal mesothelioma: CT, sonography and gallium-67 scan. AJR 1980;135:614–616.

Jeffrey RB. CT demonstration of peritoneal implants. AJR 1980;135:323–326.

Kipfer RE, Moertel CG, Dahlin DC. Mesenteric lipodystrophy. Ann Intern Med 1984;80:582–588.

Mayes GB, Chuang VP, Fisher RG. CT of pseudomyxoma peritonei. AJR 1981;136:807–808.

McLeod AJ, Zornoza J, Shirkhoda A. Leiomyosarcoma: computed tomographic findings. Radiology 1984;152:133–136.

Megibow AJ, Hulnick DH, Balthazar EJ. Ovarian metastases: computed tomographic appearances. Radiology 1985;156:161–164.

Ros PR, Olmsted WW, et al. Mesenteric and omental cysts: histologic classification with imaging correction. Radiology 1987;164:327.

Seshul MB, Coulam CM. Pseudomyxoma peritonei: computed tomography and sonography. AJR 1981;136:803–806.

Waligore MP, Stephens DH, McLeod RA. Lipomatous tumors of the abdominal cavity: CT appearance and pathologic correlation. AJR 1981;137:539–545.

chapter 9

UNKNOWNS AND
AUNT MINNIES

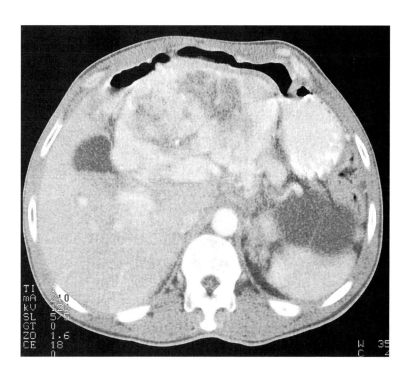

CASE 1

Clinical History: 64-year-old man with severe back pain.

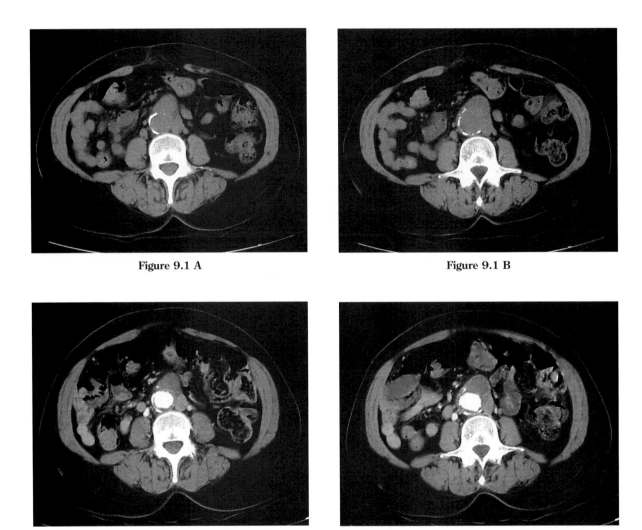

Figure 9.1 A

Figure 9.1 B

Figure 9.1 C

Figure 9.1 D

Findings: (A, B) NECT demonstrates a soft tissue mass protruding off of the anterior portion of the aorta and extending outside of the aortic calcifications. (C, D) CECT demonstrates this soft tissue mass to be outside the lumen of the aorta.

Differential Diagnosis: None.

Diagnosis: Contained rupture of the aorta.

Discussion: It is often difficult to distinguish between a mural thrombus in an aorta from a contained leak or rupture of the abdominal aorta. The problem arises because the exact location of the wall of the aorta is sometimes difficult to identify. A focal outpouching from the aorta or indistinctness of the aorta are all worrisome signs of a leaking aorta. In addition, atherosclerotic calcifications can often delineate the exact location of the wall of the aorta. In this case, a focal outpouching is seen protruding beyond the aortic calcifications, which suggests a contained leak or rupture of the aorta.

CASE 2

Clinical History: 76-year-old woman with severe epigastric pain.

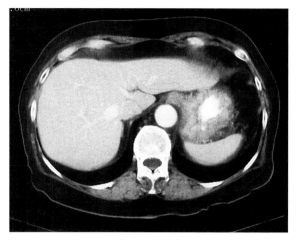

Figure 9.2 A

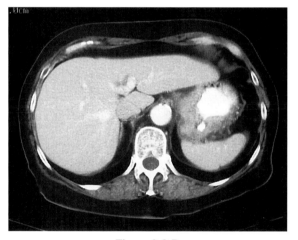

Figure 9.2 B

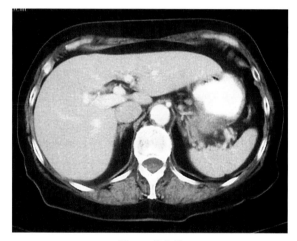

Figure 9.2 C

Findings: CECT demonstrates thickening of the distal stomach and antrum.

Differential Diagnosis: Peptic ulcer disease, gastric adenocarcinoma, gastritis, eosinophilic gastritis, metastasis.

Diagnosis: Lymphoma, stomach.

Discussion: Lymphoma of the stomach is most commonly due to non-Hodgkin disease. It can present as a diffusely infiltrating mass or as a polypoid mass with a propensity to cross the pylorus into the duodenum. Other causes of gastric thickening include neoplasms, such as gastric carcinoma and metastases (breast, melanoma). Benign causes such as peptic ulcer disease, erosive gastritis, and eosinophilic gastritis can have a similar appearance. Diagnosis is made by endoscopy and biopsy.

CASE 3

Clinical History: 51-year-old woman with a palpable pelvic mass.

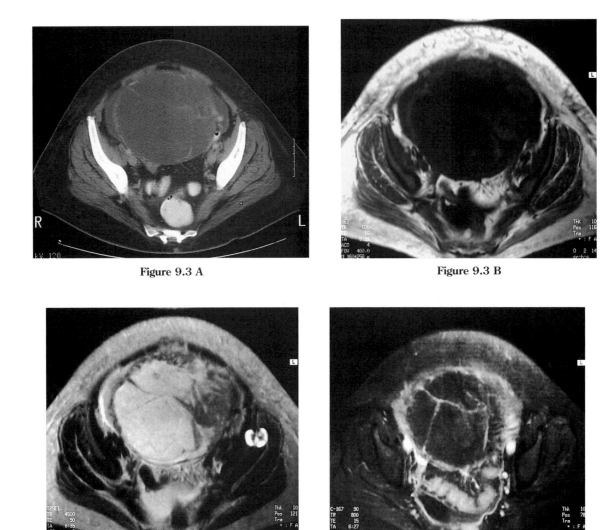

Figure 9.3 A   Figure 9.3 B

Figure 9.3 C   Figure 9.3 D

Findings: (A) CECT demonstrates a 10-cm cystic mass in the pelvis with multiple septations. (B) T1WI demonstrates the wall and septations to be isointense to muscle. (C) T2WI shows the wall and septations to be hypointense. The cystic portion follows water intensity on T1WI and T2WI. (D) Post gadolinium T1WI shows enhancement of the wall and septations.

Differential Diagnosis: Physiologic ovarian cyst, dermoid cyst, tubo-ovarian abscess, cystadenoma.

Diagnosis: Serous cystadenocarcinoma of the ovary.

Discussion: Serous cystadenocarcinoma is an epithelial neoplasm of the ovary, which is predominantly cystic in appearance with a variable amount of soft tissue. Cystadenocarcinomas tend to have thicker walls and septations with a larger soft tissue component (mural nodule) than a cystadenoma. A physiologic cyst can have a similar appearance to a cystadenocarcinoma but will typically regress following the next menstrual cycle. Fat or calcifications are usually present in a dermoid cyst (teratoma) and clinical history should exclude a tubo-ovarian abscess.

CASE 4

Clinical History: 62-year-old woman with long history of epigastric pain.

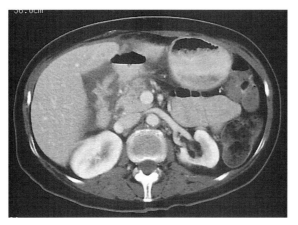

Figure 9.4 A

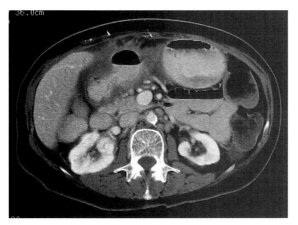

Figure 9.4 B

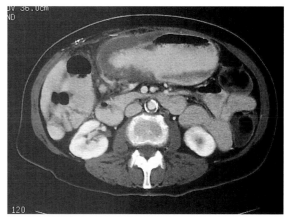

Figure 9.4 C

Findings: CECT demonstrates marked thickening of the antrum and proximal duodenum. The remainder of the stomach is spared.

Differential Diagnosis: Lymphoma, Crohn disease, tuberculosis, eosinophilic gastroenteritis, gastric adenocarcinoma.

Diagnosis: Peptic ulcer disease.

Discussion: Peptic ulcer disease is an inflammatory process that can produce mucosal thickening and ulceration in both the stomach and duodenum. The differential diagnosis of diseases that affect both the antrum and duodenum is limited. The most worrisome of these is lymphoma. Adenocarcinoma of the antrum will usually cause gastric outlet obstruction. Endoscopic biopsy should be performed to exclude a malignancy. Other entities that can involve both the gastric antrum and duodenum include Crohn disease, tuberculosis, and eosinophilic gastroenteritis.

Clinical History: 18-year-old man with acute onset of fever and right lower quadrant pain.

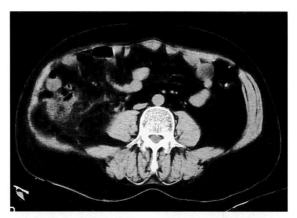

Figure 9.5 A

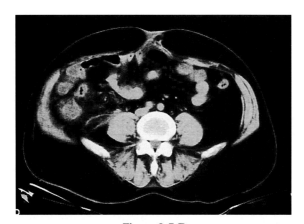

Figure 9.5 B

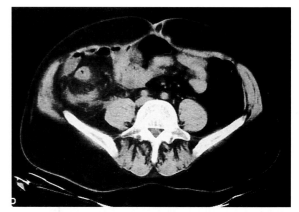

Figure 9.5 C

Findings: CECT demonstrates stranding and thickening of the cecum and pericecal fat.

Differential Diagnosis: Crohn disease, typhlitis, tuberculosis, diverticulitis, Amebiasis, Yersinia.

Diagnosis: Appendicitis.

Discussion: Causes of inflammatory changes around the terminal ileum and cecum are limited. It can be secondary to infectious causes such as tuberculosis, Amebiasis, and Yersiniis, all of which have a propensity to involve the terminal ileum and cecum. Typhlitis occurs in neutropenic patients (leukemia), which is usually known by clinical history. The patient is too young for diverticulitis. Crohn disease is a good diagnostic possibility in an 18-year-old patient, but greater terminal ileum disease would be expected than is seen in this case. The clinical history, acute onset of symptoms, and CT findings are highly suggestive of appendicitis.

CASE 6

Clinical History: 52-year-old man with a palpable mass in the right abdomen.

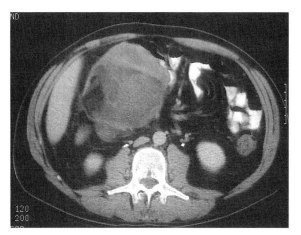

Figure 9.6 A

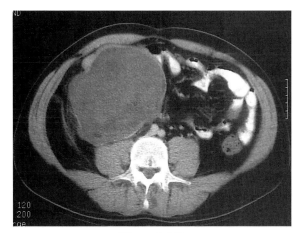

Figure 9.6 B

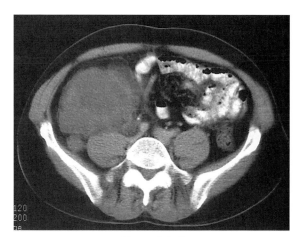

Figure 9.6 C

Findings: CECT demonstrates a large well-defined 10-cm enhancing mass in the right mid abdomen arising from the mesentery. A fat attenuation portion is present within the right side of the mass.

Differential Diagnosis: Teratoma.

Diagnosis: Liposarcoma, mesentery.

Discussion: A large well-defined mass in the mesentery is typically due to a sarcoma, lymphoma, ovarian neoplasm, abscess, or hemorrhage. The lack of fluid within the lesion excludes an abscess and hemorrhage. Lymphoma tends to have homogeneous enhancement rather than heterogeneous enhancement, as in this case. The presence of fat narrows the differential diagnosis to a liposarcoma or teratoma. Mesenteric teratomas are extremely rare and are typically seen in the pediatric population (85% in patients younger than 1 year of age). A large well-defined fat-containing lesion in the mesentery is highly suggestive of a liposarcoma.

CASE 7

Clinical History: 32-year-old man with ESRD status post left abdominal wall surgery for hernia repair.

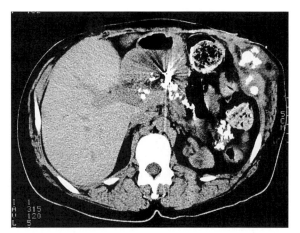

Figure 9.7 A

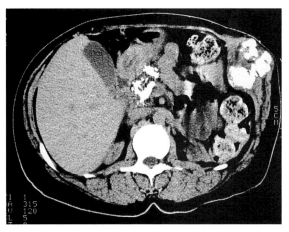

Figure 9.7 B

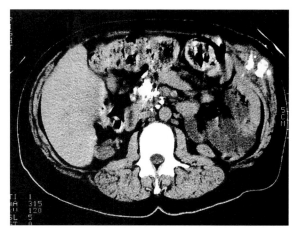

Figure 9.7 C

Findings: NECT demonstrates a 5-cm soft tissue mass in the left abdomen in the region of the prior surgery. Large chunky calcifications are seen in the lesion. Incidentally noted are pancreatic calcifications and small kidneys.

Differential Diagnosis: Desmoid tumor, osteosarcoma.

Diagnosis: Myositis ossificans.

Discussion: Myositis ossificans represents a non-neoplastic formation of fibrous tissue and bone as a response to trauma and hemorrhage. Myositis ossificans is common in young adults with male predominance. Another bone-forming neoplasm is an osteosarcoma. However, the lesion in this example does not have an aggressive appearance making this diagnosis unlikely. Desmoid tumors (fibromatosis) are also associated with trauma or surgery but rarely calcify as in this case. The history of prior surgery and large calcifications makes myositis ossificans the best diagnosis.

CASE 8

Clinical History: 65-year-old man with history of colon cancer.

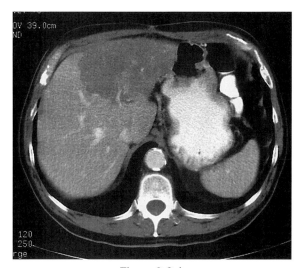

Figure 9.8 A

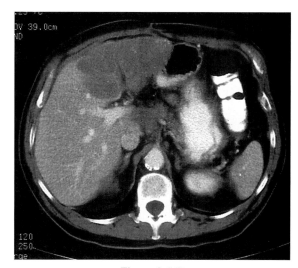

Figure 9.8 B

Findings: CECT demonstrates a low attenuation lesion in the left lobe of the liver crossing the falciform ligament.

Differential Diagnosis: Intrahepatic cholangiocarcinoma, focal fat.

Diagnosis: Metastatic adenocarcinoma of the colon, liver.

Discussion: A solitary liver metastasis is highly unusual but in a patient with a known GI primary, a metastasis must be considered. Initially, this lesion could be confused with focal fat because of the presence of vessels in the lesion. The vessels, however, are not normal in appearance. One of the vessels appears to be abruptly tapered in the periphery of the lesion, suggesting that it is being compressed. This is a finding not seen in focal fat. An intrahepatic cholangiocarcinoma is an excellent differential diagnostic choice and could easily have this appearance. Intrahepatic biliary dilatation is not present unlike in intrahepatic cholangiocarcinoma.

CASE 9

Clinical History: 35-year-old woman with chronic abdominal discomfort.

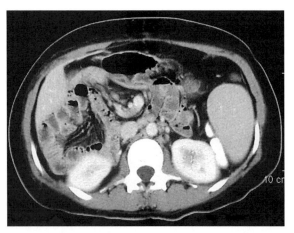

Figure 9.9 A

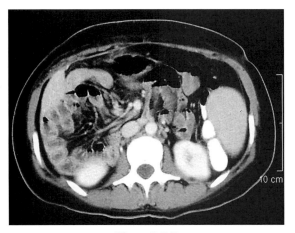

Figure 9.9 B

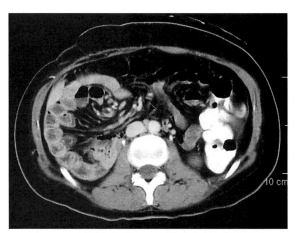

Figure 9.9 C

Findings: (A) CECT demonstrates the SMV to lie to the left of the SMA. (B) Mesenteric vessels are seen feeding a loop of small bowel in the right abdomen. No colon is seen in the right abdomen. (C) The cecum is seen in the left lower quadrant.

Differential Diagnosis: None.

Diagnosis: Malrotation (nonrotation).

Discussion: Malrotation refers to any form of rotational abnormality of the bowel, usually occurring in the second stage of rotation. In nonrotation, the small bowel rotates 90 degrees (normal 270 degrees) and reenters the abdomen. Because of the incomplete rotation, the small bowel lies to the right of the SMA and the colon and cecum to the left. The terminal ileum crosses the midabdomen to reach the left-sided cecum. Because the root of the mesentery is short, a midgut volvulus can occur. The key to the diagnosis in this case is the reversal of the normal location of the SMA and SMV and the right-sided small bowel and left-sided colon.

CASE 10

Clinical History: 65-year-old man with night sweats and weight loss.

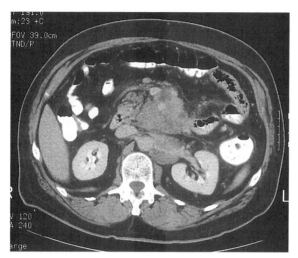

Figure 9.10 A

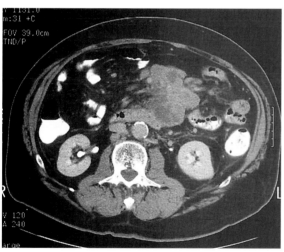

Figure 9.10 B

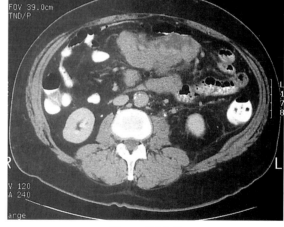

Figure 9.10 C

Findings: CECT demonstrates a 4 × 9 cm heterogeneous mass in the mid abdomen and multiple masses surrounding the left renal artery and SMA.

Differential Diagnosis: Sarcoma, desmoid, metastasis.

Diagnosis: Lymphoma.

Discussion: Lymphoma is one of the most common causes for masses occurring in the small bowel mesentery. It is most commonly non-Hodgkin lymphoma. The mass tends to surround vessels and bowel loops without causing obstruction, as in this case. Adenopathy is usually present in other parts of the abdomen (especially the retroperitoneum) to suggest the correct diagnosis. Other masses occurring in the mesentery include sarcoma, which usually displaces bowel loops and vessels, desmoid tumor (fibromatosis), and metastasis.

Clinical History: 59-year-old man with rectal discomfort and weight loss.

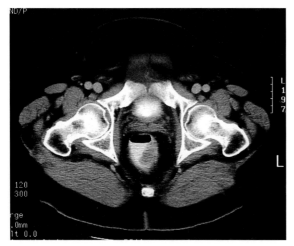

Figure 9.11 A

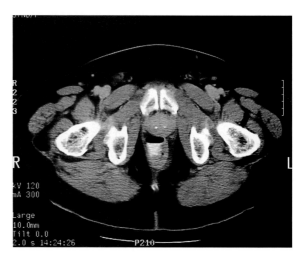

Figure 9.11 B

Findings: CECT demonstrates a soft tissue mass involving the left lateral wall of the rectum.

Differential Diagnosis: Lymphoma, metastases.

Diagnosis: Adenocarcinoma of the rectum.

Discussion: A soft tissue mass arising from the rectal mucosa, which is protruding into the lumen of the rectum, is typical of adenocarcinoma. A metastasis, on the other hand, originates in the submucosa or the serosa depending on the mode of spread (hematogenous versus intraperitoneal). These lesions will tend to be exophytic and will commonly distort the outer surface of the bowel as well as the mucosal surface. Lymphoma is more common in the cecum than the rectum and tends to be a large bulky lesion. Other entities such as tuberculosis and hemorrhage are possible but less likely than an adenocarcinoma.

CASE 12

Clinical History: 19-year-old woman with recurrent pulmonary infections.

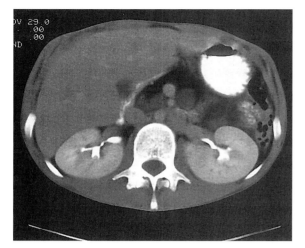

Figure 9.12 A

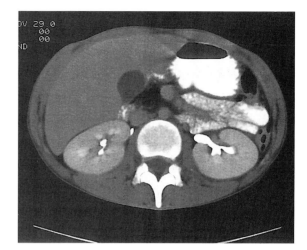

Figure 9.12 B

Findings: CECT demonstrates a fatty replaced pancreas.

Differential Diagnosis: Obesity, normal variant in elderly patients, pancreatic duct obstruction, malnutrition, Schwachman syndrome, Cushing's syndrome.

Diagnosis: Cystic fibrosis.

Discussion: Fatty replacement of the pancreas to the extent seen in this patient is most commonly due to cystic fibrosis. Very little subcutaneous fat is present to suggest obesity or Cushing's disease as an etiology. The age of the patient would exclude fatty replacement seen in the elderly. Schwachman syndrome is fatty replacement of the pancreas and metaphyseal dysplasia, which should be evident clinically. With the history of recurrent pulmonary infections and the age of the patient, cystic fibrosis is the most likely diagnosis.

CASE 13

Clinical History: 75-year-old woman with progressive jaundice and right upper quadrant pain.

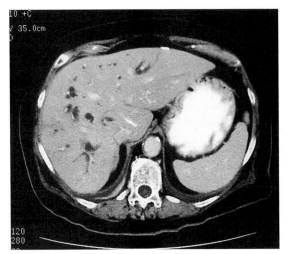

Figure 9.13 A

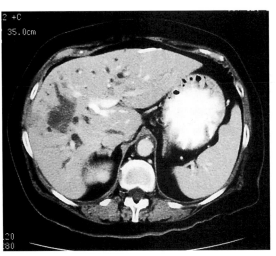

Figure 9.13 B

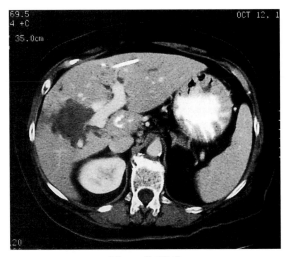

Figure 9.13 C

Findings: CECT demonstrates severe intrahepatic biliary dilatation. There is an ill-defined low attenuation lesion in the right lobe of the liver, which is encasing the right portal vein. Note the PTHD in the left lobe.

Differential Diagnosis: Metastasis, hepatocellular carcinoma.

Diagnosis: Intrahepatic cholangiocarcinoma.

Discussion: Approximately 10% of all cholangiocarcinomas are intrahepatic. They can appear as a focal ill-defined mass or as a diffusely infiltrating lesion. Because these tumors arise from the bile ducts, they commonly spread via the biliary tree causing biliary dilatation. Intrahepatic cholangiocarcinoma does not typically invade the portal vein but will encase and engulf portal and hepatic vein branches. The encasement of the portal vein and biliary dilatation helps to distinguish this lesion from HCC. Metastases rarely cause biliary dilatation and will normally be well circumscribed and multiple.

CASE 14

Clinical History: 50-year-old man with persistently elevated glucose levels.

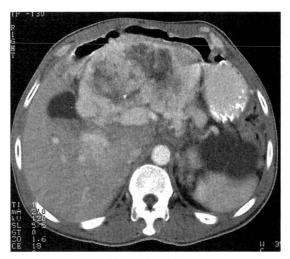

Figure 9.14 A

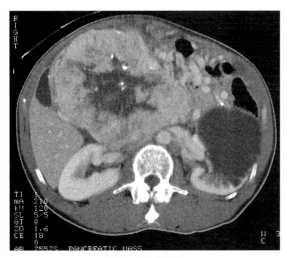

Figure 9.14 B

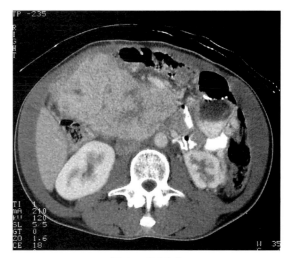

Figure 9.14 C

Findings: CECT demonstrates a large mass (13 cm) arising near the head of the pancreas. The lesion enhances with a central area of necrosis. Small calcifications are present as well as a left renal cyst.

Differential Diagnosis: Adenocarcinoma, sarcoma, metastasis, acinar cell neoplasm, nonfunctioning islet cell tumor.

Diagnosis: Glucagonoma.

Discussion: This case is unusual since glucagonomas tend to be smaller in size at the time of diagnosis. The excess glucagon causes the patient to be hyperglycemic resulting in earlier diagnosis. In addition, patients with glucagonomas present with migratory necrolytic erythema—a characteristic cutaneous lesion. This patient refused surgery, so after several years, the glucagonoma grew to this size. Other diagnostic considerations include metastasis, peripancreatic sarcoma, acinar cell neoplasm of the pancreas, and a nonfunctioning islet cell tumor.

CASE 15

Clinical History: 78-year-old woman with weight loss and left flank pain.

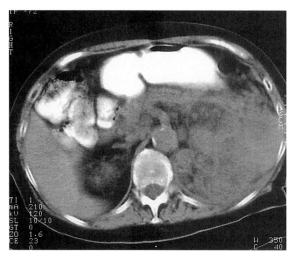

Figure 9.15 A

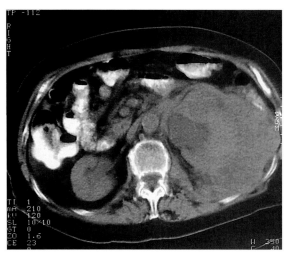

Figure 9.15 B

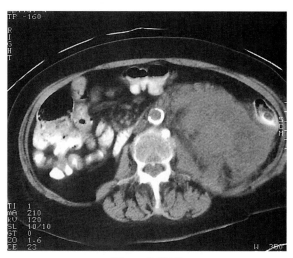

Figure 9.15 C

Findings: NECT demonstrates a large soft tissue mass in the left perinephric space. Left hydronephrosis is also present.

Differential Diagnosis: Hemorrhage, abscess, sarcoma.

Diagnosis: Perinephric lymphoma.

Discussion: The differential diagnosis for a perinephric soft tissue mass is limited. A retroperitoneal sarcoma is usually well defined and will displace the kidney rather than surround it, as in this case. Hemorrhage and abscess both are good diagnostic considerations. Clinical history (fever, trauma, anticoagulant use) is usually helpful in excluding these as possibilities. In addition, a fluid-fluid level or fluid density material is usually present within the mass, which is not seen in this example. A large perinephric soft tissue mass surrounding the kidney in the absence of pertinent history is highly suggestive of lymphoma.

CASE 16

Clinical History: 69-year-old man with increasing abdominal girth.

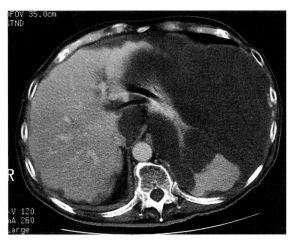

Figure 9.16 A

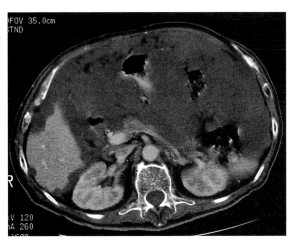

Figure 9.16 B

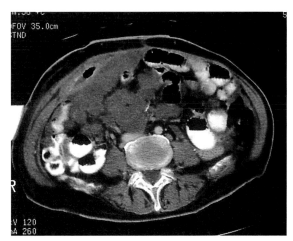

Figure 9.16 C

Findings: CECT demonstrates a low attenuation mass that fills the entire peritoneal cavity, causing mass effect on the liver, spleen, and bowel loops.

Differential Diagnosis: None.

Diagnosis: Pseudomyxoma peritonei.

Discussion: Pseudomyxoma peritonei is a result of a ruptured low-grade mucinous adenocarcinoma of appendiceal, ovarian, or colonic origin with dissemination of its contents throughout the peritoneal cavity. Slowly, these implants will grow and form gelatinous cystic lesions throughout the abdomen, which exert mass effect on the various abdominal organs. Ascites and peritonitis, on the other hand, tend to surround the bowel, liver, and spleen, without causing mass effect. They also tend to collect in dependent anatomic spaces, such as the pelvis and paracolic gutters. The appearance of this case is nearly diagnostic of pseudomyxoma peritonei.

CASE 17

Clinical History: 69-year-old woman with history of diarrhea.

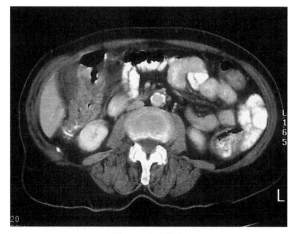

Figure 9.17 A

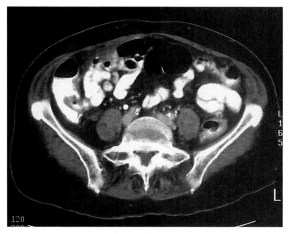

Figure 9.17 B

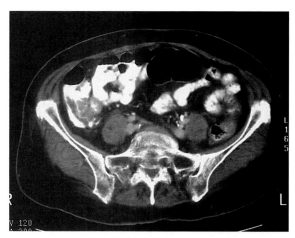

Figure 9.17 C

Findings: CECT demonstrates thickening of the terminal ileum and ascending colon with extensive inflammatory changes in the surrounding fat.

Differential Diagnosis: Lymphoma, tuberculosis, ischemia.

Diagnosis: Crohn disease.

Discussion: Thickening of the terminal ileum and proximal colon has a limited differential. Crohn disease is the first choice. Other signs of Crohn disease include fistulas, abscesses, and pronounced wall thickening averaging 13 mm. Ischemia usually involves a larger segment of the small and large bowel than is seen in this case. Pulmonary tuberculosis is frequently (approximately 50% of cases) present when tuberculosis involves the GI tract, and a chest x-ray would be helpful in further evaluating this patient. Lymphoma, which has a predilection for the right colon, is a good diagnostic choice and could easily have this appearance.

CASE 18

Clinical History: 3-week-old premature newborn presents with an enlarged liver.

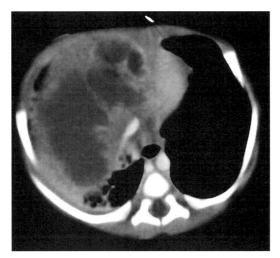

Figure 9.18 A

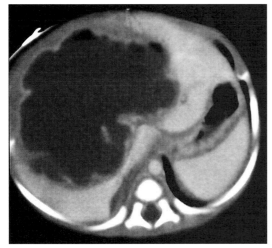

Figure 9.18 B

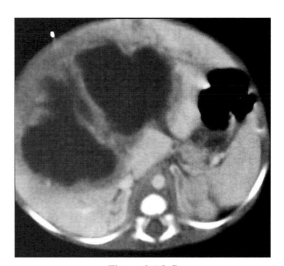

Figure 9.18 C

Findings: A large lobular cystic mass is seen in the liver with peripheral enhancement. Small pockets of air are present in the lesion.

Differential Diagnosis: Infantile hemangioendothelioma, hepatoblastoma, mesenchymal hamartoma.

Diagnosis: Hepatic abscess.

Discussion: In newborn babies, the differential diagnosis for a liver mass includes an infantile hemangioendothelioma and hepatoblastoma. Both these lesions tend to be solid rather than cystic in appearance. A mesenchymal hamartoma, which is typically cystic, can occur in the newborn, but it is extremely uncommon (usual age of presentation is 12–24 months). The key to the correct diagnosis is the presence of air in the lesion, which suggests an abscess. In this case, the patient had an infected umbilical catheter, which led to the formation of the abscess.

CASE 19

Clinical History: 70-year-old woman with history of hepatitis C.

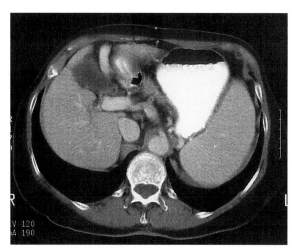

Figure 9.19 A

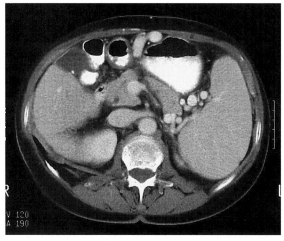

Figure 9.19 B

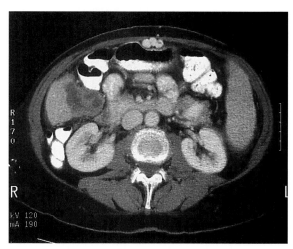

Figure 9.19 C

Findings: CECT demonstrates a small liver with splenomegaly, enlarged portal vein, and multiple collateral vessels including a recanalized paraumbilical vein. A 4-cm enhancing lesion is seen in the right lobe of the liver.

Differential Diagnosis: Metastasis.

Diagnosis: Hepatocellular carcinoma.

Discussion: This case demonstrates some of the classic findings of cirrhosis and portal hypertension. The liver is small, and the spleen is enlarged. Other signs of portal hypertension include a portal vein greater than 13 mm in diameter. The portal vein in this case is almost 2 cm. A large recanalized paraumbilical vein in the falciform ligament is seen as well as splenic hilum collaterals. A focal hypervascular mass in the liver in the setting of cirrhosis is most likely to be a hepatocellular carcinoma. A solitary metastasis without a known primary is highly unlikely.

CASE 20

Clinical History: 35-year-old man with history of epigastric pain.

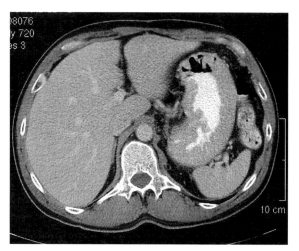

Figure 9.20 A

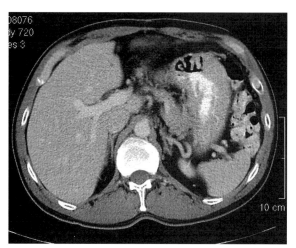

Figure 9.20 B

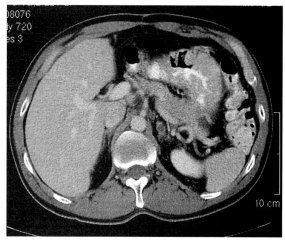

Figure 9.20 C

Findings: CECT demonstrates marked thickening of the stomach.

Differential Diagnosis: Menetrier disease, peptic ulcer disease, lymphoma, gastric carcinoma, gastritis, eosinophilic gastritis, metastases.

Diagnosis: Zollinger-Ellison syndrome.

Discussion: Zollinger-Ellison syndrome is due to a gastrinoma that causes hypersecretion of gastric acid, leading to extensive peptic ulcer disease. This will typically involve the stomach and entire duodenum (including the third and fourth portions, which are rarely involved in typical peptic ulcer disease). The CT findings are nonspecific and can be due to any entity causing gastric thickening including malignancies (lymphoma, adenocarcinoma, metastases), erosive gastritis, and Menetrier disease. Biopsy is often necessary to exclude malignancy. Treatment is resection of the gastrinoma and control of the gastric acid hypersecretion.

CASE 21

Clinical History: 57-year-old man with solid-food dysphagia.

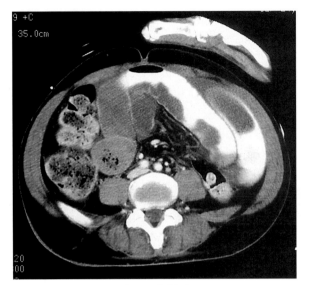

Figure 9.21 A

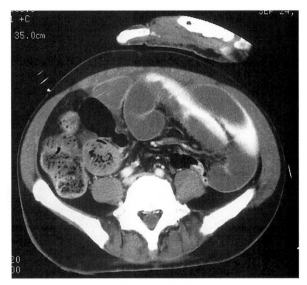

Figure 9.21 B

Findings: CECT demonstrates multiple large low attenuation filling defects in the small bowel.

Differential Diagnosis: None.

Diagnosis: "Ensuromas."

Discussion: Not to worry, "ensuroma" is not a real disorder of the GI tract. This appearance is due to inspissation of Ensure (liquid food supplement) taken by patients who cannot adequately maintain a diet to support themselves. This thick shake will coalesce in the small bowel forming the large intraluminal filling defects seen in this case before being absorbed into the bloodstream. This process appears to be intraluminal rather than mucosal or submucosal. Simple fluid is excluded since it would not be heavier than the oral contrast and would not layer out posteriorly. Hemorrhage from a GI bleed would be a consideration but hemorrhage tends to be of higher attenuation than Ensure. Other food items could have this appearance and could be included in the differential diagnosis.

CASE 22

Clinical History: 60-year-old woman with pelvic pain.

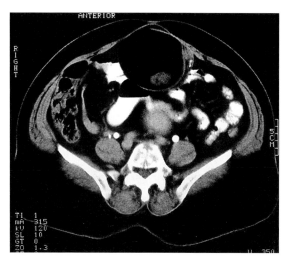

Figure 9.22 A

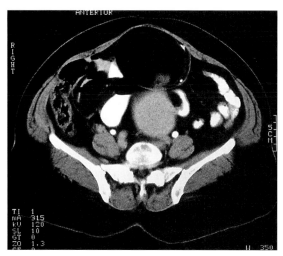

Figure 9.22 B

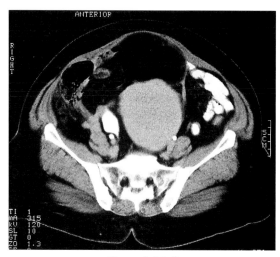

Figure 9.22 C

Findings: CECT demonstrates a 9-cm round mass composed primarily of fat in the anterior lower abdomen. There is a small soft tissue component present as well as peripheral calcifications. Note the fallopian tube on the left, which extends from the uterus to the mass.

Differential Diagnosis: None.

Diagnosis: Ovarian dermoid (teratoma).

Discussion: Ovarian dermoid (teratoma) is the most common ovarian tumor in young women. Because they are typically asymptomatic, dermoids can go undetected until late adulthood when it is found incidentally, as in this case. Diagnosis can easily be made by CT. The lesion can be predominantly cystic or fatty in composition. The presence of fat, soft tissue, and calcifications in an adnexal mass is virtually diagnostic of an ovarian dermoid. When the dermoids are large, they are usually surgically removed due to the risk of torsion.

Clinical History: 48-year-old man with gross hematuria.

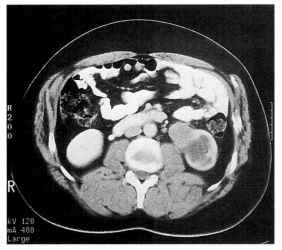

Figure 9.23 A

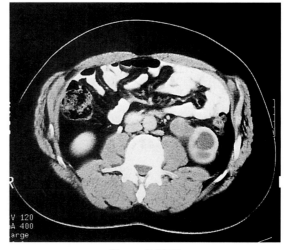

Figure 9.23 B

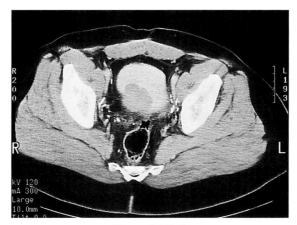

Figure 9.23 C

Findings: CECT demonstrates a soft tissue mass arising from the left renal pelvis causing hydronephrosis. A 4-cm mass is also present in the base of the bladder.

Differential Diagnosis: Metastases.

Diagnosis: Synchronous transitional cell carcinoma.

Discussion: Transitional cell carcinomas arise from the uroepithelium of the bladder and collecting system. Therefore, the greater the surface area of uroepithelium, the greater the incidence of a transitional cell carcinoma (bladder > pelvocalyceal > ureter). In up to 20% of cases of pelvocalyceal transitional cell carcinoma, a synchronous lesion will be present, as in this case. Careful examination of the entire collecting system and bladder is necessary to ensure proper staging.

CASE 24

Clinical History: 50-year-old woman post gastric surgery with fever and abdominal pain.

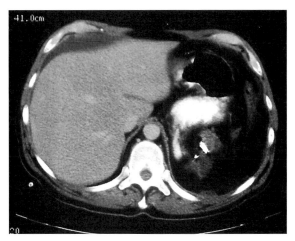

Figure 9.24 A

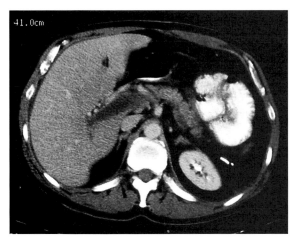

Figure 9.24 B

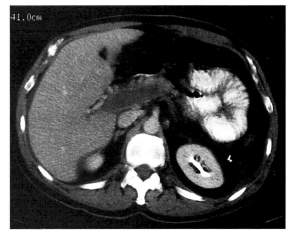

Figure 9.24 C

Findings: CECT demonstrates a small fluid collection along the anterior surface of the liver. An image more caudal demonstrates a low attenuation clot in the portal vein.

Differential Diagnosis: None.

Diagnosis: Portal vein thrombosis secondary to a subphrenic abscess.

Discussion: An area of low attenuation in the portal vein is diagnostic of portal vein thrombosis. Note also the small vessels adjacent to the portal vein, which are collaterals attempting to feed the liver. As stated previously, portal vein thrombosis can be due to many etiologies including infections leading to sepsis and phlebitis. The fluid collection around the liver represents an abscess from the patient's prior gastric surgery. This led to sepsis and phlebitis causing the thrombosis of the portal vein.

CASE 25

Clinical History: 4-month-old boy presents with increasing abdominal girth.

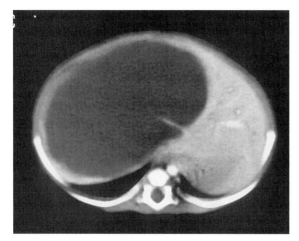

Figure 9.25 A

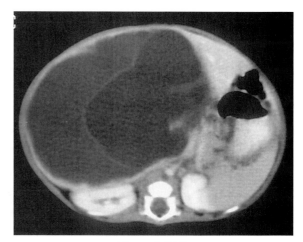

Figure 9.25 B

Findings: CECT demonstrates a large multiloculated cystic mass in the right lobe of the liver.

Differential Diagnosis: Undifferentiated embryonal sarcoma, infantile hemangioendothelioma, hepatoblastoma, metastasis.

Diagnosis: Mesenchymal hamartoma.

Discussion: The most likely diagnosis of a hepatic mass in an infant is either an infantile hemangioendothelioma, hepatoblastoma, or mesenchymal hamartoma. Of these, only mesenchymal hamartoma is predominantly cystic, with little solid component. Infantile hemangioendotheliomas can have necrosis if the tumor is large, but it is predominantly solid. In an older patient, it is often difficult to distinguish mesenchymal hamartoma from undifferentiated embryonal sarcoma. The clinical course, however, is different with the mean survival of a patient with undifferentiated embryonal sarcoma being less than 1 year.

CASE 26

Clinical History: 35-year-old man with elevated liver enzymes.*

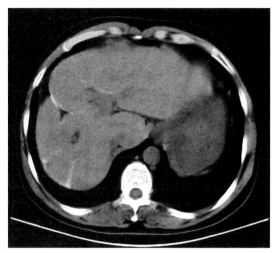
Figure 9.26 A

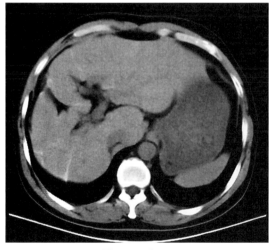
Figure 9.26 B

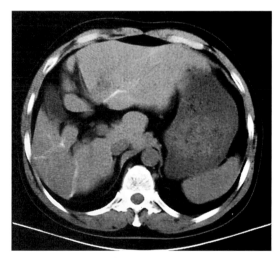
Figure 9.26 C

Findings: NECT demonstrates calcifications extending from the liver capsule toward the center of the liver.

Differential Diagnosis: None.

Diagnosis: Hepatic schistosomiasis.

Discussion: Schistosomiasis is one of the most common parasites affecting humans in the world. Various types of schistosomiasis are found including *Schistosoma japonicum,* which is prevalent in the Far East. *Schistosoma japonicum* has a classic CT appearance in the liver. It causes calcifications in the liver capsule and linear calcifications extending perpendicularly from the surface towards the center of the liver. This gives the liver the so-called "turtleback" or "tortoise shell" appearance. This is virtually diagnostic of hepatic schistosomiasis.

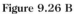

*Case courtesy of Dr. Dean Baird, Tripler Army Medical Center, Honolulu, Hawaii.

Clinical History: 65-year-old woman with weight loss.

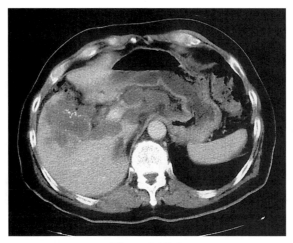

Figure 9.27 A

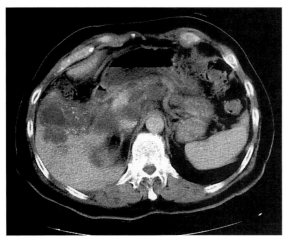

Figure 9.27 B

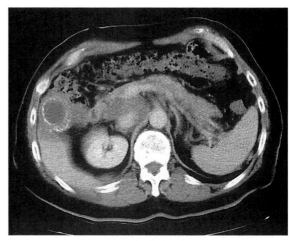

Figure 9.27 C

Findings: CECT demonstrates calcification within the wall of the gallbladder. A low attenuation mass is present infiltrating the liver.

Differential Diagnosis: None.

Diagnosis: Porcelain gallbladder with cholangiocarcinoma.

Discussion: Porcelain gallbladder is due to deposition of dystrophic calcifications within a chronically inflamed gallbladder wall. Approximately 90% of patients with porcelain gallbladder have gallstones; 10–20% of these patients progress to develop a cholangiocarcinoma of the gallbladder. Cholangiocarcinomas of the gallbladder occur in patients between the ages of 50–70 years of age. They typically extend through the gallbladder wall and infiltrate the liver. They can also spread via lymphatics to periportal and celiac lymph nodes. Prognosis is usually extremely poor. The presence of a porcelain gallbladder and an infiltrating mass is nearly diagnostic of a cholangiocarcinoma.

CASE 28

Clinical History: 78-year-old woman receiving broad-spectrum antibiotics.

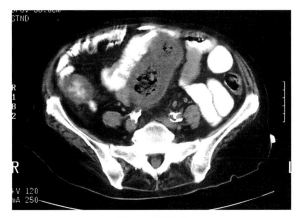

Figure 9.28 A

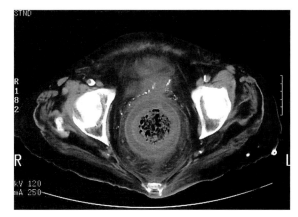

Figure 9.28 B

Findings: NECT demonstrates marked uniform circumferential thickening of the rectum and sigmoid colon. Stranding is seen in the pericolonic fat.

Differential Diagnosis: Infectious colitis, ulcerative colitis.

Diagnosis: Pseudomembranous colitis (PMC).

Discussion: The uniform circumferential thickening of the rectum and sigmoid colon is classic for pseudomembranous colitis. Typically, the bowel thickening measures about 15 mm, and the entire colon is involved. Ulcerative colitis could also affect the rectum but the amount of thickening is much less and averages about 7–8 mm. Lymphoma is usually polypoid in appearance. An infectious colitis (Shigella, Salmonella) is another good diagnostic possibility but the history of antibiotic use makes PMC the best diagnosis.